CLINICAL PROCEDURES in
VETERINARY NURSING

FOR ELSEVIER

Content Strategist: Robert Edwards

Content Development Specialist: Veronika Watkins

Project Manager: Julie Taylor

Designer: Brigette Hoette

Illustration Buyer: Narayanan Ramakrishnan

CLINICAL PROCEDURES in
VETERINARY NURSING

FOURTH EDITION

VICTORIA ASPINALL BVSc MRCVS

Retired Lecturer in Veterinary Nursing,
Hartpury College,
Gloucester, UK

ELSEVIER

Edinburgh   London   New York   Oxford   Philadelphia   St Louis   Sydney   Toronto   2019

ELSEVIER

First edition 2003
Second edition 2011
Third edition 2014

ISBN 978-0-7020-7396-0
e-ISBN 978-0-7020-7415-8

Notices

Practitioners and researchers must always rely on their own experience and knowledge in evaluating and using any information, methods, compounds or experiments described herein. Because of rapid advances in the medical sciences, in particular, independent verification of diagnoses and drug dosages should be made. To the fullest extent of the law, no responsibility is assumed by Elsevier, authors, editors or contributors for any injury and/or damage to persons or property as a matter of products liability, negligence or otherwise, or from any use or operation of any methods, products, instructions, or ideas contained in the material herein.

your source for books, journals and multimedia in the health sciences

www.elsevierhealth.com

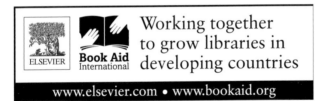

Working together to grow libraries in developing countries

www.elsevier.com • www.bookaid.org

The publisher's policy is to use paper manufactured from sustainable forests

Printed in China

Last digit is the print number: 9 8 7 6 5 4 3 2 1

CONTENTS

Nicola Ackerman, BSc(Hons) RVN CertSAN CertVNECC VTS (Nutrition) Hon MBVNA
Head Medical Nurse, The Veterinary Hospital Group, Plymouth, Devon, UK

Richard Aspinall, BVSc Cert VR MRCVS
Retired director of AAS Vets Ltd, Abbeydale, Gloucester, UK

Victoria Aspinall, BVSc MRCVS
Retired lecturer in Veterinary Nursing, Hartpury College, Gloucester, UK

Jennifer Davis, MRSPH
Retired laboratory team leader

Suzanne Easton, MSc BSc(Hons) PGCE
Associate lecturer in Veterinary Nursing

Julian Hoad, BSc(Hons) BVetMed Hon MBVNA MRCVS
Veterinary Surgeon, Crossways Veterinary Group, Storrington, West Sussex, UK

Joanna Hobbs, RVN
Locum Veterinary Nurse and co-owner of S and J Veterinary Nursing Revision

Joanne Lee, BA(Hons) GradDipVN RVN
Head Veterinary Nurse at Anderson Moores Veterinary Specialists, Winchester, UK

Lucy Middlecote, REVN Cert Ed
Lecturer in Veterinary Nursing, Hartpury College, Gloucester, UK

Rachel Mowbray, BVSc MRCVS
Veterinary surgeon, Vale Vet Group, The Animal Hospital, Stinchcombe, Dursley, Gloucestershire, UK

Georgina Parker, FdSc RVN
Referral Registered Veterinary Nurse, Cave Veterinary Specialists, Somerset, UK

Denise Prisk, DipAVN(Surgical) VTS (Anaesthesia) RVN
Anaesthesia nurse at Anderson Moores Veterinary Specialists, Winchester, UK

Trish Scorer, BSc(Hons) RVN
Quality assurance verifier

Suzanne Wildman, BAEd (Hons) RVN
Lecturer in Veterinary Nursing at Pershore College, Worcestershire, UK and co-owner of S and J Veterinary Nursing Revision

PREFACE

The third edition of *Clinical Procedures in Veterinary Nursing* was published in 2014, so it is now time to update the text in line with both changes in veterinary practice and changes in what it is expected of a newly qualified veterinary nurse, namely the Royal College of Veterinary Surgeons (RCVS) Day One Competences. These are broken down into the RCVS Day One Skills list, which describes in detail the essential clinical skills that a veterinary nurse should be capable of carrying out on the day she/he qualifies. The skills list is assessed by means of the RCVS Nursing Progress Log or similar recording system, and all licence to practice qualifications leading to entry on to the RCVS Veterinary Nurse Register must embed them within their chosen method(s) of assessment.

Armed with the list of Competences and Skills, the contributing authors have all reviewed their chapters so that the text complies with any changes and at this point can be considered to be completely up-to-date. Several of the chapters have new authors who have learned how to write using the Action/Rationale format, which is not always easy. Some of the procedures have been removed and incorporated into tasks because they were repetitious or old-fashioned and rarely used nowadays.

One of the biggest changes is the consideration of an animal's behaviour when anything is done to it. We must never forget that taking an animal into a practice, restraining it and administering any form of medication or performing any procedure is likely to be stressful – we know what is happening but the animal has no idea, and its reaction will be to run and hide or to bite and scratch or kick, if it's a horse. Recognizing these behavioural signs is vital, and steps must be taken to minimize the fear and distress that we may be causing by our actions in all the various species with which we work. These considerations have now been incorporated into the Skills list, so are also detailed in this text.

Over the years, since the first edition was published in 2003, this book has been the only textbook to describe the full range of procedures that a veterinary nurse might be expected to be able to perform, and as such is to be found on the majority of practice bookshelves. I hope that this new edition will continue to be essential reading for all nurses both in practice and in college.

Victoria Aspinall 2019

ACKNOWLEDGEMENTS

The preparation for this fourth edition was a little delayed because of my daughter's wedding, so I must thank everyone at Elsevier for allowing me to factor that in to the production timeline. Believe me, it is easier to prepare a book than it is to prepare a wedding! Thank you to the team at Elsevier and particularly to Veronika Watkins, my ever-efficient Content Development Editor, who was so supportive in my dealings with the EMSS (Elsevier Manuscript Submission System), which I never really conquered. Thank you also to all the contributing authors, some of whom are new to the whole process of writing and who quickly adapted to putting the procedures into the Action/Rationale format. I hope that between us all we have managed to produce a text that is now up-to-date and that will continue to be the standard guide for everything a veterinary nurse might encounter both in training and in practice.

ACKNOWLEDGEMENTS

Handling and restraint

Victoria Aspinall

CHAPTER CONTENTS

INTRODUCTION

No matter which procedure is to be performed, correct restraint of the patient is essential for the safety and welfare of both the animal and the handler. An animal that is securely and comfortably restrained will suffer less stress and will be less inclined to struggle and escape.

Most animals brought into a veterinary practice are used to being handled and are unlikely to bite or scratch, but you may encounter stray dogs and feral cats that are wary of human contact. Their reaction to restraint may be unpredictable and even dangerous, and you must be mindful of your own safety and take note of how the animal is responding, e.g. if it is obviously very frightened or could be about to snap. Then, having observed the animal's behavioural signs, you must take steps to minimize its fear and distress.

It is important when handling any species of animal that you approach quietly and confidently and perform the technique correctly at the first attempt, not at the third or fourth attempt – nothing upsets an animal more than clumsy, inept handling. You must know how to carry out the procedure, have all the equipment ready to hand and organize assistance if you think you are going to need it. If you need to wear some form of personal protective equipment (PPE), e.g. gauntlets, put them on before you begin the procedure. It is also important to feel confidence in yourself and confident that all this preparation will help. Animals are very sensitive to your mood and may detect your fear and bite you.

In the following descriptions of procedures, it is recognized that minimal restraint is best, if possible, but it may not always be possible, and understanding how to safely exert 'force' is an important part of a veterinary nurse's training. In some cases, restraint may inflame the animal's temper, making things worse, and it is up to you to assess the situation and behave accordingly.

After administering medication to any species of animal, take a few minutes to observe the patient for signs of any adverse reaction. If this occurs, take steps to alleviate the condition and report it to the veterinary surgeon immediately.

(For the purposes of description, the veterinary nurse restrains the patient, while the veterinary surgeon performs the task. In many cases, two nurses or a nurse and the animal's owner can perform the task.)

DOGS

Procedure: Tying a tape muzzle (Fig. 1.1)

This prevents the dog from biting the handler and diverts its attention away from the procedure being carried out.

1. **Action:** Place the dog in a sitting position on the floor.
   Rationale: In this position the dog is less likely to wriggle or bite. If the dog is small, it may be easier to place it on a table – avoid being bitten while you lift it on to the table.

2. **Action:** Ask an assistant to stand astride the dog and grasp the scruff on either side of the head just behind the ears.
   Rationale: If the dog moves its head around, the muzzle cannot be tied quickly. Be careful when scruffing a brachycephalic breed, as there is a risk of prolapsing the eyes.

3. **Action:** Using a length of cotton tape or bandage, tie a loop in it.
   Rationale: Any long strip of material can be used, e.g. a tie or even a stocking, but it must be strong enough to hold the jaws together.

4. **Action:** Approach the dog slowly and deliberately, crouching down to its level.
   Rationale: Crouching low helps to prevent fear and aggression; standing over the dog may provoke it to jump up and bite.

5. **Action:** Place the looped tape over the nose and tighten quickly and firmly with the knot over the nose.
   Rationale: Any delay in tightening the loop may allow the dog to shake its head free.

6. **Action:** Bring the long ends of the tape down and cross them over under the chin.
   Rationale: Further throws around the nose before finally crossing over will strengthen the muzzle.

7. **Action:** Take the two ends of the tape backwards and tie them in a bow behind the ears.
   Rationale: A bow allows a quick release if the dog becomes distressed.

8. **Action:** Ask the assistant holding the dog to keep the head pressed downwards.
   Rationale: This position prevents the dog from lifting its forefeet to pull off the muzzle.

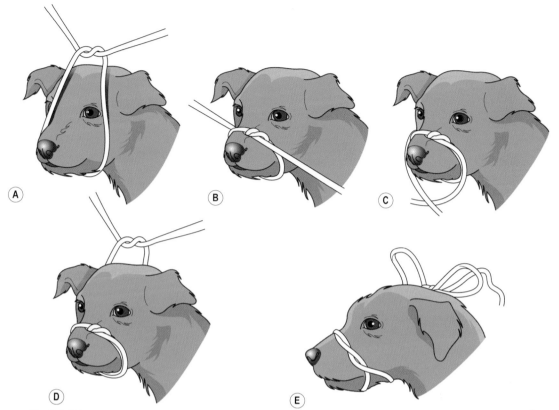

Fig. 1.1 Tying a tape muzzle. (Adapted, with permission, from Veterinary Nursing Medical Textbook, Masters and Bowden (2001), Butterworth-Heinemann.)

9. **Action:** If the dog is a brachycephalic or a short-nosed breed, insert another piece of tape under the loop over the nose and under the piece at the back of the head.
   Rationale: This prevents the muzzle from slipping off over the short nose.
10. **Action:** Bring the two ends of this piece together and tie into a bow on the bridge of the nose.
    Rationale: The dog must be carefully observed, as pressure over the nose may lead to respiratory distress.
11. **Action:** Never leave a muzzled animal unattended.
    Rationale: There is a risk of asphyxiation by vomit or saliva.

There are many types of commercial, washable muzzles on the market that are designed to fit specific sizes of dog. These are very useful and have clasps which make them quick to put on and, more importantly, quick to release if the dog becomes distressed. The downside is that it is expensive to buy a range of different sizes, so make sure you know how to use the cheaper tape muzzle. In an emergency, you can use a tie, a belt or even a stocking!

Procedure: Lifting dogs up to 15 kg bodyweight

(For example, cocker spaniels, beagles, etc.)
1. **Action:** Keep your back straight and, with your legs slightly apart, bend your knees.
   Rationale: This ensures that the weight of the dog is borne by your spine and your pelvic girdle.
2. **Action:** Place one arm around the front of the dog's chest and the other around its back end, over the tail.
3. **Action:** Hold the dog close to your chest (Fig. 1.2).
   Rationale: This will prevent the dog from struggling as it is lifted.

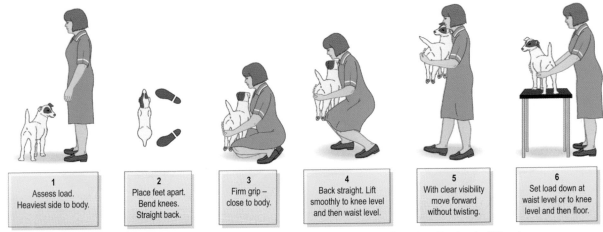

1	2	3	4	5	6
Assess load. Heaviest side to body.	Place feet apart. Bend knees. Straight back.	Firm grip – close to body.	Back straight. Lift smoothly to knee level and then waist level.	With clear visibility move forward without twisting.	Set load down at waist level or to knee level and then floor.

Fig. 1.2 The main elements of a good lifting technique. (Taken from The Complete Textbook of Veterinary Nursing, Aspinall (2011), Elsevier.)

4. **Action:** Straighten your legs, thereby raising the dog off the ground.
5. **Action:** Place it firmly on the table.
6. **Action:** Do not leave the animal unattended while it is on the table.
   Rationale: The dog may attempt to jump off the table, injuring itself, and it may then escape.

Procedure: Lifting dogs over 15 kg bodyweight (Fig. 1.3)

(For example, Labradors, springer spaniels, etc.)

1. **Action:** Arrange for another person to assist you.
   Rationale: Never attempt to lift a heavy dog by yourself. You may do permanent damage to your back!
2. **Action:** Both people stand on the same side of the dog.
3. **Action:** Keep your back straight and, with your legs slightly apart, bend your knees.
   Rationale: This ensures that the weight of the dog is borne by your spine and your pelvic girdle.
4. **Action:** Take the head end by placing one hand under the chest and the other under the neck.
   Rationale: If possible, the person lifting the head should be familiar to the dog, e.g. the owner. This reduces the risk of anyone being bitten.
5. **Action:** Hold the head close to your chest.
   Rationale: If the head is held close to you, the dog cannot turn its head round to bite.

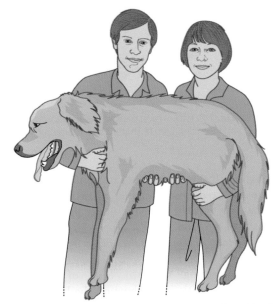

Fig. 1.3 Lifting a large dog. (Redrawn from Veterinary Nursing, Lane and Cooper (1994), Butterworth-Heinemann.)

6. **Action:** Instruct your assistant to adopt the safe lifting position (Fig. 1.2).
7. **Action:** Instruct your assistant to place one hand under the abdomen and the other around the back end.
8. **Action:** At the same time, both people straighten their legs and lift the dog on to the table.

Procedure: Lifting small dogs with spinal damage (Fig. 1.4)

(This can also be used for cats.)

1. **Action:** Approach the animal quietly and with care.
   Rationale: It may be frightened and in extreme pain, leading to unpredictable behaviour.
2. **Action:** If appropriate, apply a tape muzzle.
   Rationale: This will prevent the dog biting you as you lift it.
3. **Action:** With a straight back and bent knees, place your arms around the chest.
4. **Action:** Straighten your knees and lift the animal, allowing the legs to hang downwards.
   Rationale: This position prevents compression of the spine, which would cause acute pain and further damage.
5. **Action:** Gently place the animal on its side on a suitable non-slip surface ready for examination.
   Rationale: Care must be taken to avoid causing further pain.

Procedure: Lifting large dogs with spinal damage (Fig. 1.5)

1. **Action:** Arrange for another person to assist you.
   Rationale: Do not attempt to lift a large injured dog by yourself. You may damage your back, get bitten or cause the condition of the patient to deteriorate.
2. **Action:** Find something that can be used as a 'stretcher', such as a blanket or sheet, an ironing board or a solid plank of wood.
   Rationale: The dog must be supported on something that prevents compression of the spine, which would cause acute pain and further damage.
3. **Action:** Approach the animal quietly and with care.
   Rationale: It may be frightened and in extreme pain, leading to unpredictable behaviour.
4. **Action:** If appropriate, apply a tape or commercial muzzle (Fig. 1.1).
   Rationale: This will prevent the dog biting you as you lift it.

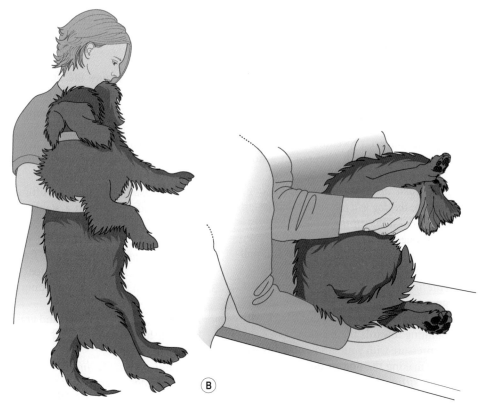

(A)　　　(B)

Fig. 1.4 Lifting a small dog with spinal damage. A, Allow the legs to hang downwards. B, Place the animal on its side on the table.

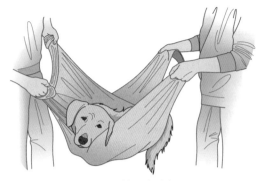

Fig. 1.5 Lifting a large dog with spinal damage.

5. **Action:** With the help of your assistant, and adopting the correct lifting position, lift the dog on to the blanket or plank.
6. **Action:** If using a plank, tie the dog on to it using tapes or bandages.
   Rationale: This will prevent the dog from falling or jumping off the 'stretcher' as you lift it, with the risk of further injury.
7. **Action:** Gently carry the dog to the table and place it on the table, still on the blanket or plank.
   Rationale: The 'stretcher' can be removed from under the dog later on.

RESTRAINT FOR GENERAL EXAMINATION

Procedure: To examine the cranial end of the body

1. **Action:** Using the correct procedure, lift the dog on to a stable examination table covered in a non-slip mat.
   Rationale: If the table does not shake and the dog's paws do not slip, the dog will feel secure and be less inclined to try and jump off the table.
2. **Action:** Stand to one side of the dog.
3. **Action:** Place one arm under the dog's neck and pull the head close to your chest with your hand.
   Rationale: If the head is held firmly against your chest, the dog cannot move to bite you.
4. **Action:** Place the other arm over the dog's back with your elbow pointing towards the far side.
5. **Action:** Apply pressure with your elbow and forearm along the spine, making the dog sit down.
   Rationale: In a sitting position, the dog will feel secure.

Procedure: To examine the caudal end of the body or take the rectal temperature

(Continuing from the previous procedure.)

1. **Action:** Keep one arm under the neck, pulling the head close to your chest.
   Rationale: If the head is held firmly against your chest, the dog cannot move to bite you.
2. **Action:** Place the other arm under the abdomen, gently lifting the dog into a standing position.
3. **Action:** Pull the body close to your chest by bringing your forearm up under the abdomen.
   Rationale: This position holds the dog securely against you, reducing the risk of it biting you and preventing it from moving during the examination.
4. **Action:** If you are required to restrain the dog for a long period of time, move your hand to lie over the spine, but be careful that the dog does not sit down again.
   Rationale: This position may be more comfortable for you, while still maintaining control over the dog.
5. **Action:** If the dog starts to move or object to the examination, quickly return to the previous position.
   Rationale: You must be aware of the dog's 'mood' and respond quickly to prevent anyone being bitten.

Procedure: To examine the dog on its side or to provide stronger control (Fig. 1.6)

1. **Action:** Apply a tape or commercial muzzle if appropriate.
   Rationale: This method is used to restrain more difficult dogs, and you should be prepared for an aggressive response.
2. **Action:** Using the correct lifting procedure, lift the dog and place it on a stable table covered in a non-slip mat.
   Rationale: If the table does not shake and the dog's paws do not slip, the dog will feel secure and be less inclined to struggle and escape.
3. **Action:** With the dog in a standing position, stand to one side of the dog.
4. **Action:** Reach over the dog and grasp the foreleg and hind leg furthest away from you at the level of the radius and tibia.
   Rationale: It may be difficult to reach over the back of larger dogs, especially if you are short or the table is high.

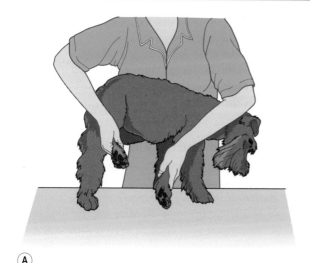
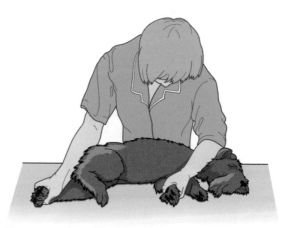
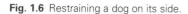
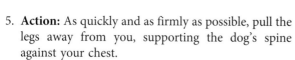

Fig. 1.6 Restraining a dog on its side.

5. **Action:** As quickly and as firmly as possible, pull the legs away from you, supporting the dog's spine against your chest.
   Rationale: This move must be done quickly before the dog begins to struggle and change position.
6. **Action:** Gently lower the body down to the table.
   Rationale: Avoid letting the body drop to the table, as this may injure or frighten the animal.
7. **Action:** Place your arm across the chest and neck and apply firm pressure to keep the dog's head on the table.
   Rationale: Most dogs will become submissive in this position, but some will try to stand up again, and you must be prepared. With large dogs, you may have to lean quite heavily, but you must always observe the behaviour and the condition of the animal.

Procedure: To examine or restrain the dog on its back

1. **Action:** Place the dog on its side as previously described.
2. **Action:** Ask an assistant to hold both the back legs while you hold both the forelegs.
   Rationale: If the dog is small, this may be performed by one person.
3. **Action:** Roll the dog over until it is lying on its back.

4. **Action:** Extend the forelegs and hind legs, presenting the ventral abdomen for examination.
5. **Action:** The sides of the neck can be grasped between the forelegs to give greater restraint if necessary.
   Rationale: Most dogs will feel quite comfortable in this position and will only struggle if they feel insecure or are in pain.

RESTRAINT FOR THE ADMINISTRATION OF DRUGS

Procedure: Administering a tablet (Fig. 1.7)

1. **Action:** Place the dog in a sitting position or in sternal recumbency on a suitable non-slip surface.
   Rationale: If the dog feels secure it will be less inclined to attempt to escape. Bending over for long periods may injure your back, so select a surface of a suitable height for you – place small dogs on a table, but dose larger dogs on the floor.
2. **Action:** If necessary, ask an assistant to hold the tail end of the dog.
   Rationale: This will prevent the dog from standing up or moving backwards.
3. **Action:** Place one hand over the top of the dog's muzzle and, using your fingers and thumb, gently raise the head and open the mouth.

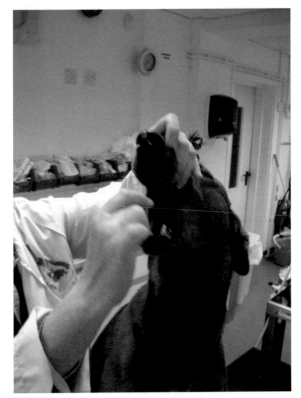

Fig. 1.7 Administering a tablet to a dog.

Rationale: Raising the head makes the lower jaw relax, making it easier to open.

4. **Action:** Hold the tablet in the fingers of your other hand, and pull down the lower jaw with your forefinger.

5. **Action:** Place the tablet on the back of the tongue.
   Rationale: If the tablet is placed as far back on the tongue as possible, the swallowing reflex is initiated, and the dog cannot spit the tablet out.

6. **Action:** Close the mouth and hold it closed with one hand.
   Rationale: This also prevents the dog from spitting the tablet out.

7. **Action:** Stroke the neck until you feel the dog swallow the tablet.
   Rationale: The dog may hold the tablet in the side of its mouth and spit it out as soon as you relax your grip. If swallowing has occurred, the tablet should be passing down the oesophagus!

8. **Action:** Observe the dog for a short time after administering the tablet.
   Rationale: Look for signs of choking or an adverse reaction such as foaming at the mouth or vomiting. Depending on the signs, take steps to control or correct the reaction.

Procedure: Administering a liquid feed or medication

1. **Action:** Place the dog in a sitting position or in sternal recumbency on a suitable non-slip surface.
   Rationale: If the dog feels secure, it will be less inclined to attempt to escape. Bending over for long periods may injure your back, so select a surface of a suitable height for you – place small dogs on a table, but dose larger dogs on the floor.

2. **Action:** If necessary, ask an assistant to hold the tail end of the dog.
   Rationale: This will prevent the dog from standing up or moving backwards.

3. **Action:** Place one hand over the top of the dog's muzzle and, using your fingers and thumb, gently tilt the head upwards and to one side.
   Rationale: This position restrains the head while encouraging the jaw to relax and open.

4. **Action:** Open the mouth slightly, creating a pocket at the angle of the jaw.
   Rationale: The pocket holds the liquid as it runs into the main part of the oral cavity.

5. **Action:** Insert a syringe filled with the liquid into the side of the mouth.
   Rationale: Try to avoid scraping the syringe over the gums, as you may damage the mucous membranes.

6. **Action:** Slowly depress the plunger so that the liquid trickles into the back of the mouth.
   Rationale: If you depress the plunger too quickly, the liquid will squirt out over you and the dog.

7. **Action:** Continue until the syringe is empty and repeat as necessary.

8. **Action:** When the procedure is complete, wipe the mouth clean and wipe up any spillage on the dog's coat.
   Rationale: Never leave the dog covered in liquid, as it will become wet and cold, and in summer dried food may attract flies.

9. **Action:** Observe the dog for a short time after you have given the liquid medication.

Rationale: Look for signs of choking and any adverse reaction such as foaming at the mouth or vomiting, then take steps to control or correct the reaction.

Procedure: Applying ear medication

1. **Action:** Place the dog in a sitting position or in sternal recumbency on a suitable non-slip surface.
   Rationale: If the dog feels secure it will be less inclined to attempt to escape. Bending over for long periods may injure your back, so select a surface of a suitable height for you. Bending over for long periods may injure your back – place small dogs on a table, but dose larger dogs on the floor.
2. **Action:** If necessary, apply a tape muzzle.
   Rationale: Some dogs may object to the application of ear medication.
3. **Action:** Stand to one side of the dog.
4. **Action:** Place one arm under the dog's neck and over the muzzle. Pull the head towards your chest.
   Rationale: This prevents the head from moving suddenly when the medication is applied. Avoid holding the head in the area of the ear, as this will interfere with the treatment.
5. **Action:** Place the other arm over the dog's back with your elbow pointing towards the far side.
   Rationale: If the dog starts to struggle, you can apply extra pressure by pressing your elbow closer to your side.
6. **Action:** The veterinary surgeon will stand on the other side of the dog and apply the medication to the nearest ear.
   Rationale: The applicator is introduced down the vertical part of the ear canal and squeezed.
7. **Action:** The ear is gently massaged to disperse the drops or ointment.
8. **Action:** To treat the other ear, exchange places.

N.B.: Many dogs do not object to the application of ear medication and can be treated single-handedly. Some dogs may shake their heads after treatment, sending the medication flying all over you!

Procedure: Applying eye medication

1. **Action:** Place the dog in a sitting position or in sternal recumbency on a suitable non-slip surface.
   Rationale: If the dog feels secure it will be less inclined to attempt to escape. Bending over for long periods may injure your back, so select a surface of a suitable height for you – place small dogs on a table, but dose larger dogs on the floor.

2. **Action:** If necessary, apply a tape or commercial muzzle.
   Rationale: Some dogs may object to the application of eye medication.
3. **Action:** Stand to one side of the dog.
4. **Action:** Place one arm under the dog's neck and over the muzzle. Pull the head towards your chest.
   Rationale: This prevents the head from moving suddenly when the medication is applied. Avoid holding the head in the area of the eye, as this will interfere with the treatment.
5. **Action:** Place the other arm over the dog's spine with your elbow pointing towards the far side.
   Rationale: If the dog starts to struggle, you can apply extra pressure by pressing your elbow closer to your side.
6. **Action:** The veterinary surgeon should stand in front of the dog and cup the head in both hands. Using the thumb of one hand, the lower eyelid can be pulled down, and the medication can be applied around the edge of the conjunctiva.
   Rationale: You must ensure that the head is held firmly, as sudden movement may result in damage to the eye.
7. **Action:** Release the tension on the eyelid and close the eyelids over the medication.
   Rationale: This allows the medication to spread over the tissues of the eye and under the eyelid.
8. **Action:** As you relax your hold on the dog, make sure that it does not rub at its eye with its paws or rub its head on the ground.
   Rationale: After about a minute, most medication will have dispersed and will no longer cause any discomfort.

N.B.: Eye medication may be applied single-handedly, but if the dog moves suddenly, there is a risk of damaging the eye.

Procedure: Restraint for a subcutaneous injection

1. **Action:** Place the dog in a sitting position or in sternal recumbency on an examination table with a non-slip surface.
   Rationale: If the dog feels secure and comfortable, it will be less inclined to move or try to escape.
2. **Action:** Apply a tape or commercial muzzle if necessary.
   Rationale: This is usually a quick and painless procedure, but some dogs may object and should be muzzled to prevent you being bitten.

3. **Action:** Grasp the scruff firmly with one hand.
   Rationale: This restrains the head and tents the skin so that it is ready for injection.

4. **Action:** Using the other hand, insert the point of the needle with the bevel uppermost into the raised skin of the scruff.
   Rationale: Be careful to avoid pushing the point of the needle through the skin on the opposite side of the raised scruff.

5. **Action:** Inject the contents of the syringe into the subcuticular space and withdraw the needle.
   Rationale: If you wish, you may draw back on the syringe before injecting to check that you have not penetrated a small blood capillary, but the blood supply to this area is relatively poor, and the risk is low.

6. **Action:** Gently massage the site of injection to disperse the drug.
   Rationale: Absorption from this site takes about 30–45 minutes.

N.B.: If the dog is likely to object to this procedure, it may be safer to arrange for an assistant to restrain the dog.

Procedure: Restraint for an intramuscular injection

1. **Action:** The dog should be placed in a standing position on the floor or on a suitable table with a non-slip surface.
   Rationale: If the dog feels secure, it will be less inclined to attempt to escape. Bending over for long periods may injure your back, so select a surface of a suitable height for you – place small dogs on a table, but dose larger dogs on the floor.

2. **Action:** Apply a tape or commercial muzzle, if necessary.
   Rationale: This injection may be slightly painful, and some dogs may object.

3. **Action:** Stand to one side of the dog.

4. **Action:** Place one arm under the neck and pull the head close to your chest.
   Rationale: If the head is firmly restrained, the dog cannot move suddenly or turn to bite.

5. **Action:** Place your other arm over the dog's chest.
   Rationale: Be prepared to restrain the dog firmly in this position, as sudden movement may cause damage and pain at the site of injection.

6. **Action:** The veterinary surgeon will stand to one side of the dog and towards the hind end of the body.

7. **Action:** The quadriceps group of muscles lies on the cranial aspect of the femur, and the veterinary surgeon will fix it between the fingers and thumb of the hand lying closest to the caudal end of the dog.
   Rationale: The quadriceps group is the most common site for intramuscular injections, but the lumbodorsal muscles and the triceps of the forelimb can also be used.

8. **Action:** Using the other hand, the needle should be introduced through the skin and the muscle mass in a direction running towards the femur and almost at right angles to the lateral aspect of the thigh.
   Rationale: At this angle the needle is unlikely to penetrate any major blood vessels or nerves.

9. **Action:** Draw back slightly on the plunger to ensure that a blood vessel has not been penetrated.
   Rationale: Muscle tissue has a good blood supply, and there is a risk of vascular penetration.

10. **Action:** If there is no blood present in the needle, inject the contents slowly.
    Rationale: Muscle tissue is very dense, and rapid injections of any volume of fluid may be very painful. Avoid giving any more than 2 ml at a time.

11. **Action:** Withdraw the needle and massage the site gently.
    Rationale: Gentle massage will help to disperse the drug into the blood stream. The effect usually takes about 20–30 minutes.

Procedure: Restraint for an intravenous injection using the cephalic vein (Fig. 1.8)

(Assume that the skin has been clipped and sterilized, ready for venepuncture.)

The cephalic vein runs over the dorsal aspect of the lower foreleg.

1. **Action:** Place the dog in sternal recumbency on a stable examination table with a non-slip surface.
   Rationale: If the dog feels secure it will be less inclined to attempt to escape. Select a surface of a suitable height for you – bending over for long periods may injure your back.

2. **Action:** Apply a tape or commercial muzzle if necessary.
   Rationale: Some dogs will object to this procedure, and a muzzle will protect you and the veterinary

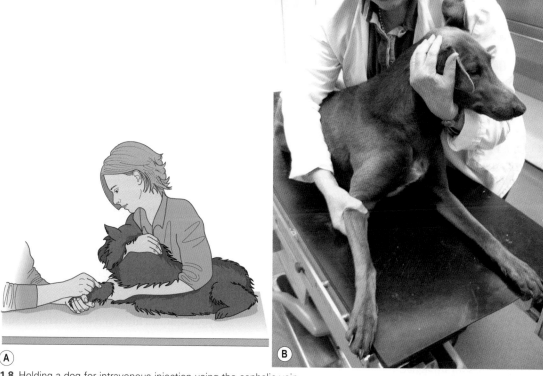

Fig. 1.8 Holding a dog for intravenous injection using the cephalic vein.

surgeon from being bitten. It also diverts the dog's attention from the injection.

3. **Action:** Stand to one side of the dog.
4. **Action:** Place one arm under the dog's chin and around the head, holding the head close to your chest.
   Rationale: If the head is held firmly and as close to you as possible, the dog is less likely to be able to bite you or the veterinary surgeon.
5. **Action:** Using your other hand, extend the foreleg on the opposite side towards the veterinary surgeon.
   Rationale: Your hand can rest on the table, ensuring that the foreleg is supported and held firmly.
6. **Action:** Cup the elbow in the palm of your hand, bringing the thumb across the crook of the elbow.
7. **Action:** Apply gentle pressure with your thumb and rotate your hand slightly outwards.
   Rationale: This pressure acts as a tourniquet, trapping blood passing up the foreleg and resulting in dilation of the vein – referred to as 'raising the vein'.

8. **Action:** Maintain this pressure while the veterinary surgeon inserts the needle through the skin and into the underlying cephalic vein.
   Rationale: The cephalic vein should be clearly visible, lying just under the skin.
9. **Action:** The veterinary surgeon should draw back on the syringe to check that the vein has been penetrated.
   Rationale: Perivascular injection may lead to tissue damage, and a check must be made that the vein has been penetrated before attempting the injection.
10. **Action:** If blood appears at the hub of the needle, raise your thumb a little. The veterinary surgeon will slowly inject the contents of the syringe into the vein.
    Rationale: Releasing the pressure allows the drug to flow into the vein.
11. **Action:** When the procedure is complete, and the needle has been slowly withdrawn, you should apply gentle pressure to the injection site for about 30 seconds.

Rationale: This prevents haemorrhage into the area around the vein.

N.B.: If a blood sample is to be collected, maintain pressure on the vein until enough blood is in the syringe.

Procedure: Restraint for an intravenous injection using the lateral saphenous vein (Fig. 1.9)

(Assume that the skin has been clipped and sterilized, ready for venepuncture.)

The lateral saphenous vein runs over the lateral aspect of the hock.

1. **Action:** Apply a tape muzzle if necessary.
   Rationale: Some dogs may object to this procedure and should be muzzled. This must be done before putting the dog into lateral recumbency.
2. **Action:** Place the dog in lateral recumbency on a stable examination table with a non-slip surface.
   Rationale: If the dog feels secure and comfortable, it will be less inclined to struggle and attempt to escape.
3. **Action:** Stand on the dorsal side of the dog, so that the legs are directed away from you.
4. **Action:** Using the arm closest to the head, place your forearm across the dog's neck, and use this hand to hold both forepaws.
   Rationale: In this position you can use the weight of your body to hold the cranial end of the body on to the table.
5. **Action:** Place the other hand around the uppermost hind leg at the level of the mid-tibia/fibula.

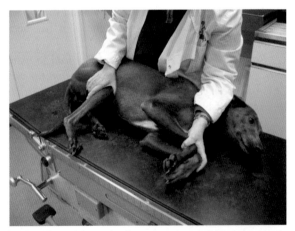

Fig. 1.9 Restraining a dog for an intravenous injection using the saphenous vein.

Rationale: The lateral saphenous vein collects blood from the hind paw and runs superficially on the caudal aspect of the hock and distal tibia. Pressure applied around the distal tibia acts as a tourniquet, trapping venous blood and causing the vein to dilate – known as 'raising the vein'.

6. **Action:** Stretch out the leg and apply gentle pressure.
7. **Action:** Maintain this pressure while the veterinary surgeon inserts the needle through the skin and into the underlying saphenous vein.
   Rationale: The saphenous vein should be clearly visible lying just under the skin.
8. **Action:** The veterinary surgeon should draw back on the syringe to check that the vein has been penetrated.
   Rationale: Perivascular injection may lead to tissue damage, and a check must be made that the vein has been penetrated before attempting the injection.
9. **Action:** If blood appears at the hub of the needle, raise your thumb a little, and the veterinary surgeon will slowly inject the contents of the syringe into the vein.
   Rationale: Releasing the pressure allows the drug to flow into the vein.
10. **Action:** When the procedure is complete and the needle has been slowly withdrawn, you should apply gentle pressure to the injection site for about 30 seconds.
    Rationale: This prevents haemorrhage into the area around the vein.

N.B.: If a blood sample is to be collected, maintain pressure on the vein until enough blood is in the syringe.

Procedure: Restraint for an intravenous injection using the jugular vein (Fig. 1.10)

(Assume that the skin has been clipped and sterilized, ready for venepuncture.)

The jugular veins run in the jugular furrow on either side of the trachea.

1. **Action:** Place the dog in a sitting position on a stable examination table with a non-slip surface.
   Rationale: If the dog feels secure and comfortable, it will be less inclined to struggle and attempt to escape.
2. **Action:** Apply a tape or commercial muzzle if necessary.

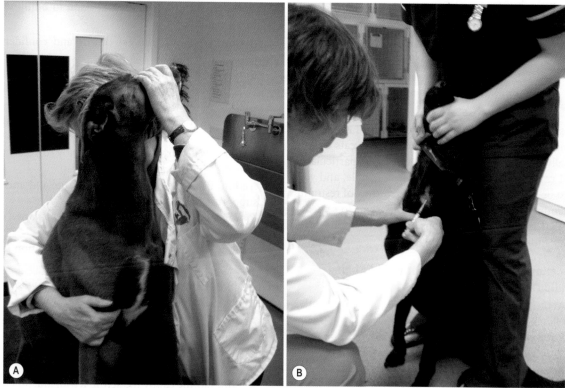

Fig. 1.10 Restraining a dog for an intravenous injection using the jugular vein.

Rationale: Some dogs may object to this procedure.

3. **Action:** Stand to one side of the dog and place one hand under the dog's chin, raising the head and bringing it close to your chest.

   Rationale: Firm restraint is essential for this procedure to prevent the dog moving suddenly and causing injury to itself or to you.

4. **Action:** Place your other arm over the dog's back and around the front of its chest, holding it close to your body.

5. **Action:** The veterinary surgeon will stand in front of the dog and apply pressure at the base of the jugular furrow with the fingers of one hand.

   Rationale: The jugular vein runs in a groove on each side of the trachea known as the jugular furrow. It collects venous blood from the head and carries it towards the heart. Pressure applied at the base of the vein will prevent the flow of blood towards the heart, causing the vein to dilate – known as 'raising the vein'.

6. **Action:** Using the other hand, the veterinary surgeon should insert the needle through the skin into the underlying vein.

   Rationale: The jugular vein should be clearly visible lying just under the skin.

7. **Action:** The veterinary surgeon should draw back on the syringe to check that the vein has been penetrated.

   Rationale: Perivascular injection may lead to tissue damage, and a check must be made that the vein has been penetrated before attempting the injection.

8. **Action:** If blood appears at the hub of the needle, raise your thumb a little, and the veterinary surgeon will slowly inject the contents of the syringe into the vein.

   Rationale: Releasing the pressure allows the drug to flow into the vein.

9. **Action:** When the procedure is complete and the needle has been slowly withdrawn, you should apply gentle pressure to the injection site for about 30 seconds.

Rationale: This prevents haemorrhage into the area around the vein.

N.B.: If a blood sample is to be collected, maintain pressure on the vein until enough blood is in the syringe.

CATS

Most cats are used to being handled and will respond to being stroked and spoken to quietly. These cats do not usually pose much of a problem, but some, particularly feral cats, can be extremely difficult to handle, and you must be prepared to exercise varying degrees of restraint depending on the individual. It is important to remember that cats have five weapons of assault – four sets of claws and a set of sharp teeth!

Procedure: Lifting a friendly cat used to being handled – method 1

1. **Action:** Approach the cat calmly and confidently, talking to it quietly.
   Rationale: Most cats are used to human noise and will be reassured by a low, quiet tone of voice.
2. **Action:** Assess whether the cat is safe to stroke.
   Rationale: A frightened or aggressive cat will warn you by hissing or growling as you approach, while a friendly cat may rub itself against your hand and even purr.
3. **Action:** If safe, gently stroke the top of the head and run your hand along its back.
   Rationale: This will reassure the cat and may elicit a purr. If the cat hisses, use another method of lifting and restraint.
4. **Action:** Gently but firmly grasp the scruff of the neck with one hand and lift the cat.
   Rationale: Picking a cat up by the scruff mimics the way in which the queen carries her kittens. It initiates an innate relaxation response, which in the wild would enable the queen to move the kittens safely from place to place without the risk of them struggling and escaping.
5. **Action:** Place the other hand under the sternum and support the cat.
   Rationale: Kittens and smaller cats may be lifted by the scruff, but heavier cats need added support.
6. **Action:** Place the cat on a stable non-slip surface.
   Rationale: If the cat feels insecure, it may try to scratch, bite or escape.

Procedure: Lifting a friendly cat used to being handled – method 2

1. **Action:** Approach the cat calmly and confidently, talking to it quietly.
   Rationale: Most cats are used to human noise and will be reassured by a low, quiet tone of voice.
2. **Action:** Assess whether the cat is safe to stroke.
   Rationale: A frightened or aggressive cat will warn you by hissing or growling as you approach.
3. **Action:** If safe, stroke the cat and gently run one hand over the chest and under the sternum.
4. **Action:** Place the other hand under the abdomen to support it from the other side.
   Rationale: In this position the cat feels supported and secure and is unlikely to struggle.
5. **Action:** Lift the cat on to a stable examination table with a non-slip surface.

Procedure: Lifting a frightened or aggressive cat (Fig. 1.11)

1. **Action:** Grasp the scruff of the cat quickly and firmly.
   Rationale: If you do not take enough scruff or if you make any mistake in handling, you are likely to get bitten or scratched.
2. **Action:** Lift the cat by the scruff, letting the hind end of the body hang down.
   Rationale: Do not leave the cat hanging for more than a few seconds, as this is unpleasant for the cat, particularly if it is large.
3. **Action:** Place the cat on a table and restrain in an appropriate way.
   Rationale: Aggressive cats may have to be restrained using equipment such as a crusher cage or a restraining bag.

Procedure: Carrying a cat (Fig. 1.12)

1. **Action:** Place the body of the cat under one elbow and forearm, holding it close to your side. Let the hind legs gently dangle.
   Rationale: The body is supported by the angle of your arm, but the hind legs are unable to push the cat's body up in order to escape. Watch out for the hind legs getting caught in side pockets.
2. **Action:** Hold the forepaws together between the thumb and fingers of the hand on that side.
   Rationale: This prevents the forelegs from scratching you.
3. **Action:** Hold the scruff of the cat firmly with your free hand.

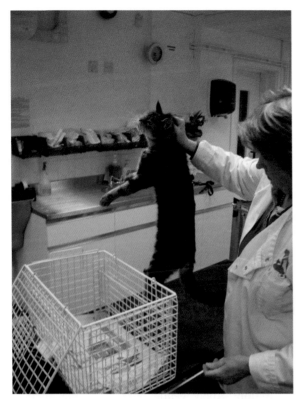

Fig. 1.11 Lifting a frightened or aggressive cat.

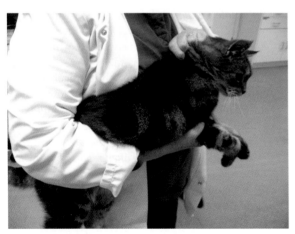

Fig. 1.12 Carrying a cat.

Rationale: In this position, the cat feels secure and comfortable. If it tries to escape, you have control of the head via the scruff and can apply stronger pressure to the body with your elbow.

N.B.: Avoid carrying aggressive or frightened cats around in your arms, as their movements are often unpredictable. They should be carried in a wire cat basket that allows them to see out whilst providing you with clear visibility of their condition.

RESTRAINT FOR GENERAL EXAMINATION

Cats that are used to being handled respond to minimal restraint, but you should be prepared to use firmer methods on more difficult cats, particularly if you are single-handed.

Procedure: To examine a friendly cat

1. **Action:** Place the cat on a stable examination table in a sitting position.
    Rationale: The cat will feel secure and comfortable and will be less inclined to try and escape.
2. **Action:** Stand to one side of the cat.
3. **Action:** Run the hand closest to the cat over its back and under its jaw, gently raising the head up a little.
    Rationale: If the cat is relaxed, this hand can be placed on the chest, but you should be ready to move to restrain the head if necessary.
4. **Action:** Place the other hand over the forelegs.
    Rationale: This prevents the cat from raising its forepaws to scratch.
5. **Action:** If the cat begins to struggle or object to examination, move the hand from under the chin and grasp the scruff.
    Rationale: This controls the head, allowing examination of the body.
6. **Action:** Use the elbow on this side to press the cat's body firmly against your side.
    Rationale: In this position, the cat is unable to move or gain enough grip to make an escape. It may be more comfortable to lift the cat, supporting it against your body, rather than leaning over the examination table.
7. **Action:** Use the other hand to hold the forelegs firmly down on to the table.
    Rationale: This controls the forepaws and prevents scratching.

N.B.: This position uses minimal restraint, allowing examination of the whole body and enabling the rectal temperature to be taken safely.

Procedure: To examine a fractious cat

1. **Action:** Firmly grasp the scruff of the cat with one hand.

   Rationale: *Some fractious cats seem to have the ability to 'use up' their scruffs by hunching their shoulders and letting their heads sink down, making the scruff very difficult to grasp. Adult toms also have thickened scruffs that are difficult to hold for any length of time.*

2. **Action:** Pick up the cat and grasp its hind legs with the other hand.

3. **Action:** Place the cat on the table in lateral recumbency, extending its head and hind legs.

   Rationale: *The cat is unable to move against the strength of the handler's arms, but a really angry cat will continue to attempt to escape, and a great deal of growling and miaowing will be heard!*

4. **Action:** As the cat struggles, make sure that you keep your arms wide apart to maintain the position.

   Rationale: *As the forelegs are not restrained, you must be careful to avoid being scratched.*

This position allows examination of most of the body, but it is inadvisable to use it to take the rectal temperature, as the cat may struggle and damage itself. For the welfare of the cat, another method of restraint should be adopted as soon as possible.

Restraint equipment available for use with more aggressive cats includes crusher cages, cat grabbers and cat bags out of which the head or legs can be extended while the rest of the body is retained inside. Wrapping an aggressive cat in a towel and extending the head or a leg is also a useful means of restraint. There are commercial cat muzzles available that extend upwards to cover the cat's eyes – being in the dark may help to calm some cats. Chemical restraint is widely used, but some form of contact with the cat will still be necessary to administer the drug.

RESTRAINT FOR THE ADMINISTRATION OF DRUGS

Procedure: Administering a tablet (Fig. 1.13)

1. **Action:** Place the cat in a sitting position on a suitable non-slip surface.

   Rationale: *The cat will feel secure and less inclined to escape.*

2. **Action:** Grasp the cat's head by placing your hand over the head and your thumb and forefinger at the angle of the jaw.

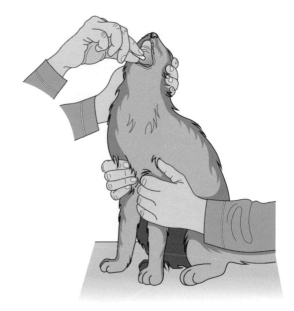

Fig. 1.13 Administering a tablet to a cat.

   Rationale: *Be aware that the cat may raise its forepaws at this point.*

3. **Action:** Apply gentle pressure at the angle of the jaw.

4. **Action:** Gently but firmly tilt the head backwards.

   Rationale: *As the head is tilted, the jaw will naturally relax, and the mouth should be easier to open.*

5. **Action:** Hold the tablet between the thumb and forefinger of your other hand.

6. **Action:** Use your second and third fingers to apply gentle downward pressure to the cat's lower jaw.

   Rationale: *At the first attempt the jaws should open easily. At later attempts, the cat may clench its jaws tightly closed, making the procedure more difficult – an experience often reported by owners!*

7. **Action:** As the jaw opens, place or drop the tablet on the back of the tongue.

   Rationale: *If the tablet is placed as far back on the tongue as possible, the swallowing reflex will be induced.*

8. **Action:** Keeping the head tilted vertically, close the mouth and hold it closed with your hand.

   Rationale: *It is important to hold the mouth closed, as this prevents the cat from spitting the tablet out.*

9. **Action:** Gently stroke the throat until the cat is seen to swallow.

Rationale: Some cats may learn to hold the tablet in the side of their cheeks until the head is released, when they then spit the tablet out.

10. **Action:** Observe the cat's behaviour for a short time after administering the tablet.

Rationale: Look for signs of choking or an adverse reaction such as foaming at the mouth and take steps to alleviate the condition.

N.B.: If you have an assistant, the cat can be further restrained by holding the forelegs while you administer the tablet as described (Fig. 1.13).

Procedure: Administering a liquid feed or medication (Fig. 1.14)

1. **Action:** Sit on a chair with a towel or other absorbent material covering your knees.

Rationale: This procedure can be messy, and the towel will absorb any spilt liquids.

2. **Action:** Take the cat on to your knee with its head pointing away from you.

Rationale: In this position, the cat will be comfortable and easy to restrain.

3. **Action:** Grasp the cat's head with one hand, with your thumb and forefinger at the angle of the jaw, and slightly tilt the head to one side.

Rationale: If the cat raises its forepaws, ask an assistant to hold them down or wrap them in the towel.

4. **Action:** Open the mouth slightly, creating a pocket at the angle of the jaw.

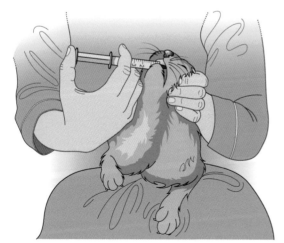

Fig. 1.14 Administering a liquid feed or medication to a cat.

Rationale: This pocket holds the liquid as it runs into the main part of the oral cavity.

5. **Action:** Using a small syringe filled with the liquid, gently insert the end of the barrel into the mouth at the angle of the jaw.

Rationale: Be as gentle as possible – rough handling can easily damage the mouth.

6. **Action:** Slowly depress the plunger so that the liquid trickles into the mouth.

Rationale: If you depress the plunger too quickly, the liquid may squirt out over you and the cat.

7. **Action:** Continue until the syringe is empty and repeat as necessary.

8. **Action:** When the procedure is complete, clean the cat's mouth, paws and any other parts which are wet or covered in liquid.

Rationale: Never leave the cat covered in liquid, as it will become wet and cold. Drying food may attract flies.

9. **Action:** Observe the cat's behaviour for a short time after administering the liquid.

Rationale: Look for signs of choking or an adverse reaction such as foaming at the mouth and take steps to alleviate the condition.

Procedure: Applying ear medication (Fig. 1.15)

1. **Action:** Place the cat in a sitting position on a stable examination table with a non-slip surface.

Rationale: The cat will feel secure and less inclined to escape.

2. **Action:** Standing to one side, place your hands on either side of the cat, bringing the hands forward to restrain the forelegs on the table.

Rationale: Cats that are used to being handled prefer minimal restraint. This procedure does not usually cause too much discomfort, and the cat is unlikely to struggle. However, if struggling does occur, be prepared to hold the scruff with one hand and restrain the forelegs with the other.

3. **Action:** The veterinary surgeon will stand in front of the cat and take hold of the ear pinna to be treated, with the finger and thumb of one hand.

Rationale: In this position, the veterinary surgeon can gain maximum access to the ear.

4. **Action:** The veterinary surgeon will gently twist the head so that it faces upwards.

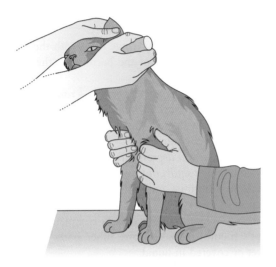

Fig. 1.15 Applying ear medication for a cat. (Redrawn from Veterinary Nursing, Lane and Cooper (1994), Butterworth-Heinemann.)

Rationale: This brings the ear uppermost so that any medication runs down the ear canal by gravity. It also helps to restrain the head.

5. **Action:** Using the other hand, the veterinary surgeon can apply the medication to the ear.

    In some cases, the cat may shake its head after administering the medication, and it will be sprayed all over you!

Procedure: Applying eye medication

1. **Action:** Place the cat in a sitting position on a stable examination table with a non-slip surface.
    Rationale: The cat will feel secure and less inclined to escape.
2. **Action:** Place one hand on either side of the cat's rump.
    Rationale: This prevents the cat from trying to go backwards and escape.
3. **Action:** The veterinary surgeon should stand in front of the cat and take the cat's head in one hand, placing the thumb over the cranium and the fingers under the chin. The affected eye should be on the far side of the head away from the palm of the hand.
    Rationale: In this position, the head is held still, reducing the risk of damage to the eye. If the cat struggles, the nozzle of the tube may scratch or penetrate the eye.

4. **Action:** The skin around the affected eye is gently stretched with the forefinger and thumb of this hand.
    Rationale: This will open the eyelids, allowing examination of the eye and conjunctiva.
5. **Action:** Using the other hand, the medication is gently applied around the edges of the conjunctiva.
    Rationale: If you are too rough, you may cause damage to the delicate conjunctiva.
6. **Action:** Relax the stretching around the eyes and eyelids.
    Rationale: This enables the eyelids to close.
7. **Action:** Gently close the eyelids over the medication.
    Rationale: This allows the drops or ointment to spread around the tissues of the eye and under the eyelids.
8. **Action:** You must maintain control of the forepaws for a short while to prevent the cat from clawing at the eye or rubbing its head on the table.
    Rationale: After a minute or so the ointment will have dissipated, and the cat should not feel any discomfort.

Procedure: Restraint for a subcutaneous injection (Fig. 1.16)

1. **Action:** Place the cat in sternal recumbency on an examination table with a non-slip surface. The cat should face away from you.
    Rationale: In this position, the cat feels secure and cannot slip.
2. **Action:** Grasp the scruff firmly with one hand.
    Rationale: This gives control of the head, as the cat is unable to turn and bite. It also tents the skin, ready for injection.

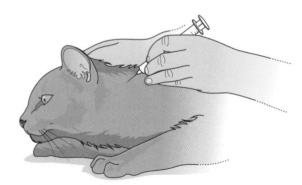

Fig. 1.16 Restraint for a subcutaneous injection of a cat. (Redrawn from Veterinary Nursing, Lane and Cooper (1994), Butterworth-Heinemann.)

3. **Action:** Using the other hand, introduce the point of the needle into the raised skin of the scruff with the bevel uppermost.

 Rationale: Be careful to avoid pushing the point of the needle through the skin on the opposite side of the raised scruff.

4. **Action:** Inject the contents into the subcuticular space and withdraw the needle.

 Rationale: If you wish, you may draw back on the syringe before injecting to check that you have not penetrated a small blood capillary, but the blood supply to this area is relatively poor and the risk is low.

5. **Action:** Gently massage the site of injection to disperse the drug.

 Rationale: Absorption from this site takes about 30–45 minutes.

N.B.: Most cats will not object to this procedure, and it can usually be performed single-handedly, provided that you give the injection quickly. However, some cats will need to be restrained by an assistant to prevent struggling.

Procedure: Restraint for an intramuscular injection (Fig. 1.17)

1. **Action:** Place the cat in a standing or lying position on an examination table with a non-slip surface.

 Rationale: In this position, the cat is held firmly but is quite comfortable. It is essential to restrain the cat adequately, as sudden movement may result in damage to the muscle tissues.

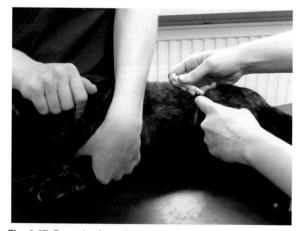

Fig. 1.17 Restraint for an intramuscular injection in a cat.

2. **Action:** Standing to one side of the cat, restrain the head firmly by grasping the scruff.

 Rationale: The head must be held tightly, as this potentially painful procedure could cause the cat to bite.

3. **Action:** The veterinary surgeon should take the nearest hind leg and locate the quadriceps group of muscles lying on the cranial aspect of the femur. The muscles should be fixed between the thumb and fingers of the hand closest to the caudal end of the cat.

 Rationale: The quadriceps group is a large muscle mass which provides easy access for injection. The hamstring group and the gluteals should not be used, as there is a risk of bone and sciatic nerve damage.

4. **Action:** Using the other hand, introduce the needle through the skin and the muscle mass in a direction running towards the femur and almost at right angles to the lateral aspect of the thigh.

 Rationale: At this angle the needle is unlikely to penetrate any major blood vessels or nerves.

5. **Action:** Draw back slightly on the plunger to ensure that a blood vessel has not been penetrated.

 Rationale: Muscle tissue has a good blood supply, and there is a risk of vascular penetration.

6. **Action:** If there is no blood present in the needle, inject the contents slowly.

 Rationale: Muscle tissue is very dense, and rapid injections of any volume of fluid may be very painful. Avoid giving any more than 2 ml at a time.

7. **Action:** Withdraw the needle and massage the site gently.

 Rationale: Gentle massage will help to disperse the drug into the blood stream. The effect usually takes about 20–30 minutes.

Procedure: Restraint for an intravenous injection using the cephalic vein (Fig. 1.18)

(Assume that the skin has been clipped and sterilized, ready for venepuncture.)

The cephalic vein runs over the dorsal aspect of the lower foreleg.

1. **Action:** Place the cat on a stable examination table with a non-slip surface, in sternal recumbency or in a sitting position.

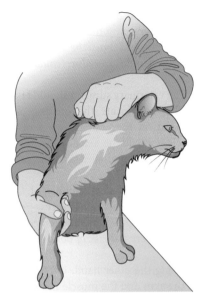

Fig. 1.18 Restraint for an intravenous injection using the cephalic vein in a cat. (Redrawn from Veterinary Nursing, Lane and Cooper (1994), Butterworth-Heinemann.)

Rationale: In this position the cat will feel secure and comfortable and will be less likely to move or try to escape.

2. **Action:** With one hand, take a firm grasp of the scruff, facing the cat towards the veterinary surgeon.
   Rationale: It is vital that the cat is held firmly, as sudden movement may cause injury to the patient, to yourself or to the veterinary surgeon.

3. **Action:** Use your forearm and elbow to hold the remainder of the body close to you.
   Rationale: Extra control can be achieved by changing the pressure exerted by your elbow.

4. **Action:** Using the other hand, extend a foreleg towards the veterinary surgeon.

5. **Action:** Support the cat's elbow in the palm of your upturned hand and place your thumb across the crook of the elbow.
   Rationale: Your hand can rest on the table, ensuring that the foreleg is supported and held firmly.

6. **Action:** Apply gentle pressure with your thumb and rotate your hand slightly outwards.
   Rationale: This pressure acts as a tourniquet, trapping blood passing up the foreleg and resulting in dilation of the vein – referred to as 'raising the vein'.

7. **Action:** Maintain this pressure while the veterinary surgeon inserts the needle through the skin and into the underlying cephalic vein.
   Rationale: The cephalic vein should be clearly visible lying just under the skin.

8. **Action:** The veterinary surgeon should draw back on the syringe to check that the vein has been penetrated.
   Rationale: Perivascular injection may lead to tissue damage, and a check must be made that the vein has been penetrated before attempting the injection.

9. **Action:** If blood appears at the hub of the needle, raise your thumb a little, and the veterinary surgeon will slowly inject the contents of the syringe into the vein.
   Rationale: Releasing the pressure allows the drug to flow into the vein.

10. **Action:** When the procedure is complete and the needle has been slowly withdrawn, you should apply gentle pressure to the injection site for about 30 seconds.
    Rationale: This prevents haemorrhage into the area around the vein.

N.B.: If a blood sample is to be collected, maintain pressure on the vein until enough blood is in the syringe.

Procedure: Restraint for an intravenous injection using the lateral saphenous vein

(Assume that the skin has been clipped and sterilized, ready for venepuncture.)

The lateral saphenous vein runs over the lateral aspect of the hock.

1. **Action:** Place the cat in lateral recumbency on a stable examination table with a non-slip surface.
   Rationale: The cat will feel secure and comfortable and will be less likely to move or try to escape.

2. **Action:** Grasp the scruff firmly with one hand.
   Rationale: The head must be restrained firmly to prevent the cat wriggling or biting.

3. **Action:** With the other hand, extend the uppermost hind leg, at the same time stretching out the body.
   Rationale: If the cat struggles or is aggressive, it may be necessary to exert extra control by wrapping the cat in a towel with the head out. The hind leg can be extended from the towel.

4. **Action:** Position your hand around the lower leg at the level of mid-tibia/fibula and apply gentle pressure.

Rationale: The lateral saphenous vein collects blood from the hind paw and runs superficially on the caudal aspect of the hock and distal tibia. Pressure applied around the distal tibia acts as a tourniquet, trapping venous blood and causing the vein to dilate – known as 'raising the vein'.

5. **Action:** Maintain this pressure while the veterinary surgeon inserts the needle through the skin and into the underlying saphenous vein.

   Rationale: The saphenous vein should be clearly visible lying just under the skin.

6. **Action:** The veterinary surgeon should draw back on the syringe to check that the vein has been penetrated.

   Rationale: Perivascular injection may lead to tissue damage, and a check must be made that the vein has been penetrated before attempting the injection.

7. **Action:** If blood appears at the hub of the needle, release the pressure a little, and the veterinary surgeon will slowly inject the contents of the syringe into the vein.

   Rationale: Releasing the pressure allows the drug to flow into the vein.

8. **Action:** When the procedure is complete and the needle has been slowly withdrawn, you should apply gentle pressure to the injection site for about 30 seconds.

   Rationale: This prevents haemorrhage into the area around the vein. Absorption of a drug from an intravenous site is instantaneous.

Procedure: Restraint for an intravenous injection using the jugular vein – method 1 (Fig. 1.19)

(Assume that the skin has been clipped and sterilized, ready for venepuncture.)

The jugular veins run in the jugular furrows on either side of the trachea.

1. **Action:** Sit on a chair and place the cat on your lap.

   Rationale: This ensures that you are comfortable and able to support and restrain the cat more easily.

2. **Action:** Turn the cat over into dorsal recumbency.

   Rationale: In this position there is easy access to the ventral part of the neck. If the cat feels secure in your lap, it will be more likely to relax.

3. **Action:** Take all four legs in one hand.

   Rationale: Control of the legs prevents the veterinary surgeon from being scratched.

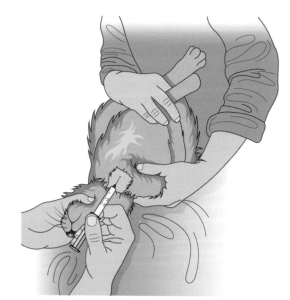

Fig. 1.19 Restraint for an intravenous injection using the jugular vein in a cat. (Redrawn from Practical Animal Handling, Anderson and Edney (1991), Pergamon.)

4. **Action:** The veterinary surgeon should gently extend the head with one hand, placing the thumb under the chin and cupping the cranium in the palm of the hand.

   Rationale: Extending the head and neck stretches out the jugular as it runs beside the trachea and tenses the overlying skin, making it easier to penetrate the vein with the needle.

5. **Action:** You can now place the thumb of your other hand at the base of the jugular furrow at the point where the trachea enters the thoracic cavity.

   Rationale: The jugular vein on each side of the trachea runs in a groove known as the jugular furrow. It collects venous blood from the head and carries it towards the heart.

6. **Action:** Apply gentle pressure.

   Rationale: Pressure applied at the base of the vein will prevent the flow of blood towards the heart, causing the vein to dilate – known as 'raising the vein'.

7. **Action:** Maintain this pressure while the veterinary surgeon inserts the needle through the skin and into the underlying jugular vein.

   Rationale: The jugular vein should be clearly visible lying just under the skin.

8. **Action:** The veterinary surgeon should draw back on the syringe to check that the vein has been penetrated.

Rationale: Perivascular injection may lead to tissue damage, and a check must be made that the vein has been penetrated before attempting the injection.

9. **Action:** If blood appears at the hub of the needle, raise your thumb a little, and the veterinary surgeon will slowly inject the contents of the syringe into the vein.

    Rationale: Releasing the pressure allows the drug to flow into the vein.

10. **Action:** When the procedure is complete and the needle has been slowly withdrawn, you should apply gentle pressure to the injection site for about 30 seconds.

    Rationale: This prevents haemorrhage into the area around the vein. Absorption of a drug from an intravenous site is instantaneous.

N.B.: The jugular vein is more often used for blood sampling because a larger volume can be collected very quickly, thus minimizing distress to the patient. During this procedure, pressure is maintained until enough blood has collected in the syringe.

Procedure: Restraint for an intravenous injection using the jugular vein – method 2

(Assume that the skin has been clipped and sterilized, ready for venepuncture.)

1. **Action:** Place the cat in a sitting position on a stable examination table with a non-slip surface.

    Rationale: The cat will feel secure and comfortable and will be less likely to move or try to escape.

2. **Action:** It may be necessary to ask an assistant to place a hand on either side of the cat's rump to maintain it in this position.

    Rationale: This should prevent the cat from struggling during the procedure. If the cat struggles, the assistant should be prepared to use extra force.

3. **Action:** You should bring one hand over the cat's back and restrain the forelegs and paws on the table.

    Rationale: If the cat struggles you may have to use the scruff to restrain and extend the head. However, this leaves the forelegs free, and the cat may scratch the veterinary surgeon.

4. **Action:** Place your other hand under the chin and raise the cat's head so that the neck and chin are in a straight line.

    Rationale: In this position, the jugular vein and overlying skin are tensed, making it easier to penetrate the vein with the needle.

5. **Action:** The veterinary surgeon should apply pressure at the base of the jugular furrow with the fingers of one hand.

    Rationale: The jugular vein on each side of the trachea runs in a groove known as the jugular furrow. It collects venous blood from the head and carries it towards the heart.

6. **Action:** Using the other hand, the veterinary surgeon should insert the needle through the skin into the underlying vein.

    Rationale: The jugular vein should be clearly visible lying just under the skin.

7. **Action:** The veterinary surgeon should draw back on the syringe to check that the vein has been penetrated.

    Rationale: Perivascular injection may lead to tissue damage, and a check must be made that the vein has been penetrated before attempting the injection.

8. **Action:** If blood appears at the hub of the needle, the veterinary surgeon will release the pressure on the vein and slowly inject the contents of the syringe into the vein.

    Rationale: Releasing the pressure allows the drug to flow into the vein.

9. **Action:** When the procedure is complete and the needle has been slowly withdrawn, you should apply gentle pressure to the injection site for about 30 seconds.

    Rationale: This prevents haemorrhage into the area around the vein. Absorption of a drug from an intravenous site is instantaneous.

N.B.: The jugular vein is more often used for blood sampling because a larger volume can be collected very quickly, thus minimizing distress to the patient. During this procedure, pressure is maintained until enough blood has collected in the syringe.

REFERENCES AND FURTHER READING

Anderson, R.S., Edney, A.T.B., 1991. Practical Animal Handling. Pergamon, Oxford.

Aspinall, V., 2011. The Complete Textbook of Veterinary Nursing, second ed. Elsevier, Oxford.

Ackerman, N., 2016. Aspinall's Complete Textbook of Veterinary Nursing, third ed. Elsevier, Oxford.

Cooper, B., Mullineaux, E., Turner, L. (Eds.), 2011. Veterinary Nursing, fifth ed. Butterworth-Heinemann, Oxford.

Lane, D., Cooper, B., 1994. Veterinary Nursing. Butterworth-Heinemann, Oxford.

Masters, J., Bowden, C., 2001. Pre-Veterinary Nursing Textbook. Butterworth-Heinemann, Oxford.

2

Measuring clinical parameters

Richard Aspinall

CHAPTER CONTENTS

INTRODUCTION

Diagnosis of a patient's condition is based on a thorough clinical examination followed by a range of diagnostic tests. Part of the clinical examination includes the measurement of certain basic indicators of the body's function, known as the clinical parameters. Among the easiest to measure, and therefore the most commonly performed, are body temperature, pulse or heart rate and respiratory rate. Once these are known, they are compared to normal values for that species, and the significance of the result is evaluated in the context of the symptoms. Later, once treatment has started, the parameters can be monitored and used as indicators of the progress of the disease.

Clinical parameters such as the percentage of blood gases or blood pressure require the use of complicated equipment but are essential measurements during anaesthesia and for monitoring the progress of the critically ill and hospitalized patient.

Measurement of clinical parameters and the monitoring of changes in their levels are essential parts of patient care. The veterinary surgeon must be able to rely on the veterinary nurse being able to perform the procedure correctly and accurately, and be confident that the nurse understands that, when the results are abnormal, some action must be taken to return them to normal.

This chapter describes the methods of measuring these parameters in detail so that the veterinary nurse can approach the process with a degree of understanding and use the more complicated pieces of apparatus without fear.

Procedure: To measure the body temperature (Table 2.1)

Equipment. Mercury or digital thermometer.

1. **Action:** Place the animal in a comfortable standing position on a table.
   Rationale: *If the patient feels uncomfortable or insecure, it will try to escape.*
2. **Action:** Ask an assistant to restrain the dog gently by placing one arm around the neck and the other around the chest. Ensure that the dog is relaxed and quiet. Hold cats lightly with both hands around the shoulders, or place one hand under its chin and the other around its chest, pulling it close to your body. Observe the patient's behaviour, taking steps to avoid causing distress.
   Rationale: *In this position, the animal will feel comfortable and unrestricted; however, the assistant will be able to react quickly if it tries to jump off the table or becomes distressed.*
3. **Action:** Select either a mercury or digital thermometer.
   Rationale: *The choice of instrument depends on availability.*
4. **Action:** Lubricate the end with K-Y jelly or a similar lubricant.
   Rationale: *Lubrication reduces the discomfort of insertion into the rectum.*
5. **Action:** Shake the mercury down to the bulb or check that the digital thermometer is switched on and displaying a reading.
   Rationale: *If the mercury is not shaken down, the reading will be inaccurate.*
6. **Action:** Gently but firmly insert the instrument into the rectum through the anus. A slight rotating action may help entrance through the rectal sphincters. Cats, particularly, may require

patient, gentle pressure before the sphincters relax.
   Rationale: *In animals, the oral route is not practical but the rectal route is easy and well-tolerated.*
7. **Action:** Leave the thermometer in position for at least 30 seconds.
   Rationale: *The mercury has to have time to warm up and expand.*
8. **Action:** Clean the end of the thermometer by wiping with a paper cloth or cotton wool.

TABLE 2.1 Normal clinical parameters in the dog and cat

Clinical parameter	Dog	Cat
Body temperature	38.3–38.7°C	38.0–38.5°C
Pulse rate	60–180 beats/min	110–180 beats/min
Respiratory rate	10–30 breaths/min	20–30 breaths/min
Capillary refill time	1–2 seconds	1–2 seconds
Oxygen saturation	Close to 99%	Close to 99%
Arterial blood pressure: systolic/diastolic	Puppy: 108/60 mmHg Adult: 141/81 mmHg	Kitten: 123/63 mmHg Adult: 129/70 mmHg
Central venous pressure	3–7 cm H_2O	3–7 cm H_2O
Carbon dioxide concentration	End-tidal: 35–54 mmHg Inspired: less than 8 mmHg	End-tidal: 32–35 mmHg Inspired: less than 8 mmHg
Volume of urine produced	1–2 ml/kg bodyweight/hour	1–2 ml/kg bodyweight/hour
Volume of tears produced	15–25 ml/min when measured using Schirmer strips	15–25 ml/min when measured using Schirmer strips
Intraocular pressure	15–25 mmHg	15–30 mmHg

Rationale: This prevents transmission of disease to another animal the next time the thermometer is used.

9. **Action:** Read the mercury thermometer by looking for the line of mercury against the scale. Read off the figures on the digital thermometer.

   Rationale: The glass of the thermometer magnifies the mercury line and makes it easier to read.

10. **Action:** Record the reading on the hospital record or clinical record.

    Rationale: To monitor rises or falls in the body temperature.

11. **Action:** Shake down the mercury or reset the digital reading.

    Rationale: To prepare the thermometer for use in the future.

12. **Action:** Place the bulb of the instrument in the disinfectant container.

    Rationale: This prevents transmission of disease to another animal the next time the thermometer is used.

Procedure: To measure the pulse rate by palpation of the femoral artery (Table 2.1)

1. **Action:** Place the animal in a comfortable standing position on a table.

   Rationale: If the patient feels uncomfortable or insecure, it will try to escape.

2. **Action:** Ask an assistant to restrain the dog gently by placing one arm around the neck and the other around the chest. Ensure that the dog is relaxed and quiet. Hold cats lightly with both hands around the shoulders, or place one hand under its chin and the other around its chest, pulling it close to your body. Observe the patient's behaviour, taking steps to avoid causing distress.

   Rationale: In this position, the animal will feel comfortable and unrestricted; however, the assistant will be able to react quickly if it tries to jump off the table.

3. **Action:** Standing on one side of the animal, place the fingers of one hand on the medial aspect of the thigh. Locate the femoral artery where it runs down the medial aspect of the femur (Fig. 2.1).

   Rationale: The pulse can be palpated at any point where an artery runs over a bone and close to the body surface. The femoral pulse is the easiest to detect.

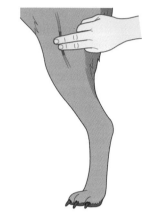

Fig. 2.1 Medial view of the hind leg of a dog to show the finger position used to measure the pulse rate by palpation of the femoral artery.

4. **Action:** Press gently against the artery with the second and third fingers and feel the pulse.

   Rationale: The tips of the fingers are sensitive to touch. The thumb and the forefinger have a pulse of their own, which may be mistaken for the dog's pulse.

5. **Action:** Count the beats of the pulse for 60 seconds.

   Rationale: Sixty seconds is enough time in which to detect any abnormalities.

6. **Action:** Record the pulse rate.

   Rationale: If there are any irregularities in rate and rhythm, inform the veterinary surgeon.

Procedure: To measure the pulse rate using a stethoscope (Table 2.1)

1. **Action:** Place the animal in a comfortable standing position on a table.

   Rationale: If the animal is quiet and comfortable, the heart can be heard more easily.

2. **Action:** Ask an assistant to restrain the dog gently by placing one arm around the neck and the other around the chest. Ensure that the dog is relaxed and quiet. Hold cats lightly with both hands around the shoulders, or place one hand under its chin and the other around its chest, pulling it close to your body. Observe the patient's behaviour, taking steps to avoid causing distress.

   Rationale: In this position, the animal will feel comfortable and unrestricted; however, the assistant will be able to react quickly if it tries to jump off the table or it becomes distressed.

3. **Action:** Place the earpieces of the stethoscope in your ears and place the stethoscope head on the lower left chest caudal to and just dorsal to the elbow – between the third and sixth ribs.
   Rationale: This is close to the left ventricle, where the heart beat can be best heard.
4. **Action:** Listen to the rhythm of the heart and count the heart beats for 60 seconds.
   Rationale: Sixty seconds is enough time in which to detect any abnormalities.
5. **Action:** Record the pulse rate.
   Rationale: If there are any irregularities in rate or rhythm, inform the veterinary surgeon.

Procedure: To measure the pulse rate by palpation of the chest (Table 2.1)

1. **Action:** This method is best used for narrow-chested breeds of dog, such as whippets, greyhounds or lurchers, and for most cats.
   Rationale: The hand will reach across the sternum more easily with such animals.
2. **Action:** Place the animal in a comfortable standing position on a table.
   Rationale: If the animal is quiet and comfortable, the heart can be heard more easily.
3. **Action:** Ask an assistant to restrain the dog gently by placing one arm around the neck and the other around the chest. Ensure that the dog is relaxed and quiet. Hold cats lightly with both hands around the shoulders, or place one hand under its chin and the other around its chest, pulling it close to your body. Observe the patient's behaviour, taking steps to avoid causing distress.
   Rationale: In this position, the animal will feel comfortable and unrestricted; however, the assistant will be able to react quickly if it tries to jump off the table or becomes distressed.
4. **Action:** Either put the flat of the hand on the lower left chest caudal to and just dorsal to the elbow or stretch the hand across to the other side over the sternum and feel the heart beating.
   Rationale: To feel the heart beating within the chest.
5. **Action:** Count the beats over 60 seconds.
   Rationale: Sixty seconds is enough time in which to count the rate.
6. **Action:** Record the pulse rate.
   Rationale: If there are any irregularities in rate or rhythm, inform the veterinary surgeon.

Procedure: To measure the pulse rate using an oesophageal stethoscope (Table 2.1)

1. **Action:** The patient is anaesthetized with a cuffed endotracheal tube in place.
   Rationale: A conscious animal will not tolerate the placing of the tube through the mouth and into the oesophagus.
2. **Action:** Select the correct diameter of oesophageal stethoscope.
   Rationale: Small animals require a smaller bore of tube than larger animals.
3. **Action:** Lay the stethoscope tube on the outside of the dog or cat and measure the approximate length from the mouth to the heart. Mark the tube with a pen or adhesive bandage at the mouth end.
   Rationale: This ensures that the tube is best placed to hear the heart when inside the oesophagus.
4. **Action:** Lubricate the end of the stethoscope with K-Y jelly and introduce it through the patient's mouth and into the oesophagus using gentle pressure. Push it in up to the pre-marked part of the tube.
   Rationale: Gentle pressure enables the tube to enter the oesophagus. Pushing the tube up as far as the mark ensures that the end of the tube lies close to the heart.
5. **Action:** Insert the earpieces of the stethoscope into your ears and listen to the rhythm of the heart.
   Rationale: If there are any irregularities in rate or rhythm, inform the veterinary surgeon.
6. **Action:** Count the heart beats for 60 seconds.
   Rationale: Sixty seconds is enough time in which to count the rate and detect any abnormalities.
7. **Action:** Record the pulse rate on the patient's anaesthetic chart.
   Rationale: The use of the oesophageal stethoscope helps to monitor any cardiac changes during administration of the anaesthetic.

Procedure: To measure the respiratory rate by direct observation (Table 2.1)

1. **Action:** Place the animal in a comfortable standing position on a table.
   Rationale: If the patient feels uncomfortable or insecure, it will try to escape.
2. **Action:** Observe the movement of the rib cage.
   Rationale: The chest expands and contracts once with each breath.
3. **Action:** Count the number of breaths taken over 60 seconds.

Rationale: Sixty seconds is enough time to obtain an accurate measurement of the rate.

4. **Action:** Record the respiration rate on the patient's hospital chart or clinical case record.
   Rationale: This helps produce a permanent record of any changes, which may indicate a need for treatment.

Procedure: To measure the respiratory rate using a stethoscope (Table 2.1)

1. **Action:** Place the animal in a comfortable standing position on a table.
   Rationale: If the patient feels uncomfortable or insecure, it will try to escape.
2. **Action:** Place the earpieces of the stethoscope in your ears and place the diaphragm of the stethoscope on the upper half of the chest, just caudal to the scapula.
   Rationale: This position ensures that the diaphragm of the stethoscope lies over the trachea and bronchi. This is the best place to hear air movement into and out of the lungs.
3. **Action:** Count the breaths taken over 60 seconds.
   Rationale: Sixty seconds is enough time to obtain an accurate measurement of the rate.
4. **Action:** Record the respiration rate on the patient's hospital chart or clinical case record.
   Rationale: This helps produce a permanent record of any changes, which may indicate a need for treatment.

Procedure: To measure the respiratory rate using an oesophageal stethoscope (Table 2.1)

1. **Action:** The patient is anaesthetized with a cuffed endotracheal tube in place.
   Rationale: A conscious animal will not tolerate the placing of the tube through the mouth and into the oesophagus.
2. **Action:** Select the correct diameter of oesophageal stethoscope.
   Rationale: Small dogs require a smaller bore of tube than larger dogs.
3. **Action:** Lay the stethoscope tube on the outside of the dog and measure the approximate length from the mouth to the heart. Mark the tube with a pen or adhesive bandage at the mouth end.
   Rationale: This ensures that the tube is best placed to hear the heart when inside the oesophagus.
4. **Action:** Lubricate the end of the stethoscope with K-Y jelly and introduce it through the patient's mouth and into the oesophagus, using gentle pressure. Push it in up to the pre-marked part of the tube.
   Rationale: Gentle pressure enables the tube to enter the oesophagus. Pushing the tube up as far as the mark ensures that the end of the tube lies close to the heart.
5. **Action:** Insert the earpieces of the stethoscope into your ears and listen to the rhythm of the heart.
   Rationale: If there are any irregularities in rate or rhythm, inform the veterinary surgeon.
6. **Action:** Record the respiration rate on the patient's anaesthetic chart.
   Rationale: The use of an oesophageal stethoscope helps to monitor depth of anaesthetic.

Procedure: To assess capillary refill time (CRT) (Table 2.1)

1. **Action:** Ask an assistant to hold and gently restrain the animal on the table.
   Rationale: If the animal is held securely, it will not try to jump off the table or become stressed.
2. **Action:** Keeping the animal's mouth closed, raise the lip and look at the gum over the upper dental arch.
   Rationale: To assess the colour and general appearance of the gum.
3. **Action:** Gently press on the gum with the ball of your thumb.
   Rationale: Pressure will push all the blood out of the squeezed area.
4. **Action:** Lift your thumb and observe the time it takes for the gum to become pink again.
   Rationale: Releasing the pressure allows the blood to flow back into the gum capillaries.
5. **Action:** The gum should take approximately 1–2 seconds to return to normal.
6. **Action:** Report any abnormalities to the veterinary surgeon.
   Rationale: So that prompt action can be taken, e.g. a dehydrated dog may have an increased CRT, which indicates a need for intravenous fluids.

CRT is a quick and useful way of assessing the circulation. Generally, a dehydrated animal will have a prolonged CRT because of the reduction in circulating blood volume. This technique also allows assessment of the colour of the mucous membranes – paler gums might indicate anaemia, a blue tinge or cyanosis might indicate respiratory problems and yellow coloration or jaundice might indicate liver problems or haemolytic anaemia.

Procedure: To measure the electrical activity of the heart using an electrocardiogram

An electrocardiogram (ECG) trace (Fig. 2.2) measures the electrical activity of the heart muscle and is produced by attaching electrical contacts to two set points on the outside of the body (Fig. 2.3). One of the leads is the earth wire, which is clipped onto the right hind leg. In animals, the other contacts are on each of the other three limbs and provide three different measurements of the electrical waves produced as the heart muscle contracts.

Equipment. ECG machine and leads, surgical spirit.

1. **Action:** Place the animal in left lateral recumbency. Some cats may resent this position, and it may be

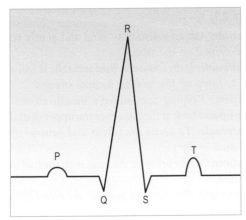

Fig. 2.2 A normal lead II ECG trace.

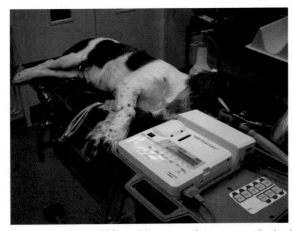

Fig. 2.3 Use of an ECG machine to monitor an anaesthetized dog in left lateral recumbency.

better to have them in a normal upright sitting position. Do not sedate the animal. Observe the patient's behaviour, taking steps to avoid causing distress.

Rationale: This is the standard position for performing ECG recordings. The use of sedatives may affect the ECG trace. Some animals may become distressed and begin to struggle, which may affect the trace.

2. **Action:** Ask an assistant to hold the animal's front and back legs so that it lies comfortably on the table.

Rationale: If the patient is comfortable, it will not struggle and affect the resulting trace.

3. **Action:** Attach the four leads to the four limbs as follows: **red** to the right foreleg; **yellow** to the left foreleg; **black** to the right hind leg; **green** to the left hind leg.

Rationale: The clips should be attached just below the elbows and below the hocks and should be allowed to hang down to minimize movement.

4. **Action:** Soak the crocodile clips with surgical spirit.

Rationale: This ensures good electrical contact.

5. **Action:** Make sure that the room is quiet and stress-free. Set the ECG machine to manual control and switch it on.

Rationale: Any noise or movement will affect the ECG trace.

6. **Action:** Using the markings on the machine, select lead I and do a test trace. Set the electrical filters if required.

Rationale: The filters reduce excessive electrical interference from other electrical circuits in the room, e.g. electric lights or plugged-in appliances, which would affect the trace.

7. **Action:** Record a 1 mV deflection on the test trace.

Rationale: This helps to calibrate the measurements of the actual trace.

8. **Action:** Set the paper speed to 2.5 mm/second and record traces from leads I, II, III, AVR, AVL and AVF. Record each lead for 30 seconds.

Rationale: This routine forms a standard initial survey for the detection of any obvious irregularities. Thirty seconds provides enough time for frequent abnormalities to be identified.

9. **Action:** Increase the paper speed to 5 mm/second and record lead II for a further 30 seconds.

Rationale: The most useful and diagnostic measurement is taken across the heart on lead II, from the left foreleg to the right hind leg. Faster paper speed will show abnormalities of rhythm or waveform more clearly by stretching the recording over a longer piece of paper.

10. **Action:** Read the trace and look for abnormalities of rhythm and abnormalities in the PQRST waves.

    Rationale: Arrhythmias, chamber size irregularities and blocks of the cardiac conduction pathways can be diagnosed by the use of an ECG.

11. **Action:** The veterinary surgeon may require longer traces if an abnormality does not appear in the allocated time.

    Rationale: Some arrhythmias may be intermittent, e.g. in an animal showing signs of fainting. In some cases, special small, ambulatory ECG units, known as Holter monitors, may have to be worn by the animal when exercised. These record digitally and can be used to recall the trace from the time when the dog showed symptoms (e.g. fainting).

12. **Action:** Label the trace with the client's name, date of the recording, name, age and sex of the animal and the case number.

    Rationale: This enables the trace to be identified. If traces are taken at a later date, it enables them to be related to the earlier readings.

Procedure: To measure the percentage of oxygen (oxygen saturation) in the blood using a pulse oximeter (Table 2.1)

The pulse oximeter works by transmitting a pulsed infrared light across a thin flap of tissue to a sensor on the other side of a clip. Small pulsing arterioles within this tissue alter the passage of the light and allow the machine to record a pulse rate. Oxygen tension is calculated by using the difference in the light absorption of deoxygenated blood compared with that of oxygenated blood. The machine expresses this difference as a percentage.

Equipment. Portable pulse oximeter and sensor lead (Fig. 2.4).

1. **Action:** Set up the pulse oximeter near to the patient and either plug it in to the mains or, if battery-operated, ensure that the battery is charged.

    Rationale: The pulse oximeter must be clearly visible to the anaesthetist.

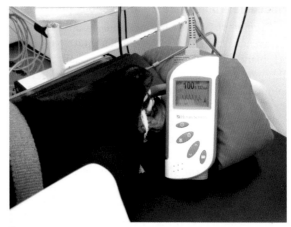

Fig. 2.4 A pulse oximeter.

2. **Action:** Set the pulse oximeter to sound its alarm if the pulse rate and oxygen tension go above or below the normal range.

    Rationale: This ensures that action can be taken if the oxygen level falls or if the heart rate is too slow or too fast.

3. **Action:** Select the correct sensor for the size of the patient.

    Rationale: Smaller animals require smaller clips.

4. **Action:** Select the correct site on which to attach the sensor.

    Rationale: Sites include the tongue, interdigital web, lip, vulva or prepuce.

5. **Action:** Select a site that does not interfere with the surgical procedure.

    Rationale: For instance, using the tongue would interfere with a dental extraction.

6. **Action:** Switch the machine on and monitor the oxygen tension and pulse rate.

    Rationale: To identify and correct any reduction in blood oxygen levels or changes in the pulse rate.

7. **Action:** Record the readings on the patient's anaesthetic chart.

    Rationale: Pulse oximetry is used to monitor any changes in anaesthetic level. The heart rate may rise if the depth of anaesthesia is decreasing or start to slow if the depth is increasing. Oxygen tension may fall if there is a problem with the anaesthetic machine or if the blood in pulmonary circulation is unable to take up the gas, e.g. in cases of pulmonary oedema.

Procedure: To measure central venous pressure

Equipment. A 1 litre bag of saline, an infusion set, an intravenous catheter (14 G or smaller) and a No. 15 scalpel blade. You may also need a specially designed 'through the needle' jugular catheter, chlorhexidine solution, swabs, spirit and bandaging materials, a three-way tap, 2 × 0.5 m of sterile drip tubing to connect to the catheter and to the three-way tap, a metric ruler and a stand to hold the ruler vertically.

1. **Action:** Assemble the apparatus required (Fig. 2.5).
   Rationale: *Central venous pressure (CVP) can be measured by using simple apparatus usually found in a veterinary practice. Manometers are available but are not a necessity.*

2. **Action:** Ask an assistant to restrain the animal for a jugular puncture. At all stages, you must observe the patient's behaviour.
   Rationale: *A calm, gentle approach will prevent the animal struggling, but you must be aware of signs of distress in the patient, e.g. struggling, growling and/or biting or breathing more rapidly, and take steps to alleviate the distress.*

3. **Action:** Clip, swab and wipe with spirit an area of the jugular furrow near the thoracic inlet on the selected side of the neck.
   Rationale: *To ensure maximum sterility. The site is at a similar level to the right atrium of the heart, which is where the CVP is measured.*

4. **Action:** Put on disposable gloves.
   Rationale: *To ensure maximum sterility.*

5. **Action:** Ask your assistant to raise the jugular vein by applying digital pressure to the base of the jugular furrow at the thoracic inlet (see Chapter 1).
   Rationale: *This will cause the vein to engorge by blocking blood return to the heart – known as 'raising the vein'.*

6. **Action:** When the vein is raised, gently push the needle and catheter into the vein with the point towards the head. Check that blood is flowing out of the needle hub and remove the needle while holding the catheter firmly in place.
   Rationale: *This will leave the flexible plastic catheter inside the vein. A rigid needle would be likely to dislodge and lacerate the vein if the animal were to move.*

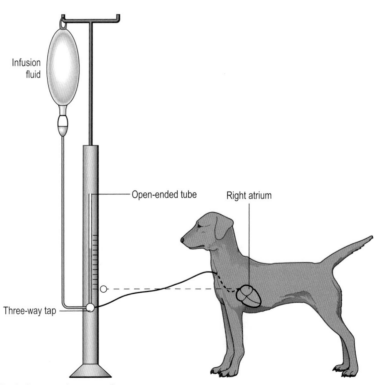

Fig. 2.5 Method of measuring central venous pressure.

7. **Action:** An alternative method is to make a small stab incision through the skin over the vein. If you go too deep, you may cut into the vein itself. It can be helpful to mark the spot over the vein and then ask the assistant to release pressure. Move the skin (and spot mark) away from the vein and make the incision.

   Rationale: Cutting the skin allows the thin through the needle catheter to be placed in the vein with minimal resistance. If the skin is not cut first, the catheter may fray or roll back over the needle and may damage the vein.

8. **Action:** Set the three-way tap to allow saline to flow out of the free end of the infusion set, allowing air bubbles in the saline to disperse. Connect the tubing to the end of the catheter once all air bubbles have dispersed.

   Rationale: Air bubbles might cause an air embolism or a block in the circulation and threaten the patient's life. Check that the tube has no blockages or kinks.

9. **Action:** Fix the catheter in place using a bandage or adhesive tape strips.

   Rationale: Under local anaesthetic, a butterfly bandage could be placed around the catheter hub or tubing and sutured to the animal's skin.

10. **Action:** Turn the three-way tap to exclude the patient and allow saline to flow up the vertical tubing until halfway up its length (25 cm).

    Rationale: This primes and checks the patency of the tubing and removes any possibility of air entering the patient.

11. **Action:** Check that there are no air bubbles in the pressure tube.

    Rationale: This prevents air from inadvertently entering the patient's blood stream. Bubbles will reduce the accuracy of the measurement.

12. **Action:** Set the three-way tap to exclude the drip bag so that the catheter is now connected, via the tubing and the tap, to the vertical open tubing stretched over the ruler.

    Rationale: This allows the patient's blood pressure to be measured.

13. **Action:** The level in the vertical tube will fall rapidly and settle at a certain mark, where it will oscillate up and down in time with the patient's breathing.

    Rationale: This is the CVP. The pressure of the column of water will equal the pressure in the patient's right atrium.

14. **Action:** Make sure that the zero line on the ruler is level with the right atrium of the heart in the chest.

    Rationale: This is only a rough guide. A spirit level can be used for greater accuracy.

15. **Action:** Read the CVP in centimetres of water (cm H_2O) against the ruler.

    Rationale: Ask the veterinary surgeon for an interpretation.

16. **Action:** Reconnect the drip to the animal by turning the three-way tap to exclude the pressure arm of the tubing.

17. **Action:** Repeat the readings hourly using the procedure as described from point 10.

    Rationale: This is used to monitor the CVP during the day – usually with an animal on prolonged intravenous therapy.

The CVP is the pressure of the blood entering the right atrium. The jugular catheter must be level with the right atrium of the heart at the time of the measurement. CVP measurement can be useful to determine whether too much fluid is being given to an animal being kept on a drip for a long time:

- A raised CVP may indicate over-perfusion and a raised blood volume.
- A lowered CVP might reflect a failing heart or loss of blood pressure due to shock or blood loss. A faster drip rate is required to increase blood volume.
- Monitoring such a case might show an increase in CVP as shock improves or blood volume increases.

The absolute measurement is less important than the trend shown by the CVP results.

Procedure: To measure arterial blood pressure using a non-invasive technique (Table 2.1)

Invasive (direct) techniques of blood pressure measurement, where arteries are catheterized and linked to a pressure transducer, are more accurate and may be a more common method of blood pressure measurement in university and referral practices. In general veterinary practice, non-invasive (indirect) measurement techniques are more likely to be used.

1. **Action:** Place the animal in a comfortable standing position on a table. Observe the patient's behaviour, taking steps to avoid causing distress.

   Rationale: If the animal feels uncomfortable or insecure, it will try to escape. A distressed animal may have an artificially raised blood pressure. This is particularly important in conscious cats.

2. **Action:** Set up the instrument.
3. **Action:** Choose a cuff of an appropriate size for the animal (Fig. 2.6).

   Rationale: If the cuff is the wrong size, the measurement will be inaccurate. Too large a cuff will produce a lower blood pressure reading than the actual pressure in the animal, and too small a cuff will produce a higher blood pressure reading than the actual pressure.
4. **Action:** Choose a suitable site on a distal limb or the tail (see below).

   Rationale: The cuff is placed over a peripheral artery where a pulse can be palpated. The chosen site must be almost cylindrical for the cuff to sit comfortably and to maximize the accuracy of the measurements.
5. **Action:** Shave the transducer site or wet thoroughly with spirit. Lubricate with gel and place the transducer over the artery while listening for the pulse on the instrument's loudspeaker or earphones. Inflate the cuff until the pulse stops, then, while looking at the pressure dial, slowly deflate the cuff until the pulse restarts.

   Rationale: Shaving and the use of gel reduce air interference between the transducer and the skin and improve the signal. The cuff pressure at which the pulse restarts is the systolic pressure. Note: it is not necessary to shave cats, as this causes distress and may potentially cause an artificial rise in blood pressure.

6. **Action:** Take a number of readings over several minutes.

   Rationale: This allows for variations caused by anxiety or movement, which can produce an artificially raised result.
7. **Action:** Record the measurement on the patient's anaesthetic chart or clinical case record.

   Rationale: Blood pressure measurement is used to monitor the effect of an anaesthetic or as part of a health check.

   Cuff positioning sites include (Fig. 2.7):
   - Tail base (coccygeal artery) – best in conscious dogs and cats
   - Forelimb proximal to carpus (median artery)
   - Forelimb distal to carpus (common palmar digital artery)
   - Hindlimb proximal to hock (saphenous artery) – best in anaesthetized dogs
   - Hindlimb distal to hock (medial plantar artery).

   In dogs, blood pressure measurement is usually part of anaesthetic monitoring (Fig. 2.8). Anaesthetic drugs can cause a lowered pressure (hypotension), and fluctuations in the pressure can reflect change in the depth of anaesthesia or blood volume. Monitoring allows necessary action to be taken to correct the altered blood pressure.

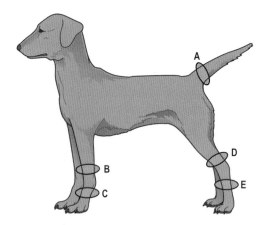

Cuff positions

A   Tail base (coccygeal artery)
B   Proximal to carpus (median artery)
C   Distal to carpus (common palmar digital artery)
D   Proximal to hock (saphenous artery)
E   Distal to hock (median plantar artery)

Fig. 2.7 Cuff positioning sites for the measurement of blood pressure.

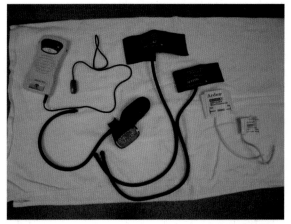

Fig. 2.6 Blood pressure monitoring kit with a range of cuff sizes.

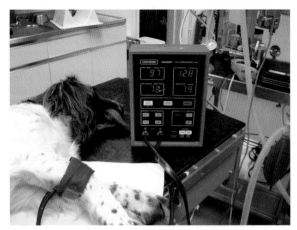

Fig. 2.8 Automatic blood pressure monitoring device – purchased from a hospital and adapted for veterinary use.

In cats, raised blood pressure (hypertension) is reasonably common in older animals and is often a consequence of diseases such as renal failure. Routine monitoring of older cats may detect hypertension and allow corrective treatment. Conditions such as retinal haemorrhage and blindness can be directly caused by a raised blood pressure.

Procedure: To measure carbon dioxide levels using a mainstream capnograph (Table 2.1)

A mainstream capnograph measures end-tidal carbon dioxide (CO_2) levels (i.e. it samples the last bit of expired air from each breath). The technique is used during anaesthesia to monitor the inspired and expired CO_2.

1. **Action:** Set up the capnograph.
2. **Action:** After turning off the anaesthetic gas supply, disconnect the endotracheal tube from the gas delivery tube.
   Rationale: This is done in order to insert the mainstream sensor into the gas flow to and from the animal. Turning off the gas first will help prevent spillage of anaesthetic gases into the environment.
3. **Action:** Connect the CO_2 sensor between the endotracheal tube and the gas delivery tube.
   Rationale: Inspired and expired gases pass through the sensor.
4. **Action:** Restart the anaesthetic gases and set the vaporizer to the correct concentration, as required by the veterinary surgeon.
   Rationale: To maintain the level of anaesthesia.
5. **Action:** Read the CO_2 levels from the digital display.

6. **Action:** Record the levels on the patient's anaesthetic record or print a graph directly from the machine.
   Rationale: To allow monitoring of anaesthesia and enable early corrective action to be taken if the levels start to rise.
7. **Action:** Take readings every 60 seconds throughout the anaesthetic procedure.
   Rationale: To identify any trends and allow early corrective treatment.

Procedure: To measure carbon dioxide levels using a sidestream capnograph (Fig. 2.9)

A sidestream capnograph measures end-tidal CO_2 and inspired CO_2 concentrations.

1. **Action:** Set up the capnograph.
2. **Action:** Without disconnecting the endotracheal tube, attach the small tube leading to the instrument to the special port on the end of the gas delivery tube.
   Rationale: This machine sucks a small sample of gas out of the gas flow, rather than being positioned in the midst of the flow.
3. **Action:** Read the levels of inspired and expired CO_2 from the digital display. They are displayed as a scrolling graph showing the changes of CO_2 concentration with each breath.
   Rationale: Both inspired and end-tidal CO_2 levels are measured.

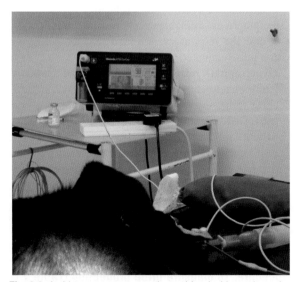

Fig. 2.9 A sidestream capnograph combined with a pulse oximeter. 'Please note that the capnograph (lower reading) was not working at the time of this photograph'.

4. **Action:** Record the levels on the patient's anaesthetic record or print a graph directly from the machine.

   Rationale: To allow monitoring of anaesthesia and enable early corrective action to be taken if the levels start to rise.

5. **Action:** Take readings every minute throughout the anaesthetic procedure.

   Rationale: To identify any trends and allow early corrective treatment.

The sidestream capnograph is more accurate than the mainstream capnograph, and is useful in monitoring both the patient's anaesthetic progress and the efficiency of the anaesthetic equipment. The mainstream type of capnograph has several disadvantages compared with the sidestream type:

- It is more vulnerable to accidental damage as the sensor lies close to the animal during use. The sidestream capnograph can be placed a safe distance away and is less likely to be disturbed.
- It only measures expired end-tidal CO_2, and is primarily useful for identifying a pulmonary problem and a consequent rise in CO_2. However, if the level of CO_2 in the inspired gases is high (e.g. exhausted soda lime in a circuit), the mainstream machine cannot specify whether the cause of the problem is the patient or the apparatus. In a dangerous, life-threatening situation, time may be lost trying to determine the cause of the problem.

Capnographs are available which measure both the CO_2 level and the respiratory rate, and may be combined with a pulse oximeter.

   Hypercapnia – raised CO_2 levels – may be caused by:
- faulty anaesthetic equipment, e.g. blocked endotracheal tube, excessive dead space, faulty valves, exhausted soda lime
- patient problems, e.g. hypoventilation (reduced respiratory rate, breath holding), any lung condition that prevents the normal exchange of oxygen and carbon dioxide.

   Hypocapnia – lowered CO_2 levels – may be caused by:
- patient problems, e.g. hyperventilation caused by panting, or excessive respiratory rate.

Procedure: To measure urine production (Table 2.1)

Equipment. Sterile urinary catheter, empty used drip bag, infusion set.

1. **Action:** Catheterize the patient as described in Chapter 3.
2. **Action:** Drain the bladder with a 50 ml syringe until it is empty.

   Rationale: To get an accurate measure of future urine production.

3. **Action:** Connect the needle end of the infusion set to the urinary catheter.
4. **Action:** Make sure that the empty drip bag is level with, or preferably below, the level of the animal's bladder.

   Rationale: This uses gravity to fill the bag and to prevent inadvertent reflux of stale urine back into the bladder.

5. **Action:** Once an hour, **either** weigh the bag on accurate scales **or** empty it with a 50 ml syringe and note the volume.

   Rationale: One millilitre of urine weighs approximately 1 g. Thus, the volume can be calculated by determining the weight of the urine in grams. This gives the volume of urine produced per hour.

Hourly urinary output is a useful indicator of renal function. Normal kidneys will produce 1–2 ml urine/kg bodyweight/hour. If urine production is less than 0.5 ml/kg bodyweight/hour, then the animal may be severely dehydrated or in renal shutdown.

This procedure is most likely to be performed in hospitalized and recumbent patients. The catheter may be left in place for more than 24 hours, and it is very important that a sterile approach is taken. Bladder infection in a patient that is already ill may cause its condition to deteriorate.

Procedure: To measure tear production (Table 2.1)

Equipment. Schirmer tear measurement strips.

1. **Action:** Ask an assistant to restrain the animal on the table. Observe the patient's behaviour, taking steps to avoid causing distress.

   Rationale: The animal needs to be comfortable to allow the measurement to be made.

2. **Action:** Remove two Schirmer test strips from their sterile plastic envelope.

   Rationale: These are packaged to keep the strips dry and sterile.

3. **Action:** Fold the end of one strip at the notch near the end. Try not to touch the paper with your fingers.

   Rationale: Touching the strip may cause moisture to be absorbed from your fingers, and this may affect the accuracy of the result.

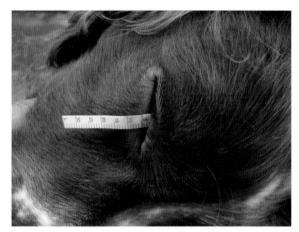

Fig. 2.10 Use of Schirmer strips to measure tear production.

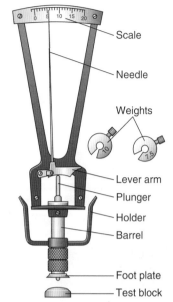

Fig. 2.11 A Schiotz tonometer.

Scale
Needle
Weights
Lever arm
Plunger
Holder
Barrel
Foot plate
Test block

4. **Action:** Gently roll out the lower eyelid and hook the short end of the strip so that it rests against the junction of the cornea and the conjunctiva (Fig. 2.10).
   Rationale: *This ensures that the strip makes good contact with the area of tear production.*
5. **Action:** Gently close the eyelids.
   Rationale: *This will hold the strip in place.*
6. **Action:** Hold in place for 1 minute.
   Rationale: *This is the standard time of the test.*
7. **Action:** Remove the strip and measure the length of the blue-stained area of wet paper.
   Rationale: *The longer the length of the stain, the greater the volume of tears produced.*
8. **Action:** Repeat the measurement in the other eye using the second strip.
   Rationale: *To compare the two eyes.*

This simple test is a useful method of assessing tear production. Keratoconjunctivitis sicca (or 'dry eye') is a distressing problem in certain breeds, and the Schirmer test can be used to diagnose and monitor the effectiveness of treatment.

Procedure: To measure intraocular pressure (Table 2.1)

Intraocular pressure (IOP) rises if the eye begins to suffer from glaucoma. This increase in pressure can be very destructive to the internal structures of the eye, and can cause severe pain, blindness and eventual collapse of the eye. Tonometry readings are a useful method of assessing any rise in pressure and indicating whether drugs should be used to reduce the pressure. Serial readings can indicate how effective treatment has been. The

mechanical tonometer (Fig 2.11) is less accurate and should be used only as a guide. The Tono-Pen™ (Fig 2.12) is much more accurate and reliable. The Tono-Vet™ (Fig 2.13) is the easiest to use, requires a minimum of restraint and does not require the application of local anaesthetic.

Equipment. Either a mechanical IOP instrument (Schiotz) or a digital instrument such as a Tono-Pen or a Tono-Vet.

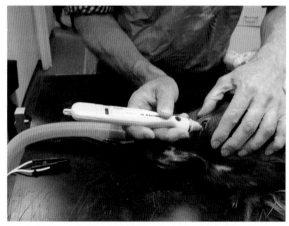

Fig. 2.12 Use of a Tono-Pen™ to measure intraocular pressure.

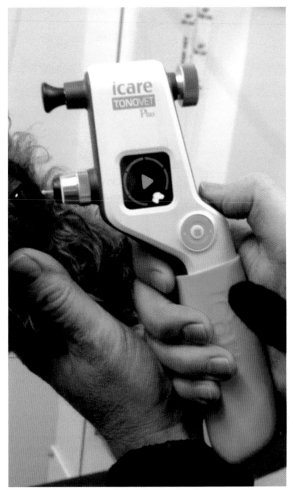

Fig. 2.13 A Tono-Vet™ in use – note the minute probe 'hitting' the cornea.

1. **Action:** Ask an assistant to restrain the animal on the table. Observe the patient's behaviour, taking steps to avoid causing distress.
   Rationale: *The animal needs to be comfortable and firmly restrained to allow the measurement to be taken.*
2. **Action:** Put local anaesthetic drops in both eyes. (Proxymetacaine disposable drops are suitable.)
   Rationale: *This desensitizes the cornea so that it can be touched without the animal blinking or reacting.*
3. **Action:** Select the appropriate piece of equipment.
   Using a Schiotz Tonometer (Fig 2.11)
1. **Action:** Calibrate the machine (Fig 2.11) by pressing it gently onto the metal test block. Different weights can be added to the plunger.
   Rationale: *This sets the zero pressure level.*

2. **Action:** Ask the assistant to hold the animal's head up so that the cornea is horizontal.
   Rationale: *Readings depend on gravity, so the instrument must be held as vertically as possible.*
3. **Action:** Gently rest the instrument on the cornea and take a reading from the needle.
   Rationale: *A soft eyeball will only deflect the probe a little, thus producing a reading closer to the zero baseline. Conversely, a harder eyeball will deflect the probe more, producing a higher reading.*
4. **Action:** Take at least two readings from both eyes.
   Rationale: *This allows comparison of the pressure in both eyes and, by repetition, checks the accuracy of the instrument. Each reading should be the same as the previous measurement.*
5. **Action:** Record the readings on the clinical case record or hospitalization chart.
   Rationale: *To allow comparison with later measurements and enable monitoring of the efficacy of treatment.*
   Using a Tono-Pen™ (Fig 2.12)
1. **Action:** Put a new latex sheath over the end of the Tono-Pen™ using the cardboard applicator supplied by the manufacturers.
   Rationale: *This protects the sensitive end of the instrument and prevents cross-infection.*
2. **Action:** Calibrate the machine by pushing the button near the tip, with the head of the Tono-Pen™ held downwards. When it beeps, point the head vertically upwards. The machine should read 'good' on the display bar, and readings can now be taken. If the display says 'bad', the process has to be repeated until the correct response is obtained.
   Rationale: *This calibrates the tonometer and ensures the accuracy of the readings.*
3. **Action:** Gently touch the latex-covered tip to the anaesthetized cornea of the patient. This should be done several times until a beep is heard.
   Rationale: *The machine works by gentle corneal contact, not by deforming the surface by pressure.*
4. **Action:** Repeat the readings more than once, and take them from both eyes.
   Rationale: *This allows comparison of the pressure in both eyes and, by repetition, checks the accuracy. Each reading should be the same as the previous measurement.*
5. **Action:** Discard the latex sleeve.
   Rationale: *To prevent cross-infection.*

6. **Action:** Record the readings in the clinical case record or on the hospitalization chart.

   Rationale: *To allow comparison with later measurements and enable monitoring of the efficacy of treatment.*

   Using a Tono-Vet (Fig 2.13). The principle of the Tono-Vet's action is that it bounces a small plastic rod (the probe) off the surface of the eye, measures the deceleration of the probe and the rebound time and calculates the IOP from these parameters.

   It is simpler to use than the Tono-Pen, and does not require the application of a local anaesthetic to the cornea or any prior calibration. The instrument can be used to measure IOP in dogs, cats and other species.

1. **Action:** Place the wrist strap around your wrist and secure it.

   Rationale: *The wrist strap protects the tonometer from accidentally dropping onto the floor.*

2. **Action:** Turn it on by pushing either the 'Select' or the 'Measure' button.

3. **Action:** Remove the red probe base cover and open the probe tube by removing the cap. Do not dispose of the cover. Insert the probe into the probe base.

   Rationale: *The disposable probe is used to take the measurement. It is disposable to prevent cross-infection with other animals.*

4. **Action:** The display will now show a play symbol and a species picture.

   Rationale: *This indicates that the instrument is ready to take a measurement.*

5. **Action:** The species symbol can be changed by pressing the 'Select' button from the menu and finding the relevant setting for the species being assessed.

   Rationale: *Different species have different types of corneas, and the machine is preset to take into account those differences.*

6. **Action:** Make sure the animal's head is horizontal, i.e. not tipped up or down.

   Rationale: *This improves the accuracy of the measurement.*

7. **Action:** Make sure that the probe is also horizontal. A red probe light will show if the machine is tipped, and a green light indicates that it is level.

   Rationale: *This improves the accuracy of the measurement.*

8. **Action:** Use minimal restraint of the animal and observe the animal's behaviour to ensure that it is not distressed.

   Rationale: *Distress may raise the IOP.*

9. **Action:** Bring the probe tip close to the eye (4–8 mm is the optimum distance) and aim for the centre of the cornea.

   Rationale: *The probe should contact the centre of the cornea to get an accurate reading.*

10. **Action:** Press the 'Measure' button and keep it pressed. The machine will then take six rapid measurements.

    Rationale: *A series of six readings gives the most accurate average result.*

11. **Action:** After six readings, a long beep will sound.

    Rationale: *This indicates that the readings are finished.*

12. **Action:** The display will show the reading. A green light indicates that the measurement is good; a red or yellow light indicates that the process must be repeated.

13. **Action:** Discard the probe and record the IOP.

    Rationale: *Discarding the probe will prevent infection of the next patient.*

REFERENCES AND FURTHER READING

Ackerman, N., 2016. Aspinall's Complete Textbook of Veterinary Nursing, third ed. Elsevier, Oxford.

Aspinall, V., 2011. The Complete Textbook of Veterinary Nursing, second ed. Elsevier, Oxford.

Chandler, E.A., Thompson, D.J., Sutton, J.B., Price, C.J., 1995. Canine Medicine and Therapeutics. Blackwell Science, Oxford.

Cooper, C., Mullineaux, E., Turner, L., 2011. Textbook of Veterinary Nursing, fifth ed. BSAVA, Gloucester.

Hall, L.W., Clarke, K.W., Trim, C.M., 2001. Veterinary Anaesthesia. W.B. Saunders, London.

Hotson-Moore, A. (Ed.), 1999. Manual of Advanced Veterinary Nursing 1999. BSAVA, Gloucester.

Moore, M. (Ed.), 1999. Manual of Veterinary Nursing 1999. BSAVA, Gloucester.

3

Medical nursing procedures

Jo Masters and Nicola Ackerman

CHAPTER CONTENTS

INTRODUCTION

Medical conditions can be divided into those that are caused by microorganisms and are infectious, e.g. feline infectious respiratory disease or canine parvovirus, and those that develop as a result of an upset in the normal processes of the body, e.g. renal failure, diabetes mellitus or exocrine pancreatic insufficiency. Many patients may not require hospitalization and may be treated during a consultation or at home, but some will require further diagnostic tests and, if critically ill, will require observation and skilled nursing care. Those patients that have an infectious disease must be isolated to prevent the spread of infection, and barrier nursing procedures must be instigated either at home or within the practice.

The aim of nursing the medical patient is to help the animal to return to a state of normal health as soon as possible. Whilst in the hospital it must be kept warm and comfortable, free from pain and, remembering that this is an animal removed from its normal surroundings, free from fear and apprehension. Veterinary nurses play an extremely important part in the recovery process, and the care that they give must be based on an understanding of the disease process and the aims of the treatment regime.

This chapter describes the general techniques used in medical nursing and relates them to some of the more common conditions seen in practice. It is important to understand that most of the techniques can be used in a range of conditions, and examples of their use are listed before each procedure.

MEDICAL TECHNIQUES

Procedure: General examination of the dog or cat

1. **Action:** Observe the patient in its kennel and record any abnormalities.
   Rationale: Handling the patient will involve some stress, which may influence clinical signs; observing the animal first might give you some insight into its mental status before you interact with it.
2. **Action:** Remove the patient (if required) and place in a comfortable position suited to a full examination.
   Rationale: If the patient feels comfortable it is less likely to try to escape. A cat or small dog should be examined on a table, whereas a larger dog may be more suited to an examination on the floor.
3. **Action:** Ask an assistant to reassure and restrain the patient.
   Rationale: Reassuring the patient will help it to relax. An assistant should be ready to restrain the patient if it tries to escape or becomes aggressive during the examination.
4. **Action:** Examine the patient. In the dog, start at the cranial end and work systemically towards the tail. In the cat, start at the tail and work cranially. Identify any abnormalities, including discharges, wounds, lumps and painful areas.
   Rationale: Examining a patient in a set systematic pattern as a routine will limit the likelihood of any area being excluded. Any abnormalities should be noted, however minor or unrelated to the treatment the patient is receiving.

5. **Action:** The five vital assessments should be taken. These are temperature, pulse and respiration (TPR) parameters; a pain score; and a nutritional assessment. The nutritional assessment should include weight, body condition score (BCS) and muscle condition score (MCS).
   Rationale: The five vital assessments should be noted whenever the patient is examined as a measure of the patient's progress.
6. **Action:** Record all findings on the patient's hospitalization sheet and clinical history.
   Rationale: All findings must be recorded to help identify any abnormalities and communicate the patient's progress to all staff. Report any abnormalities to the veterinary surgeon.

Procedure: Barrier nursing – avoidance of cross-infection

1. **Action:** Ideally, staff should be allocated solely to the isolation facility and not allowed to nurse patients in the general ward. If this is not possible, isolation patients should always be attended to last.
   Rationale: Staff may potentially transmit infection from the patient they are nursing to others of the same species or those susceptible to infection, such as immunologically challenged patients and paediatric or geriatric patients.
2. **Action:** Personal protective equipment (PPE) includes clothing such as disposable gloves, aprons and foot covers. Ideally, whole body protective suits should be worn. Everything should be placed in the hazardous waste bin after use. Foot baths should also be provided and used.
   Rationale: Protection from zoonotic disease is a high priority. The wearing of protective clothing will prevent disease being spread via staff clothing.
3. **Action:** Patients that are most likely to spread disease should be cleaned out and treated after all other patients in the isolation facility.
   Rationale: This will prevent disease being spread from the most infectious patient by the nursing staff.
4. **Action:** Each patient in the isolation facility should be allocated its own equipment, i.e. food bowl, water bowl, litter tray. These may be described as fomites and should be washed and disinfected, or sterilized separately from others. Bedding should all be disposable and should be placed in the hazardous waste bin after use.

Rationale: Infection can be spread from fomites such as kennel equipment. Allocation of equipment to specific kennels will limit this, as will cleaning the items separately. Keep track of equipment by numbering kennels and their related equipment. Most bedding cannot be sterilized satisfactorily and may pass infection on during the cleaning process.

5. **Action:** All findings must be recorded on the patient's hospitalization record and clinical history. Report all abnormalities to the veterinary surgeon. Barrier nursing notices should be displayed.

   Rationale: The veterinary surgeon should be made aware of the patient's progress. It is the veterinary surgeon who is ultimately responsible for the case. Barrier nursing notices can prevent inadvertent cross-contamination by warning personnel entering the isolation area. Personnel entering the area should be kept to a minimum.

Procedure: Application of an enema (dogs)

Enemas can be used to empty the rectum and distal colon, to aid in diagnostics or to administer drugs. In situations where solutions are to be used to empty the rectum of faecal matter, the animal should be sedated or anaesthetized for the procedure to be effective. Examples of solutions that can be used include water (rectal lavage), soapy water (chlorhexidine solutions), oily substances (such as liquid paraffin/mineral oil) and phosphate enemas (proprietary brands). The manual breaking down of compacted faeces is normally required.

1. **Action:** Prepare all equipment – including enema solution at body temperature and associated tubing, catheters, Higginson's syringe as required, disposable gloves, aprons and absorbent tissue (Fig. 3.1). Lubricant will also be required.

   Rationale: As with all procedures, the preparation of the equipment before beginning the procedure is both an efficient and a practical method of working. The solution should be warmed to prevent shock and promote tolerance.

2. **Action:** As the patient is anaesthetized, it is important to ensure that the core body temperature is monitored and maintained. In this case, the rectal temperature cannot be monitored.

   Rationale: Hypothermia is the most common cause for delayed recovery from anaesthesia. Monitoring body temperature and providing external heating such as a heat mat will help to prevent this.

3. **Action:** The end of the tubing to be inserted into the rectum should be lubricated before insertion. The assistant should raise the patient's tail, and the anal area should be cleaned with some warm water to remove any faecal material or debris.

   Rationale: Lubricating the tube end will allow easy access and prevent damage to the rectal mucosa. The anal area should be cleaned to prevent infection being introduced from the outside.

4. **Action:** Place the end of the tubing in the patient's anus and gently twist until it is in the rectum. The enema solution should be introduced slowly, either by gravity or by pump, depending on the method

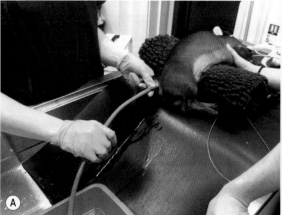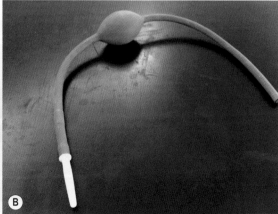

Fig. 3.1 Use of a Higginson's syringe to perform an enema in a dog. (From Clinical Procedures in Small Animal Practice, Aspinall and Aspinall (2013), Saunders, p. 190, Fig 7.9)

used. The solution may be administered until a back flow is seen.

Rationale: *Gently twisting the tube end will encourage the anal sphincter to relax and allow passage of the tube into the rectum. This is more difficult in cats. A back flow will indicate that the rectum is full of enema solution.*

5. **Action:** When bowel evacuation is complete, the patient should be cleaned appropriately and a note made of the amount and type of excreta passed.

Rationale: *The patient should be thoroughly clean, dry and comfortable before being put back into its kennel. The type of excreta passed may indicate the reason for a constipation problem, e.g. bones.*

Procedure: Catheterization of the dog

- Two people are required.
- Examples of procedures include short-term catheterization to obtain a sterile urine sample, or indwelling catheterization, which is useful in recumbent patients.

- Examples of catheter types include conventional plastic or Foley silicone dog catheters (Fig. 3.2).

1. **Action:** Prepare all the equipment, including sterile catheter and any application equipment, e.g. stylets to assist with introduction, lubricant, disposable gloves, apron, sterile sample container or collecting vessel such as a kidney dish, syringe and three-way tap or bung. If measurement of urine output is required, a urine collection bag will need to be prepared. Absorbent material such as swabs/tissue will be useful, and suture material may be required for indwelling catheters.

Rationale: *As with any procedure, the preparation of the equipment before beginning the procedure is both an efficient and a practical method of working. Ensure that you understand why the catheter is being introduced and any procedures that will*

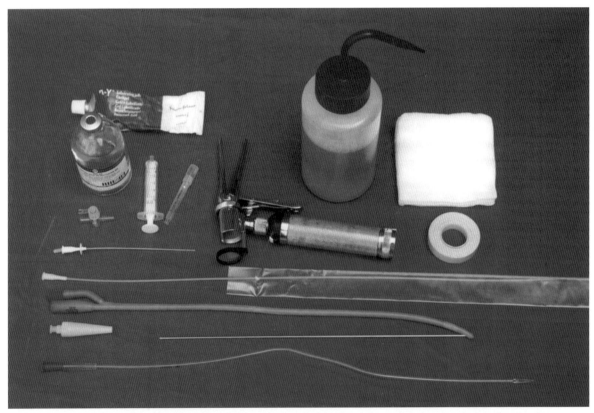

Fig. 3.2 Equipment required for general catheterization. Catheters are, from top to bottom: Jackson's cat catheter, conventional dog catheter, latex Foley catheter with stylet correctly placed, Tiemann catheter.

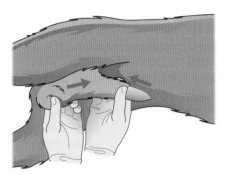

Fig. 3.3 Extruding the penis of a dog (From Clinical Procedures in Small Animal Practice, Aspinall and Aspinall (2013), Saunders, p. 186, Fig 7.6.)

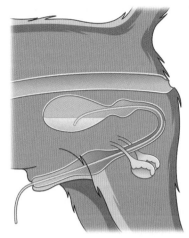

Fig. 3.4 Passing a urethral catheter into the bladder of a dog. (From Clinical Procedures in Small Animal Practice, Aspinall and Aspinall (2013), Saunders, p. 187, Fig 7.7.)

be carried out after its introduction. This will enable all necessary equipment to be prepared. The catheter and collection bag should be sterile to prevent infection being introduced into the urinary tract.

2. **Action:** The assistant should restrain the patient. Gloves and aprons should be put on. The preputial area should be cleaned and the penis extruded (Fig. 3.3).

    Rationale: The patient may be standing or in lateral recumbency, depending on personal preference. Protective clothing should be worn to prevent the spread of zoonoses and introduction of infection to the patient.

3. **Action:** Remove the catheter from its outer packaging, and cut the end from the inner packaging, which is used as a feeder sleeve.

    Rationale: The use of a feeder sleeve allows the catheter to be fed into the urethra without having to touch the sterile tubing.

4. **Action:** The catheter tip should be lubricated, introduced into the urethra and then advanced using gentle pressure (Fig. 3.4). Urine will flow back down the catheter when the bladder is reached and may require collection. The bladder may need flushing, depending on the procedure to be carried out. Suturing or sticking the catheter to the prepuce will be required if the catheter is to be indwelling.

    Rationale: Gentle pressure should enable the catheter to pass the narrowing of the urethra at the ischial arch or around an enlarged prostate gland. If resistance is met, the catheter size may need to be reassessed. The application of zinc oxide tape to the

catheter enables it to be sutured to the preputial area.

5. **Action:** Remove the catheter slowly and dispose of it correctly. Clean and dry the patient.

    Rationale: Removing the catheter slowly will help prevent tissue damage and urine splashes, which could be a zoonotic risk. All catheters and associated equipment should be disposed of in the offensive waste. Keeping the patient clean will prevent urine scalds.

Procedure: Catheterization of the bitch

- Two people are required.
- Examples of procedures include short-term catheterization to obtain a sterile urine sample, or indwelling catheterization, which is useful in recumbent patients.
- Examples of catheter types include Foley indwelling catheters for the bitch and Tiemann catheters for the bitch. A vaginal speculum (sterile) will be required unless the insertion is to be carried out using the sterile digital method (Fig. 3.2).

1. **Action:** Prepare all the equipment, including sterile catheter and any application equipment (such as vaginal speculum and stylets to assist with introduction if required), lubricant, disposable gloves, apron, sterile sample container/collecting vessel (such as a kidney dish) and three-way tap or bung. If measurement of urine output and input is required, a urine collection bag will need to be prepared.

Rationale: As with all procedures, preparing the equipment before you begin is both an efficient and practical method of working. Ensure that you understand why the catheter is being introduced and any procedures that will be carried out after its introduction. This will enable all necessary equipment to be prepared. The catheter and collection bag should be sterile to prevent infection being introduced to the urinary tract. Foley catheters must not be reused, as the balloon weakens after each use.

2. **Action:** Put on gloves and an apron. Ask the assistant to restrain the patient, either in lateral or dorsal recumbency or in a standing position, depending on the insertion method used. If the catheter is to be inserted using the digital method, sterile gloves should be worn by the person carrying out the procedure.

    Rationale: Protective clothing should be worn to prevent the spread of zoonoses and introduction of infection to the patient. For insertion in dorsal recumbency, the patient should be in a straight position with the hind legs flexed and drawn cranially. For all methods, the tail must be firmly restrained.

3. **Action:** The vulval area should be cleaned and free from debris.

    Rationale: Cleaning the area will prevent introduction of infection to the urogenital tract.

4. **Action:** The catheter should be removed from its outer wrapping, exposing the tip from the inner sleeve, and lubricated. Do not use petroleum-based lubricants on latex catheters. If using a Foley catheter, the stylet should be placed and the balloon checked for easy inflation (Fig. 3.2).

    Rationale: Aseptic technique is necessary to prevent introduction of infection. Stylets aid with the introduction and placement of the catheter and should be sterile. Most stylets are placed through the tubing, but stylets used with Foley catheters should be laid alongside the tubing with the stylet placed in a drainage hole at the catheter's tip.

5. **Action:** Place the speculum blades between the vulval lips. If working with the patient in dorsal recumbency, the blades should be inserted as far caudally as possible, and the speculum should then be inserted vertically into the vestibule, turning the handles cranially. If working with the patient in a standing position, the speculum should be inserted at a slight angle towards the spine, then horizontally.

    Rationale: In dorsal recumbency the blades should be inserted to avoid the clitoral fossa.

6. **Action:** Once the speculum is in place, open the blades and identify the urethral orifice.

    Rationale: The urethral orifice should be visible halfway between the vulva and the cervix. If the patient is standing, it will be on the floor of the vestibule; if in dorsal recumbency, it will be on the uppermost side.

7. **Action:** If using the sterile digital method (Fig. 3.5), the first finger of one hand (usually the non-writing hand) should be lubricated and placed into the vestibule, feeling along the ventral surface for a raised area.

    Rationale: The urethral orifice is just cranial to this raised area and can be identified with the finger to guide the catheter in.

8. **Action:** The tip of the catheter should be inserted into the urethral orifice and gradually advanced until it reaches the bladder.

    Rationale: With the patient in dorsal recumbency, the hind legs should now be extended caudally to allow straightening of the urethra for easier catheter introduction.

9. **Action:** If a Foley catheter is to be indwelling, the balloon should be inflated, the stylet removed and

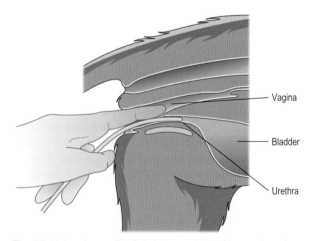

Fig. 3.5 Using the sterile digital approach to urinary catheterization of the bitch. (From Clinical Procedures in Small Animal Practice, Aspinall and Aspinall (2013), Saunders, p. 188, Fig 7.8.)

a collection bag attached. An Elizabethan collar may be used.

Rationale: The inflated balloon keeps the catheter secure in the bladder without the need for suturing.

10. **Action:** When the appropriate procedure has been completed, remove the catheter slowly, having first deflated the balloon in the Foley catheter, and dispose of it correctly. Ensure that the patient is clean and dry before being returned to its kennel.

    Rationale: Removing the catheter slowly will prevent tissue damage and reduce the risk of urine splashes, which could carry a zoonotic disease. All catheters and associated equipment should be disposed of in the clinical waste. Keeping the patient clean will prevent urine scalds.

Procedure: Catheterization of the tomcat

This procedure is normally carried out under a general anaesthetic, as it may be painful, and struggling may cause penetration of the urethra.

- Two people are required.
- Examples of procedures include short-term catheterization to obtain a sterile urine sample, indwelling catheterization (which is useful in recumbent patients) or hydro propulsion (using water pressure to dislodge blockages).
- Examples of catheter types (Fig. 3.2) include conventional cat catheters, Jackson catheters and silicone catheters for use in the cat.

1. **Action:** Prepare all the equipment, including sterile catheter and any application equipment, e.g. stylets to assist with introduction if required, sterile lubricant, disposable gloves, apron, sterile sample container or collecting vessel (such as a kidney dish) and three-way tap. If measurement of urine output is required, a urine collection bag will need to be prepared.

   Rationale: As with all procedures, preparing the equipment before you begin is both an efficient and practical method of working. Ensure that you understand why the catheter is being introduced and any procedures that will be carried out after its introduction. This will enable all necessary equipment to be prepared.

2. **Action:** Put on gloves and apron. Position the anaesthetized cat in lateral or dorsal recumbency, ensuring

that the tail is out of the way. Clip and fully clean the area.

Rationale: In this position, the perineal area and the penis can be easily accessed. Cleaning is required to reduce the risk of bacteria being introduced into the bladder.

3. **Action:** Remove the catheter from its outer packaging and cut the end from the inner packaging, which is used as a feeder sleeve. Lubricate the tip of the catheter.

   Rationale: The use of a feeder sleeve allows the catheter to be fed into the urethra without touching the sterile tubing. Lubrication of the tip will ensure ease of introduction and will prevent tissue damage.

4. **Action:** Extrude the penis by applying gentle pressure on either side of the prepuce and introduce the catheter into the urethra (Fig. 3.6). If a Jackson cat catheter is used, remove the metal stylet.

   Rationale: Gentle preputial pressure should result in extrusion of the penis.

5. **Action:** Continue with the procedure – collection of sample, drainage of bladder, hydro propulsion, etc.

   Rationale: If an indwelling Jackson or silicone cat catheter is used, suture it to the prepuce. Attach a collection bag and use an Elizabethan collar.

6. **Action:** Remove the catheter slowly and dispose of it in the clinical waste. Return the cat to its kennel when it is clean and dry and fully recovered from the anaesthesia.

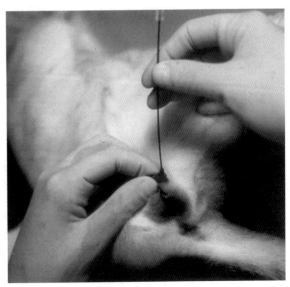

Fig. 3.6 Catheterization of a tomcat.

Rationale: Removing the catheter slowly will prevent tissue damage and urine splashes, which could be a zoonotic risk. All catheters and associated equipment should be disposed of in the clinical waste. Keeping the cat clean and dry will prevent urine scalds.

Procedure: Catheterization of the queen

This procedure is normally carried out under a general anaesthetic, as it may be painful, and struggling may cause penetration of the urethra.

- Two people are required.
- Examples of procedures include short-term catheterization to obtain a sterile urine sample, indwelling catheterization (which is useful in recumbent patients) or hydro propulsion (using water pressure to dislodge blockages).
- Examples of catheter types include conventional cat catheters, Jackson catheters and silicone catheters for use in the cat.

1. **Action:** Prepare all the equipment, including sterile catheter and any application equipment, e.g. stylets to assist with introduction, sterile lubricant, disposable gloves, apron, sterile sample container or collecting vessels such as a kidney dish and three-way tap. If measurement of urine output is required, a urine collection bag will need to be prepared.

   Rationale: As with all procedures, preparing the equipment before you begin is both an efficient and practical method of working. Ensure that you understand why the catheter is being introduced and any procedures that will be carried out after its introduction. This will enable all necessary equipment to be prepared.

2. **Action:** Remove the catheter from its outer packaging and cut the end from the inner packaging, which is used as a feeder sleeve. Lubricate the tip of the catheter.

   Rationale: The use of a feeder sleeve allows the catheter to be fed into the urethra without touching the sterile tubing. Lubrication of the tip will ensure ease of introduction and will prevent tissue damage.

3. **Action:** Place the catheter between the vulval lips and introduce into the urethra by angling the catheter ventrally, using gentle pressure until the catheter enters the urethral orifice.

   Rationale: The use of a vaginal speculum is not necessary for this procedure. Queen catheterization is not often performed, as blockages are rare.

4. **Action:** Continue with procedure – collection of sample, drainage of bladder, hydro propulsion, etc.

   Rationale: If an indwelling Jackson or silicone cat catheter has been used, suture it in place, attach a collection bag and use an Elizabethan collar.

5. **Action:** Remove the catheter slowly and dispose of it correctly. Return the cat to its kennel when it is clean and dry.

   Rationale: Slowly removing the catheter will prevent tissue damage and urine splashes, which could be a zoonotic risk. All catheters and associated equipment should be disposed of in the clinical waste. Keeping the cat clean and dry will prevent urine scalds.

Procedure: Manual expression of the bladder

- Two people are required.

Manual expression of the bladder may be required in recumbent patients or those suffering from bladder paralysis. Natural elimination of the bladder is preferable to urinary catheterization but it should not be attempted where there is any possibility of urethral obstruction.

1. **Action:** Put on gloves and apron and prepare urinary collection equipment (if required) and absorbent tissue.

   Rationale: Protection of staff from zoonotic diseases transmitted by urine is essential. Urinary collection equipment, such as a kidney dish or a sterile sample pot, may be required if the urine requires analyzing.

2. **Action:** An assistant should restrain the patient in a standing position in a suitable area that is clean and easy to disinfect (Fig. 3.7).

   Rationale: Restraining the patient in the standing position will ensure easy access to the bladder. The area in which the patient urinates should be easy to disinfect to prevent contamination. Dogs will often feel happier urinating outside.

3. **Action:** Isolate the bladder by palpation of the caudal abdomen, and place one hand on either side of it on the external abdominal wall.

   Rationale: A full bladder should be easy to palpate, as it will feel like a distended sac in the caudal abdomen. If you have difficulty isolating the bladder, ask a veterinary surgeon to examine the patient for you.

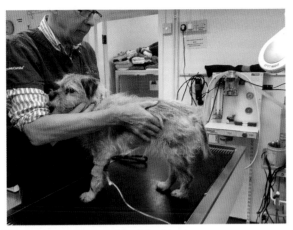

Fig. 3.7 Manual expression of the bladder.

4. **Action:** Apply gentle pressure to the abdominal wall on either side of the bladder to encourage urination. Urine should flow freely and be directed into a collection container (Fig. 3.7). Do not be tempted to squeeze the bladder – if there is any resistance and no urine flow, stop the procedure.

    Rationale: Gentle pressure either side of the bladder will mimic the action of the abdominal muscles and should produce a flow of urine. If there is an obstruction in either the bladder or the urethra, no urine will flow. A full bladder may rupture if pressure is put on it.

5. **Action:** When the flow ceases, release the pressure. Measure the volume of urine expressed, and note its colour, turbidity, smell and the time at which it was passed. Record your results on the patient's hospital record.

    Rationale: Records should be kept of all procedures. Measuring fluid output is vital in patients on fluid therapy, and a comparison of these details will enable accurate assessment of the patient's progress.

6. **Action:** Ensure that the patient is clean and dry before replacing it in its kennel. All areas where urination has occurred should be cleaned and disinfected, and disposable clothing placed in the offensive waste.

    Rationale: Ensuring that the patient is clean and dry will prevent urine scalds. Protection of staff and other patients from contamination is vital – disinfection should be a high priority.

Procedure: Cystocentesis

• Two people are required.

This technique should only be carried out by a veterinary surgeon on a palpable bladder. It may be the only practical method of draining the bladder when it is obstructed and is utilized when wanting to obtain a urine sample for bacterial culture.

1. **Action:** Prepare all the equipment, including disposable aprons and gloves, sterile gloves for the veterinary surgeon, a sterile syringe (5–20 ml) and needle of appropriate size (usually 23G × 2.5 cm), three-way tap and sterile urinary collection vessel as required. Clippers and skin preparation solution should be at hand.

    Rationale: As with all procedures, preparing the equipment before you begin is both an efficient and practical method of working. For the welfare of the patient, choose a syringe of suitable size and a long needle with a narrow gauge – this should ensure adequate flow. Urine collection may include the preparation of a sterile sample, so a suitable pot may be required.

2. **Action:** Put on gloves and apron and restrain the patient in lateral recumbency with the abdomen angled slightly dorsally.

    Rationale: The patient should be restrained to allow easy access to the bladder. Raising the bladder also reduces the risk of inappropriate puncture of the abdominal organs.

3. **Action:** An area of about 5 cm² should be clipped on the midline of the caudal abdomen. Prepare the area in an aseptic fashion using a suitable surgical preparation scrub.

    Rationale: This area needs to be treated as a surgical site, and an aseptic technique should be used.

4. **Action:** The veterinary surgeon will put on the sterile gloves and manually locate and immobilize the bladder through the abdominal wall. Using the syringe with needle attached, the veterinary surgeon will insert the needle through the abdominal wall and into the bladder. When the syringe plunger is drawn back, the urine should start to flow.

    Rationale: The aim is to insert the needle into the bladder, causing as little trauma as possible, and to prevent the introduction of infection by utilizing an aseptic technique.

5. **Action:** Gentle pressure should be applied at the injection site as the needle is removed.

   Rationale: Gentle pressure around the injection site will encourage natural tissue recoil around the pierced area and prevent leakage.

6. **Action:** Collect the urine for analysis or dispose of it in the clinical waste. A note should be made of the volume, colour, smell and turbidity for the patient's records. All equipment used should be disposed of in the offensive waste.

   Rationale: Urine should be carefully disposed of in the offensive waste to protect staff and other patients from contamination. A record of urinary output should be noted on the patient's records to enable assessment of its progress.

7. **Action:** The patient should be thoroughly cleaned and dried before it is placed back in its kennel.

   Rationale: Prevention of infection is a high priority.

Procedure: Peritoneal dialysis

• Two people are required – this technique should only be carried out by a veterinary surgeon.

Peritoneal dialysis is used to filter waste products from the blood in patients suffering from conditions such as acute renal failure. In these cases, the use of osmotic diuretics may fail to stimulate urine production. Peritoneal dialysis can also be used to reduce body temperature in hyperthermic animals.

1. **Action:** Prepare all the equipment, including disposable aprons and gloves, sterile gloves for the veterinary surgeon, a small sterile surgical pack, local anaesthetic, peritoneal catheter, trocar, giving set and dialysis fluid warmed to body temperature. A collection vessel for the waste fluid should be available. Clippers and skin preparation solution should be at hand.

   Rationale: As with all procedures, preparing the equipment before you begin is both an efficient and practical method of working. A strict aseptic technique should be used. Dialysis fluid is specific to this procedure and should be warmed to body temperature to prevent shock.

2. **Action:** Put on gloves and apron and restrain the patient in dorsal recumbency. The hair should be clipped from the ventral abdomen and the site aseptically prepared.

   Rationale: Restraining the patient in dorsal recumbency will result in ease of access to the ventral abdomen. The ventral area should be treated as a surgical site and aseptic technique should be maintained.

3. **Action:** The veterinary surgeon will inject local anaesthetic into the midline umbilical area.

   Rationale: A general anaesthetic can be contraindicated in some patients.

4. **Action:** The surgical site should be draped and a small incision made in the skin so that the catheter can be inserted into the abdomen with the aid of a trocar.

   Rationale: The site should be draped to aid in asepsis. A trocar is a needle-like instrument which can be used to pierce the abdominal wall.

5. **Action:** When the catheter is in place, the giving set and the bag containing dialysis fluid should be attached and allowed to flow into the abdominal cavity.

   Rationale: The nitrogenous waste flowing through the capillary bed of the peritoneum diffuses into the dialysis fluid.

6. **Action:** After a specified period of time (usually 30 minutes), the dialysis fluid is removed under gravity. This procedure may be repeated until the blood chemistry improves. Suture placement of the catheter may be required.

   Rationale: The dialysis fluid carries the nitrogenous waste out with it, thus benefiting the patient by reducing urea levels. Removing the fluid by gravity can sometimes be difficult and slow, and allowing the patient to move around can aid the flow. If necessary, repeat the procedure whilst monitoring the blood urea and creatinine levels of the patient.

7. **Action:** Ensure that the wound is clean and dry and there is no leakage from the wound, before the patient is placed back in its kennel. The patient should be closely monitored, as there is a high risk of peritonitis and shock.

   Rationale: A patient in acute renal failure may be immunologically compromised, and it is easy for infections such as peritonitis to develop.

PHYSIOTHERAPY

Procedure: Passive physiotherapy – massage

Physiotherapy is used to maintain and improve peripheral circulation and is useful in recumbent patients. Massage is especially useful for the limbs.

1. **Action:** Restrain the patient in a comfortable position that enables access to the limbs.

   Rationale: For the procedure to be beneficial, the patient needs to feel relaxed and comfortable. It may be preferable to use the patient's kennel rather than an examination table, which it may associate with pain and discomfort.

2. **Action:** Examine each limb in turn to check for wounds and any other abnormalities.

   Rationale: Massage should not be carried out if any abnormalities are present – check with the veterinary surgeon.

3. **Action:** Massage each limb in turn by briskly rubbing from the feet towards the body for at least 5 minutes per limb.

   Rationale: Massaging from the feet towards the trunk of the body encourages venous return.

4. **Action:** Reassure the patient whilst the procedure is being carried out.

   Rationale: Talking to the patient will help it to relax, and the massage will become not only beneficial for the circulation but also a source of comfort and attention for the animal.

5. **Action:** Regular massage should be part of the patient's daily care.

   Rationale: For full benefit, massage should be carried out regularly during the patient's treatment.

Procedure: Passive physiotherapy – coupage

Physiotherapy is used to maintain and improve peripheral circulation and is useful in recumbent patients. Coupage promotes thoracic circulation and helps to prevent hypostatic pneumonia.

1. **Action:** Restrain the patient in sternal recumbency (or standing).

   Rationale: The sternal position allows access to either side of the thorax and facilitates the greatest possible lung expansion.

2. **Action:** Examine the patient for signs of abnormality – such as wounds, tumours and fractures.

   Rationale: Coupage may be contraindicated in some conditions such as fractured ribs, where further damage could be caused. If in doubt, consult the veterinary surgeon.

3. **Action:** Cup your hands and slap either side of the thorax from the most caudal part of the area to the cranial part. Repeat for up to 5 minutes.

   Rationale: This slapping promotes coughing and improves the thoracic circulation. It also assists in the removal of bronchial secretions.

4. **Action:** This procedure should be carried out up to 4–5 times daily or as recommended by the veterinary surgeon.

Rationale: Coupage must be carried out regularly to maintain thoracic circulation in a recumbent patient.

Procedure: Passive physiotherapy – supported exercise (dogs)

Physiotherapy is used to maintain and improve peripheral circulation and is useful in recumbent patients. Supported exercise can be carried out using proprietary frames, but 'towel walking' is the most common method used for paraplegic patients in a practice (Fig. 3.8). Specialized slings and hoists can be purchased. Use of a harness rather than a lead will give you better control of the dog and help support the weight in the front if needed.

1. **Action:** Depending on the size of dog, 'towel walking' can be carried out by one or two people. A strong towel or sling and dog harness will be required – the size is dependent on the size of the patient.

   Rationale: For large dogs, one person will be needed to support the hindquarters and one to support and control the front of the patient. In giant breeds, two people may be required to support the hindquarters alone. Health and safety should always be taken into consideration, and the procedure should not be attempted without sufficient staff available.

2. **Action:** Restrain the dog and attach a harness. Roll the towel into a 'sausage' shape and pass under the caudal abdomen. Hold the towel at each end, supporting the body so that the feet are on the ground (Fig. 3.8).

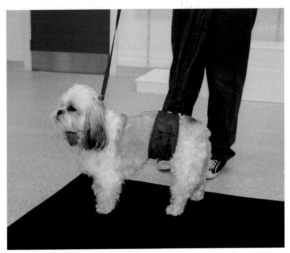

Fig. 3.8 Abdominal support sling or towel walking using one person. (From Aspinall's Complete Textbook of Veterinary Nursing, Ackerman, N., 2016, Elsevier, p. 310, Fig 18.17.)

Rationale: The towel is used to support the hindquarters of the patient and mimic its usual stance (Fig. 3.8). In a small dog, one person may be able to hold the ends of the towel with one hand and the patient's lead with the other.

3. **Action:** Encourage the dog to walk, while supporting the hindquarters.

   Rationale: Supported walking encourages circulation and gives the patient confidence to try and use its limbs whilst they are being supported.

4. **Action:** Encourage urination and defecation and improve the patient's mental attitude by carrying out this procedure in an outside environment.

   Rationale: The opportunity to be outside is often invaluable in changing the patient's mental attitude and will encourage normal behaviour such as urination and defecation.

5. **Action:** The opportunity for a supported walk should be offered to the patient at least three times a day as part of a physiotherapy technique.

   Rationale: This procedure needs to be carried out regularly to promote improvement in the patient's condition.

Procedure: Passive physiotherapy – hydrotherapy (dogs)

Physiotherapy is used to maintain and improve peripheral circulation and is useful in recumbent patients. Hydrotherapy can be carried out for small dogs in sinks or baths available in the practice. For larger patients, referral to specialized facilities may be necessary. Hydrotherapy causes more stress than benefit in most cats!

1. **Action:** Fill a sink or bath of suitable size with warm water – ideally slightly above body temperature.

   Rationale: The water should be deep enough to force the patient to move or swim and should be warm enough to be inviting and not chill the patient.

2. **Action:** Gradually lower the patient into the water, supporting the patient's body. Ideally, the patient should start to move the limbs in a swimming action. Do not leave the patient – it will require constant support and reassurance.

   Rationale: Support the patient's body at all times to prevent panic or drowning. The swimming action provides excellent physiotherapy to the limbs without requiring weight bearing and will help build muscle tissue and increase its strength.

3. **Action:** The length of time required will vary from patient to patient, but as a general rule start with approximately 5 minutes, building up the time as the patient becomes more confident.

   Rationale: Initially the patient will tire quickly, but as its strength builds, it will tolerate a longer session in the water.

4. **Action:** The patient should be dried properly and placed in a warm kennel when each session is over.

   Rationale: Do not allow the patient to become chilled as it goes back into an environment in which it cannot move.

5. **Action:** As with all physiotherapy techniques, hydrotherapy sessions need to be regular to have a beneficial effect on the patient.

   Rationale: Regular exercise of the limbs will build up muscle mass.

Hydrotherapy is now commonly carried out in commercial pools, of which there are two main types:
- Underwater treadmills – consist of a tank that is filled or emptied according to use and through which the treadmill runs. The water level and the speed of the treadmill can be altered to suit the patient.
- Pools – consist of a large pool entered by means of a ramp. Some pools also have jets that may be used to increase the workload of swimming.

Procedure: Passive physiotherapy – passive joint movement

Physiotherapy is used to maintain and improve peripheral circulation and is useful in recumbent patients. Passive joint movement will improve limb circulation and helps prevent stiffness of the joints.

1. **Action:** Ensure the patient is comfortable and relaxed – you may wish to carry out this procedure with the patient in its kennel rather than on an examination table.

   Rationale: A relaxed patient will benefit more from the procedure than a patient that is anxious and tense.

2. **Action:** An assistant may be required to restrain the patient's head until the patient becomes familiar with the process. It may be possible to carry out the procedure single-handed if the patient is in lateral recumbency in its kennel.

   Rationale: The patient may be supported in a standing position or in lateral recumbency in its kennel. This will depend on its condition.

The help of an assistant may be required in some cases.

3. **Action:** Slowly flex and extend the joints, one limb at a time, starting with the carpal/tarsal joints and then moving upwards to the next joint.

   Rationale: Slowly flexing and extending the joints will enable them to become more flexible. If a patient has been recumbent for a few days, the joints may have become very stiff. Be careful to keep within the normal range of movement to prevent joint damage. Working upwards along the limb encourages venous return.

4. **Action:** The amount of time spent working on each joint should be related to the patient's condition and the degree of joint degeneration. It is usual to increase the length of the sessions as the patient's condition improves.

   Rationale: Always seek advice from the veterinary surgeon.

5. **Action:** As with all physiotherapy techniques, joint movement sessions need to be regular to have a beneficial effect on the patient.

   Rationale: Regular movement of the joints will improve circulation and prevent stiffness.

NURSING MEDICAL CONDITIONS

Procedure: Nursing the patient with diarrhoea

A patient with diarrhoea of unknown aetiology should always be treated as a possible source of infection. Infectious diseases that may have diarrhoea as a clinical sign include canine parvovirus and feline infectious enteritis. Diseases that are also zoonotic include campylobacteriosis and salmonellosis. If an infectious disease is suspected, barrier nursing should be maintained throughout the patient's stay (see earlier in the chapter).

1. **Action:** If no definite diagnosis has been made, provide isolation facilities or choose a kennel that is easy to clean and disinfect.

   Rationale: Always suspect an infectious disease if no diagnosis has been made or whilst diagnostic tests are being carried out. It is likely that the kennel occupied by a diarrhoeic patient will require regular cleaning and disinfection, so management of this should be taken into account.

2. **Action:** If an infectious disease is suspected, instigate barrier nursing techniques.

   Rationale: Barrier nursing should be employed to protect both staff and other patients from the spread of infection.

3. **Action:** Provide a comfortable environment for the patient, including absorbent bedding and warmth. For cats, ensure that a clean litter tray is available at all times.

   Rationale: These patients will be feeling uncomfortable and insecure. They may defecate frequently, and therefore will require bedding that is absorbent and disposable. Most cats will prefer to use a clean litter tray, so make sure it is cleaned every time it is used.

4. **Action:** Ensure that the medical treatment prescribed by the veterinary surgeon is carried out and recorded on the patient's record (Fig. 3.9).

   Rationale: The veterinary surgeon may have prescribed drugs, which must be given at the advised times to have maximum effect. The administration of any drug should be noted on the patient's clinical history to ensure that all members of staff are aware that the treatment has been given.

5. **Action:** Monitor any fluid therapy that is being given. This is likely to be administered intravenously. An example of a fluid commonly used for diarrhoeic patients is Hartmann's solution. Intravenous catheters should be examined and checked twice daily for any inflammation or phlebitis. Fluid therapy giving sets should be wiped down daily with a disinfectant to prevent ascending infections. Any gross contamination should be removed as soon as noted.

   Rationale: Patients with diarrhoea lose water and electrolytes, which need to be replaced by the appropriate fluid. Infection control procedures should be instigated for the care of intravenous cannulas.

6. **Action:** Monitor and record the five vital assessments for patient parameters, i.e. TPR; pain score; and nutrition assessment (weight, BCS and MCS, see Fig. 5.10). An assessment of the patient's hydration status should be made and recorded.

   Rationale: Patient parameters are required to assess progress. Clinical signs of dehydration include slightly sunken eyes, dry mucous membranes and a loss of skin elasticity.

7. **Action:** Monitor and record the patient's fluid intake and output, i.e. the rate and volume of fluid

Kennel Chart						

Kennel Chart

Animal	Owner	Case Number
Species	Clinician	Student
Breed	Clinical Summary	
Colour		
Sex		
Age		

Date	Day No.	Date	Day No.
Weight	Diet	Weight	Diet

	AM	PM		AM	PM
Temp			Temp		
Pulse			Pulse		
Resp			Resp		
Fed			Fed		
Ate			Ate		
Drank			Drank		
Taken Out				Taken Out			
Urine				Urine			
Faeces				Faeces			

MEDICATION		MEDICATION	
PROCEDURES		PROCEDURES	
COMMENTS		COMMENTS	

Fig. 3.9 Example of a hospitalization kennel chart. (Adapted, with permission, from Pre-Veterinary Nursing Textbook, Masters and Bowden (2001), Butterworth-Heinemann.)

the patient is given, as well as the amount and type of urine and faeces it produces.

Rationale: Monitoring fluid intake and output provides the information needed to gauge the hydration status and progress. The amount, colour and type of faeces passed should be recorded to assess the recovery process.

8. **Action:** A soiled patient should be bathed immediately with warm water and dried with disposable absorbent towel before being placed back in the clean kennel. Disposable aprons and gloves should be worn throughout the procedure and should be disposed of in the offensive or hazardous waste after use.

Rationale: Clip away heavily soiled hair, ensuring that it is easy to clean the area if further diarrhoea occurs. Wrapping the tail in a bandage will also aid in cleaning. The patient may be sore in places; check this with the veterinary surgeon. Thoroughly drying the patient before returning it to its kennel will prevent further soreness, and the patient will not become chilled. All contaminated equipment should be regarded as a possible source of infection and be disinfected or placed in the hazardous waste. Non-infectious faecal material should be disposed of in the offensive waste, unless required for analysis.

9. **Action:** Diagnostic tests may be planned for this patient. Blood samples may be taken to measure the patient's hydration status. Faecal material may be required to aid in the diagnosis of the condition and may require collection at regular intervals. Check with the veterinary surgeon before disposing of any faecal material from the patient.

Rationale: Packed cell volume (PCV) and blood electrolyte levels will help monitor the hydration status of the patient. Analysis of the components of the faecal material may include bacteriology.

10. **Action:** The nutritional requirements of the patient will depend on the severity of the condition. Nil by mouth should not be advised, as this will potentially prolong the length of illness, as the gastrointestinal system will be devoid of essential nutrients required. A highly digestible diet is typically offered, with a gradual reintroduction of the patient's usual food.

Rationale: The use of a highly digestible diet is less likely to inflame the gastrointestinal tract – a proprietary diet may be used in the practice. Once this diet is being tolerated without causing diarrhoea, the patient's usual diet can be slowly reintroduced.

11. **Action:** If you have any concern over the condition of the patient, notify the veterinary surgeon immediately.

Rationale: These patients can develop problems very rapidly and require constant veterinary care.

Procedure: Nursing the vomiting patient

A patient with vomiting of unknown aetiology should always be treated as a possible source of infection. Infectious diseases that have vomiting as a clinical sign include canine parvovirus and feline infectious enteritis. Zoonotic diseases include leptospirosis. If an infectious disease is suspected, barrier nursing should be maintained throughout the patient's stay (see earlier in the chapter). Vomiting can range from a minor episode, such as that resulting from scavenging, to a major attack, as occurs with some forms of poisoning. Each type will require different degrees of nursing.

1. **Action:** If no definite diagnosis has been made, provide isolation facilities or choose a kennel that is easy to clean and disinfect.

Rationale: Always suspect an infectious disease if no diagnosis has been made or whilst diagnostic tests are being carried out. It is likely that the kennel occupied by a vomiting patient will require regular cleaning and disinfection, so management of this should be taken into account.

2. **Action:** If an infectious disease is suspected, use barrier nursing techniques.

Rationale: Barrier nursing should be employed to protect both staff and other patients from infection.

3. **Action:** Provide a comfortable environment for the patient, including absorbent bedding and warmth.

Rationale: These patients will be feeling uncomfortable and insecure. Vomiting may occur frequently and will require efficient cleaning. The patient may be clinically shocked and must be kept warm.

4. **Action:** Ensure that the medical treatment prescribed by the veterinary surgeon is carried out and recorded in the patient's clinical history (Fig. 3.9).

Rationale: The veterinary surgeon may have prescribed drugs for this patient, which must be given at the advised times to have maximum effect. The administration of any drug should be noted on the patient's records to ensure that all members of staff are aware that the treatment has been given.

5. **Action:** Monitor any intravenous fluid therapy that is being administered. Intravenous cannulas should be inspected twice daily and re-dressed using aseptic techniques. Giving set lines should be wiped down with a disinfectant daily.

   Rationale: *Patients that are persistently vomiting will lose water and electrolytes, which need to be replaced by an appropriate fluid. It is important to adhere to good infection control procedures so that no nosocomial infections occur.*

6. **Action:** Monitor and record the five vital assessments of the patient, i.e. TPR; pain score; and nutritional assessment (weight, BCS and MCS, see Fig. 5.10). An assessment of the patient's hydration status should be made and recorded.

   Rationale: *Patient parameters are required to assess progress. Clinical signs of dehydration include slightly sunken eyes, dry mucous membranes and a loss of skin elasticity.*

7. **Action:** Monitor and record the patient fluid intake and output, i.e. the rate and volume of fluid the patient is given and the amount and type of vomit, urine and faeces it produces.

   Rationale: *Monitoring fluid intake and output provides the information needed to gauge the animal's hydration status and progress. The amount, colour and type of vomit should be recorded to make an assessment of progress.*

8. **Action:** Diagnostic tests may be planned for this patient. Blood samples may be taken to measure the patient's hydration status. Prepare equipment as required.

   Rationale: *PCV and blood electrolyte levels will help monitor the hydration status of the patient.*

9. **Action:** The nutritional requirements of the patient will depend on the severity of the condition. If anti-emetics are not contraindicated, administer and then offer food as soon as possible. If still vomiting, micro-enteral nutrition should be instigated. Semi-elemental diets can be given, and, if tolerated, highly digestible diets can be offered.

   Rationale: *Enteral nutrition is required in order for the gastrointestinal system to receive required nutrients. Once this diet is being tolerated without causing vomiting, the patient's usual diet is gradually reintroduced.*

10. **Action:** If you have any concern over the condition of the patient, notify the veterinary surgeon immediately.

    Rationale: *These patients can develop problems very rapidly and require constant veterinary care.*

Procedure: Nursing the paraplegic or recumbent patient

Examples of conditions that may result in paraplegia include spinal trauma, spinal neoplasia, head injuries and pelvic fractures.

1. **Action:** Choose a kennel of a size in which the patient can lie comfortably on its side. Waterproof bedding such as a foam mattress is ideal, with absorbent bedding material placed on top. Try to prop the patient in sternal recumbency with foam pads or sandbags. Remember that these patients may be lying in the same kennel for some time, so try to place them in an area where they can see some activity to keep them stimulated.

   Rationale: *The patient must be able to lie comfortably but the kennel should not be so large that the patient could move around and damage itself. Sternal recumbency will help to prevent hypostatic pneumonia. Foam mattresses are comfortable for the patient and help to prevent the formation of decubitus ulcers. Absorbent bedding is required, as these patients are often incontinent.*

2. **Action:** Monitor and record the five vital assessment, i.e. TPR; pain score; and nutritional assessment (weight, BCS and MCS, see Fig. 5.10). Urinary and faecal outputs should be recorded, as well as any progress. Any abnormalities should be recorded, and the veterinary surgeon notified.

   Rationale: *Patient parameters are required to assess progress. Recumbent patients will lose heat quickly and may require covering with blankets or the use of an infrared lamp or other heating device. Heat pads are not recommended for patients that are unable to move, as they may be burnt.*

3. **Action:** Provide a suitable diet for the life stage and clinical condition of the animal. Ensure that food and water are placed within reach of the patient. Some of these patients may refuse to eat and tempting them with their usual favourite foods may stimulate the appetite. Water must be available at all times – intake should be measured.

   Rationale: *Energy requirements are low but recumbent patients require a diet that will supply enough* energy for tissue repair and the stress of being kennelled over a long period. It is important to keep the appetite stimulated.

4. **Action:** Even if the patient is incontinent, dogs should be taken outside for a change of environment on a regular basis using 'towel walking' techniques (Fig. 3.8).
   Rationale: A change in the patient's environment will be stimulating. Supported exercise techniques promote good circulation and enable the patient to gain confidence.

5. **Action:** Turn the patient in its kennel at least every 4 hours to prevent hypostatic pneumonia and decubitus ulcers. Apply padding to bony prominences to prevent decubitus ulcers. Make sure that the patient is clean and dry every time it is turned to prevent urine scalding. The patient may have an indwelling catheter, and this should be cared for accordingly.
   Rationale: Hypostatic pneumonia occurs when there is pooling of the blood in the lungs and is seen in patients left in lateral recumbency for long periods without turning them. Decubitus ulcers occur on the bony prominences and are extremely slow in healing. Urine scalds are easily prevented with good nursing. The patient must be kept clean and dry at all times – barrier creams can be applied to the most susceptible areas.

6. **Action:** Carry out physiotherapy techniques.
   Rationale: Simple physiotherapy such as supported exercise, passive joint movement and massage should be carried out. If equipment is available, hydrotherapy may be used.

Procedure: Nursing the seizuring patient

Seizures can occur for a number of different reasons, including epilepsy, toxicity and neoplasia in the central nervous system. The seizure consists of three phases – pre-ictal, ictal and post-ictal, with collapse occurring during the ictal phase. These seizures, or 'fits', will often take place at home, and advice will initially be given to the owner (often over the telephone). Personal safety must be taken in account – an animal that is fitting may inadvertently bite.

1. **Action:** Advise the owner to not touch the animal and to ask all people to leave the room. Move all furniture away from the animal to prevent injury. Reduce noise and darken the environment. Observe the animal until the fit is over, leaving the dog with as little stimulus as possible.

Rationale: All stimulation should be removed from the animal, i.e. people, noise, light, as these can promote another fit. A quiet environment will help the animal recover more quickly.

2. **Action:** If the fit becomes continuous (any fitting longer than 5 minutes) or the animal experiences repeated fits that occur one after the other (known as a cluster), the animal must be brought to the surgery as soon as possible. This must be explained to the owner and its importance emphasized.
   Rationale: Prolonged fitting is known as status epilepticus, and there is a high risk of brain swelling and subsequent brain damage These patients will require anticonvulsant therapy and steps must be taken to reduce the body temperature. Violent fitting activity raises the body temperature.

3. **Action:** The veterinary surgeon may wish to give intravenous anticonvulsants but be unable to due to the seizure activity. Rectal or intranasal medication can be initially administered, and an intravenous cannula then placed. The patient's temperature, pulse, respiration and mucous membrane colour should be monitored frequently. An oxygen supply should be readily available in case of respiratory difficulties.
   Rationale: Anticonvulsants will depress the central nervous system and control the fit; however, they may also cause respiratory problems, so constant observation is required.

4. **Action:** The progress and continuing nursing care of these patients depends on the aetiology of the fit. Some patients, e.g. those with idiopathic epilepsy, can be stabilized and may be discharged with anticonvulsive therapies. Other patients may have signs of an underlying disease of which the fit is one of the symptoms – diagnostic tests may be required to confirm this.
   Rationale: Idiopathic epilepsy can be treated with oral anticonvulsants, and the cause may never be identified, but other fits may be part of a metabolic condition such as renal disease, hepatic disease or poisoning, and will be treated differently.

Procedure: Nursing the patient with cardiac failure – congestive heart failure

Congestive heart failure occurs when the heart fails to function effectively – it compensates by changing its rate, leading to clinical signs which indicate the side of the heart that is affected. Right-sided heart failure will result in poor venous return to the heart, congestion of organs such as the liver and spleen and possibly the development of ascites. Left-sided heart failure will result in poor venous return from the lungs, causing pulmonary congestion and oedema, tachypnoea and coughing.

1. **Action:** Choose a kennel of a size in which the patient can lie comfortably. Bedding should be comfortable and absorbent. The kennel should be in a quiet area.

   Rationale: The patient needs to be able to lie comfortably. It may be on drug therapy that results in an increase in urination, so acrylic bedding or incontinence pads may be useful in case of leakage. These patients require a stress-free environment.

2. **Action:** Monitor and record the five vital assessments, i.e. TPR; pain score; and nutrition assessment (weight, BCS and MCS, see Fig. 5.10). Urinary and faecal output should be recorded. Note any progress. Any abnormalities should be recorded (Fig. 3.9), and the veterinary surgeon notified. Take the patient out to urinate frequently.

   Rationale: Patient parameters are required to assess progress. Geriatric patients will lose heat quickly and may require covering with blankets or the use of an infrared lamp or other heating device. Heat pads are not recommended for patients that are unable to move away from the heat, as they may be burnt. The patient may be under treatment with diuretics and therefore need to urinate more frequently.

3. **Action:** Cardiac patients need a diet that is low in salt, contains protein of high biological value and is highly digestible. Cardiac patients are often overweight, and a diet with reducing capabilities may be utilized at the discretion of the veterinary surgeon. Potassium supplementation may be required. Water must be available at all times – intake should be measured.

   Rationale: A diet that is low in salt will help to reduce pulmonary oedema and ascites, which occur as a result of hypertension and venous congestion. The lack of salt decreases the palatability of the diet, so these patients must be prevented from becoming anorexic. Potassium levels may drop in patients on diuretic therapy, as potassium is being lost in the urine.

4. **Action:** Ensure that the medical treatment prescribed by the veterinary surgeon is carried out and recorded on the patient's record. Cardiac drug therapy includes diuretics, bronchodilators, vasodilators and glycosides.

   Rationale: The veterinary surgeon may have prescribed drugs for this patient that must be given at the advised times to have the maximum effect. The administration of any drug should be noted on the patient's records to ensure that all members of staff are aware that the treatment has been given.

5. **Action:** Canine patients must be taken outside on a lead to urinate or defecate. Cats must have access to a clean litter tray at all times.

   Rationale: The patient must be rested as much as possible and not over-exercised, so keep on a lead.

Procedure: Nursing the patient with renal disease

Renal diseases include acute renal failure (complete/almost complete lack of renal function), chronic renal failure (progressive loss of renal function) and nephrotic syndrome, associated with the development of glomerulonephritis. Leptospirosis – a zoonotic disease – can be a differential in acute renal failure, and barrier nursing (see earlier in the chapter) may be instigated until a diagnosis is made.

1. **Action:** Choose a kennel that is of a size in which the patient can lie comfortably. Bedding should be comfortable and absorbent.

   Rationale: The patient needs to be able to lie comfortably. Acrylic bedding or incontinence pads may be useful in cases of incontinence. White bedding is useful in identifying the colour of the urine absorbed – the presence of blood will be especially noticeable.

2. **Action:** Monitor and record the five vital assessments, i.e. TPR; pain score; and nutritional assessment (weight, BCS and MCS, see Fig. 5.10). Urinary and faecal output should be recorded. Note any progress. Any abnormalities should be recorded (Fig. 3.9), and the veterinary surgeon notified.

   Rationale: Patient parameters are required to assess progress of treatment. Measure urinary output and fluid intake.

3. **Action:** Renal patients require a diet that is low in protein and phosphorus. The protein used must be of high biological value. Patients may have oral ulceration and may require much encouragement to eat. Hand feeding or tube feeding may be considered.

   Rationale: Low protein levels will help to reduce levels of nitrogenous waste. The protein must be of a high biological value to enable it to be utilized for maintenance and repair. Phosphorus levels will be elevated in uraemic patients so the diet must contain low phosphorus levels.

4. **Action:** Ensure that the medical treatment prescribed by the veterinary surgeon is carried out and recorded on the patient's record. Drugs that may be used include antiemetics, hypertension drugs and angiotensin converting enzyme (ACE) inhibitors/blockers.
   Rationale: *Drugs prescribed for this patient by the veterinary surgeon must be given at the advised times to have maximum effect. The administration of any drug should be noted on the patient's records to ensure that all members of staff are aware that the treatment has been given.*

5. **Action:** The continuing nursing care will be dependent on the disease condition. Patients with renal failure will require intravenous fluid therapy, and this must be carefully monitored. Treatment for patients with acute renal failure may include peritoneal dialysis. Monitoring of electrolyte levels is required for all animals receiving fluid therapy.
   Rationale: *Fluid therapy will be given to correct electrolyte loss and maintain hydration. There is a potential for large losses during diuresis.*

6. **Action:** Monitor the intravenous catheter site twice daily and re-dress accordingly. The intravenous fluid giving set should be wiped down daily with a disinfectant.
   Rationale: *The site should be inspected for any subcutaneous swelling or inflammation. Stringent infection control procedures should be instigated to prevent ascending infections.*

7. **Action:** It is likely that the veterinary surgeon will require blood and urine samples for diagnostic assessment of the patient's progress.
   Rationale: *Blood and urine contain various parameters which change as the patient progresses.*

8. **Action:** Canine patients must be taken outside to urinate or defecate. Cats should have access to a clean litter tray at all times.
   Rationale: *Urine may require collection to assess progress. Check with the veterinary surgeon.*

Procedure: Nursing the patient with hepatic disease

Hepatic disease is usually caused by a bacterial or viral infection. Examples include adenovirus, which causes infectious canine hepatitis, and *Leptospira icterohaemorrhagiae*, which causes leptospirosis. Both of these are infectious diseases and, if they are suspected, barrier nursing should be instigated until a definitive diagnosis is made. Leptospirosis is a zoonosis, so extra care should be taken to protect all personnel involved. Toxic damage caused by poisoning or prolonged drug therapy can sometimes result in hepatitis.

1. **Action:** Choose a kennel that is of a size in which the patient can lie comfortably. Bedding should be comfortable and absorbent.
   Rationale: *The patient needs to be able to lie comfortably. Acrylic bedding or incontinence pads may be useful in cases of incontinence.*

2. **Action:** Monitor and record the five vital assessments, i.e. TPR; pain score; and nutritional assessment (weight, BCS and MCS, see Fig. 5.10). The mucous membranes may be jaundiced, and ascites may develop. Urinary and faecal output should be recorded. Note any progress. Any abnormalities should be recorded (Fig. 3.9), and the veterinary surgeon notified.
   Rationale: *Patient parameters are required to assess progress. Jaundice occurs where there are excessive levels of bilirubin in the blood – a result of the hepatitis affecting the biliary system. Ascites is the result of fluid accumulation (due to portal hypertension) in the abdomen – this could include blood, urine, transudates and exudates.*

3. **Action:** Most hepatic patients need an energy-dense diet with moderate amounts of protein with a high biological value and increased levels of water-soluble vitamins. These patients are often anorexic, and good nutritional support is essential. Hand feeding or tube feeding may be required.
   Rationale: *Protein is required to supply the patient's basic needs and support regeneration of damaged tissue.*

4. **Action:** Ensure that the medical treatment prescribed by the veterinary surgeon is carried out and recorded on the patient's record. Drugs that may be used are of a supportive nature.
   Rationale: *Drugs prescribed for this patient by the veterinary surgeon must be given at the advised times to have maximum effect. The administration of any drug should be noted on the patient's records to ensure that all members of staff are aware that the treatment has been given.*

5. **Action:** The continuing nursing care will depend on the cause of the disease. Patients are likely to require intravenous fluid therapy, and this must be carefully

monitored. Monitor the intravenous catheter site twice daily and re-dress accordingly. The intravenous fluid giving set should be wiped down daily with a disinfectant.

Rationale: *Fluid therapy will be given to correct electrolyte loss and maintain hydration.*

The site should be inspected for any sub-cutaneous swelling or inflammation. Stringent infection control should be instigated to prevent ascending infections.

6. **Action:** It is likely that the veterinary surgeon will require blood samples to be taken. Diagnostic imaging techniques may be also used. If a liver biopsy is required, the patient will have to be prepared for surgery.

Rationale: *Blood biochemistry will be used to make the diagnosis and assess the patient's progress. Diagnostic imaging will be used to assess the liver size. A biopsy will enable the histopathology of the liver tissue to be examined.*

7. **Action:** Canine patients must be taken outside to urinate or defecate. Cats must have access to a clean litter tray at all times.

Rationale: *Supportive therapies must include good nursing techniques.*

Procedure: Nursing the patient with pancreatic disease

Disease conditions of the exocrine part of the pancreas include pancreatitis and exocrine pancreatic insufficiency.

1. **Action:** Choose a kennel that is of a size in which the patient can lie comfortably. Bedding should be comfortable and absorbent.

Rationale: *The patient needs to be able to lie comfortably. Acrylic bedding or incontinence pads may be useful in cases of incontinence.*

2. **Action:** Monitor and record the five vital assessments, i.e. TPR; pain score; and nutritional assessment (weight, BCS and MCS, see Fig. 5.10). Any abnormalities should be recorded (Fig. 3.9), and the veterinary surgeon notified.

Rationale: *Patient parameters are required to assess progress. Care should be taken when handling the patient, as there is likely to be pain in the cranial abdomen.*

3. **Action:** Patients with pancreatitis can vomit persistently and quickly become dehydrated. Intravenous fluid therapy is required and should be monitored closely. Monitor the intravenous catheter site twice daily and re-dress accordingly. The intravenous fluid giving set should be wiped down daily with a disinfectant.

Rationale: *The site should be inspected for any sub-cutaneous swelling or inflammation. Stringent infection control procedures should be instigated to prevent ascending infections. The fluid and electrolytes that have been lost must be replaced with a suitable fluid, such as Hartmann's.*

4. **Action:** Nutritional support is very important in these patients. Micro-enteral nutrition may have to be instigated in some cases. A semi-elemental diet or a low fat highly digestible food might be required.

Rationale: *As soon as vomiting is controlled, nutritional support should be instigated to replace lost electrolytes and protein.*

5. **Action:** Pancreatitis is an extremely painful condition, and peritonitis may develop as a complication. Ensure that the medical treatment prescribed by the veterinary surgeon is carried out and recorded on the patient's record. Drugs that may be used include analgesics and gastro-protectants.

Rationale: *Drugs prescribed for this patient by the veterinary surgeon must be given at the advised times to have maximum effect. The monitoring of the analgesic regime is vital as these patients will be in extreme pain if the dose is insufficient. The administration of any drug should be noted on the patient's records to ensure that all members of staff are aware that the treatment has been given.*

6. **Action:** Tests will be carried out to confirm the diagnosis and to assess the patient's progress. Blood and faecal samples may be required.

Rationale: *Diagnostic tests for pancreatitis include haematology (leucocytosis may be present), biochemistry (to assess serum amylase and lipase) and abdominal ultrasonography (to assess the degree of peritonitis). Canine and feline pancreatic-specific lipase tests may be run for confirmation of pancreatitis.*

7. **Action:** Once hospital treatment has finished, the patient will require strict dietary management.

Rationale: *Once the pancreas has been damaged, it is unlikely to return to normal function. Nutritional management with a low-fat diet may help to prevent acute or chronic attacks recurring.*

Procedure: Nursing the patient with diabetes mellitus

Diabetes mellitus is caused by degeneration of the endocrine part of the pancreas. This normally secretes the hormone insulin, which stimulates glucose uptake by the cells as a source of energy and storage of excess glucose in the liver as glycogen. In patients with type 1 diabetes mellitus, insufficient amounts of insulin are released, resulting in hyperglycaemia (raised blood glucose levels) and excretion of excess glucose in the urine.

1. **Action:** The patient may be admitted with ketoacidosis and will require immediate intravenous fluid therapy and insulin treatment to lower blood glucose levels. The choice of fluid therapy will depend on the presenting electrolyte levels and acid-base balance. The veterinary surgeon will decide on the type of insulin and route of administration, depending on these levels.

   Rationale: Insulin is required to enable the passage of glucose, derived from the breakdown of carbohydrates in the diet, into the cells to be used to provide energy. Fats are broken down to create an energy source. Ketones are a by-product of this process, and when they start to build up in the blood (ketoacidosis), a metabolic acidosis occurs. Insulin is also required to aid in the removal of ketones.

2. **Action:** Choose a kennel that is of a size in which the patient can lie comfortably. Bedding should be comfortable and absorbent.

   Rationale: The patient needs to be able to lie comfortably.

3. **Action:** Monitor and record the patient's five vital assessment parameters, i.e. TPR; pain score; and nutritional assessment (weight, BCS and MCS, see Fig. 5.10). Any abnormalities should be recorded and the veterinary surgeon notified.

   Rationale: Patient parameters are required to assess the progress. Body weight will have to be closely monitored as these animals can be dehydrated when presented and body weight will change once rehydrated.

4. **Action:** Maintenance of a patient with diabetes mellitus requires a strict routine. At-home blood sampling should be actively promoted.

   Rationale: At-home blood sampling has proven to be more reflective of the animal in its normal state. Hospitalization is stressful (particularly in cats) and produces different blood glucose results.

5. **Action:** Before administering insulin, always feed the patient. If the patient eats this, inject the prepared dose of insulin. Insulin is usually given subcutaneously in proprietary insulin syringes or in insulin pens. Ensure that the subcutaneous injection has been given correctly to enable the insulin to work. If the patient does not eat its food, seek advice from the veterinary surgeon and do not administer the insulin.

   Rationale: Hypoglycaemia could occur if food is not eaten and insulin is then administered. The dose of the insulin must be administered accurately using the correct dosage syringe. Proprietary syringes are calibrated in international units (IU), either 40 IU/ml or 100 IU/ml.

6. **Action:** All treatments must be noted on the patient's record.

   Rationale: If the patient does not respond, or if there is an excessive response to the insulin injection, the record can be checked and used to adjust the dose.

7. **Action:** Nutritional support of the diabetic patient is important. The diet will depend on species and BCS. It is vital that the patient is kept to a strict regime and that no extra food or titbits are offered.

   Rationale: The amount of food consumed each day must balance the amount of the insulin that is administered.

8. **Action:** Hypoglycaemia (low blood glucose) can be a complication. Clinical signs include disorientation, tremors, weakness, ataxia, collapse and coma. A conscious patient should be given oral glucose in the form of glucose powder, sugar or honey. An unconscious patient will require intravenous glucose as soon as possible.

   Rationale: Hypoglycaemia may occur when too much insulin has been given in comparison to the amount of carbohydrates consumed, or when other clinical disease is present.

9. **Action:** The owner of a diabetic animal must understand that the patient must continue with a strict regime in order to keep the condition stable. This includes a constant amount of food and of a constant composition. In addition, exercise must be monitored: the same amount of exercise should occur at the same time each day. Once the patient is stabilized, the dose of insulin must remain constant. Some cases of diabetes mellitus are transient, whereas other patients may require insulin for the remainder of their lives.

   Rationale: High levels of blood glucose due to ingestion of large amounts of food or in response to low levels of insulin may cause the condition of the patient to become unstable. Unusual energy demands, such as a very long walk, can also result in instability. Some patients may have diabetes as a secondary condition, e.g. a bitch may develop diabetes after her 'season'. If she is spayed, thus stabilizing the hormone fluctuations of the oestrous cycle, she may not require insulin in the future.

Procedure: Nursing the patient with diabetes insipidus

Diabetes insipidus results from either a failure of the pituitary gland to produce antidiuretic hormone (ADH) or of the kidneys to respond to ADH. ADH controls the permeability of the collecting ducts of the renal nephron and affects the volume and concentration of the resulting urine. Prolonged production of dilute urine results in extreme thirst and potentially fatal dehydration.

1. **Action:** The patient will present with marked polydipsia and polyuria.
   Rationale: The patient is unable to concentrate the urine, so will pass dilute urine frequently. A secondary polydipsia develops as a result of dehydration.

2. **Action:** Choose a kennel that is of a size in which the patient can lie comfortably. Bedding should be comfortable and absorbent. Water must be available, and canine patients must be frequently taken outside to urinate.
   Rationale: The patient needs to be able to lie comfortably. If the patient is not offered water, it will dehydrate quickly as it will still exhibit polyuria.

3. **Action:** Monitor and record the five vital assessment parameters, i.e. TPR; pain score; and nutritional assessment (body weight, BCS and MCS, see Fig. 5.10). Fluid intake and output should be noted. Any abnormalities should be recorded, and the veterinary surgeon notified.
   Rationale: Patient parameters are required to assess progress. Fluid intake and output will indicate the degree of the problem.

4. **Action:** Diagnosis of diabetes insipidus involves the use of the water deprivation test. The patient must be well hydrated and have good renal function.
   Rationale: The water deprivation test assesses the ability of the patient to concentrate its urine.

The patient can become dehydrated quickly and this test should only be carried out by a veterinary surgeon. Assessment of the patient's hydration status should be made throughout the test. The renal function of the patient should be taken into consideration as further complications could occur.

5. **Action:** Empty the patient's bladder and measure the specific gravity using a refractometer (see Chapter 11). Record the results.
   Rationale: The specific gravity measurement will assess the concentration of the urine before water deprivation.

6. **Action:** The patient should be weighed, and 5% of its bodyweight calculated. It should then be placed in a kennel without food and water for 1 hour.
   Rationale: This provides a measurement on which to base the subsequent results.

7. **Action:** After an hour the patient's bladder should be emptied, the patient weighed and the urine specific gravity measured. Repeat this process until 5% of the patient's bodyweight is lost.
   Rationale: When a normal patient loses 5% of its bodyweight, it will concentrate its urine to a specific gravity of more than 1.020. If the patient has diabetes insipidus, it will still produce dilute urine of a specific gravity of less than 1.007, and a diagnosis can be made.

8. **Action:** When the testing is finished the patient should be allowed free access to water.
   Rationale: The patient may become severely dehydrated if water is withheld for too long.

9. **Action:** Ensure that the medical treatment prescribed by the veterinary surgeon is carried out and recorded on the patient's record.
   Rationale: The veterinary surgeon may have prescribed drugs for this patient, which must be given at the advised times to have maximum effect. The administration of any drug should be noted on the patient's records to ensure that all members of staff are aware that the treatment has been given.

REFERENCES AND FURTHER READING

Ackerman, N., 2016. Aspinall's Complete Textbook of Veterinary Nursing, third ed. Elsevier, Oxford.

Aspinall, R., Aspinall, V., 2013. Clinical Procedures in Small Animal Practice. Saunders, London.

Aspinall, V., 2011. The Complete Textbook of Veterinary Nursing, second ed. Elsevier, Oxford.

Blood, D.C., Studdert, V.P., 2000. Comprehensive Veterinary Dictionary. W.B. Saunders, London.

Cooper, B., Mullineaux, E., Turner, L., 2011. BSAVA Textbook of Veterinary Nursing, fifth ed. BSAVA, Gloucester.

Masters, J., Bowden, C., 2001. Pre-Veterinary Nursing Textbook. Butterworth-Heinemann, Oxford.

4

Administration of fluid therapy

Georgina Parker and Carole Brown

CHAPTER CONTENTS

INTRODUCTION

The healthy body contains between 60% and 70% water, which is found inside and surrounding all the cells. This fluid maintains a balanced state within the body so that the normal metabolic processes can function efficiently – a process known as homeostasis. Dissolved in the body fluids are chemical materials that are essential for the body's metabolism and which play a part in controlling the movement of fluid around the body. Many medical conditions and surgical procedures cause an upset in fluid balance and if nothing is done to correct this, the animal may become severely dehydrated or go into shock and die. The purpose of fluid therapy is to replace any deficit so that the circulating fluid volume is restored and renal function is improved.

There are many types of fluid used in fluid therapy and the fluid replaced must be as close as possible, in terms of the chemical constituents and volume, to that lost from the general circulation. This chapter explains the theory that underpins the selection of fluids and describes in detail the procedures involved in supplying the fluid to the patient.

Procedure: Appreciation of water content in the body (Fig. 4.1)

1. **Action:** 100% total bodyweight.
   Rationale: 60% water + 40% other body structures.
2. **Action:** Intracellular fluid (ICF) = 2/3 of body fluid.
   Rationale: ICF is located within the cells.
3. **Action:** Extracellular fluid (ECF) = 1/3 of body fluid.
   Rationale: ECF is located outside the cells; plasma – water contained within blood, interstitial fluid bathing cells, transcellular fluid within specialized areas.
4. **Action:** Body fluids contain electrolytes, which yield ions.
   Rationale: It is important to know the electrolyte and ion composition of body fluids to ensure the correct fluid is administered.
5. **Action:** Ions are small water-soluble particles carrying one or more negative or positive charges. Sodium chloride (NaCl) is an electrolyte that dissociates into sodium ions and chloride ions when dissolved in water.

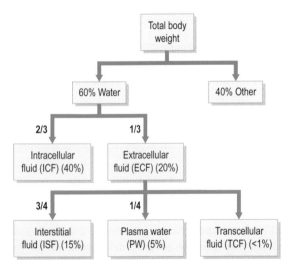

Fig. 4.1 The distribution of body water into its principal compartments. (Adapted, with permission, from Veterinary Nursing, Lane and Cooper (2003), Butterworth-Heinemann.)

Rationale: It is important to know which ions are in ICF and ECF to ensure that the correct fluid therapy is administered. Cations are ions that are positively charged; the main cations in ICF are potassium (K^+) and magnesium (Mg^{2+}), and the main cation in ECF is sodium (Na^+). Anions are ions that are negatively charged; the main anions in ECF are chloride (Cl^-) and bicarbonate (HCO_3^-).

6. **Action:** Water balance and concentration need to be maintained equally within the body.
   Rationale: Osmosis is the process by which water moves from a low concentration to a high concentration through a semipermeable membrane represented by the cellular membranes. Osmotic pressure is the pressure needed to prevent osmosis from happening. Osmotic pressure is maintained in the healthy animal by various homeostatic mechanisms.

Procedure: Appreciation of water balance in the body

1. **Action:** Water intake – ingestion.
   Rationale: Ingestion of fluids and foods.
2. **Action:** Water intake – metabolism
   Rationale: Metabolism of fats and carbohydrates.
3. **Action:** Average rate of water loss – 50 ml/kg/24 h.
   Rationale: This is the amount that needs to be replaced daily to ensure water balance.
4. **Action:** Sensible water loss – 25 ml/kg/24 h. This can be regulated by homeostatic mechanisms in the body.
   Rationale: Sensible loss via urine.
5. **Action:** Insensible water loss – 25 ml/kg/24 h. This cannot be directly regulated.
   Rationale: Insensible losses – respiratory, cutaneous and faeces.
6. **Action:** Water replacement = 50 ml/kg/24 h.
   Rationale: To balance water loss.
7. **Action:** Electrolyte replacement:
   Sodium 1 mmol/kg/24 h
   Potassium 2 mmol/kg/24 h
   Rationale: To balance electrolyte loss.
8. **Action:** Acidosis = high levels of H^+ ions in the blood, i.e. pH falls. May be a metabolic acidosis as can occur in advanced diabetes mellitus or ketosis, or a respiratory acidosis as can occur if the animal holds its breath, e.g. during anaesthesia, which results in high levels of carbon dioxide in the blood.

Rationale: Correct the acid/base imbalance with fluid containing alkaline ions.

9. **Action:** Alkalosis = low levels of H^+ ions, i.e. pH rises. May be a metabolic alkalosis as a result of prolonged vomiting and diarrhoea, or a respiratory alkalosis, e.g. due to excessive panting.
   Rationale: Correct the acid/base imbalance with fluid containing acidic ions.

Procedure: Assessing level of dehydration of the patient

1. **Action:** Normal physical appearance despite a history of fluid loss.
   Level (degree of dehydration as a percentage of bodyweight): Slight >5%.
2. **Action:** Mild to dry mucous membranes, slight decrease in skin turgor.
   Level: Mild 5–6%.
3. **Action:** Decrease in skin turgor; dry mucous membranes; mild tachycardia; sunken eyes; slight increase in capillary refill time.
   Level: Mild 6–8%.
4. **Action:** Marked decrease in skin turgor; dry mucous membranes; sunken eyes; weak pulse; increased capillary refill time; oliguria; cold extremities.
   Level: Moderate 10–12%.
5. **Action:** Very marked decrease in skin turgor; pale and dry mucous membranes; sunken eyes; tachycardia; cold extremities; muscle weakness; collapse; depression; anuria.
   Level: Severe 12–15%.

Procedure: Selection of fluids in relation to their action in the body

1. **Action:** Isotonic fluid.
   Rationale: Equal osmotic pressure to plasma – no fluid movement, thereby maintaining equilibrium.
2. **Action:** Hypertonic fluid.
   Rationale: Greater osmotic pressure than plasma – thereby encouraging movement of fluid from cells into circulation.
3. **Action:** Hypotonic fluid.
   Rationale: Lower osmotic pressure than plasma – thereby encouraging movement of fluids into cells.
4. **Action:** Crystalloids.
   Rationale: These fluids contain small dissolved molecules that enter the bloodstream and temporarily increase the blood volume before passing into the cells and equilibrating with the ICF.

5. **Action:** Colloids.
   Rationale: These fluids contain large molecules that remain within the circulation, thereby increasing osmotic pressure and expanding plasma volume.
6. **Action:** Blood product – plasma.
   Rationale: This helps to expand plasma volume and treat hypoproteinaemia.
7. **Action:** Whole blood.
   Rationale: Used in cases where red blood cell replacement and plasma volume expansion are required.

Procedure: Selection of fluid for specific needs

1. **Action:** 0.9% NaCl – normal saline (isotonic crystalloid).
   Rationale: Replace ECF. Gastric losses or loss of acidic ions from vomiting.
2. **Action:** 0.18% NaCl + 4% dextrose (isotonic crystalloid).
   Rationale: Maintenance requirements; primary water deficit replacement; neonatal ECF replacement.
3. **Action:** 5% dextrose (isotonic crystalloid).
   Rationale: Primary water deficit replacement.
4. **Action:** Hartmann's solution (isotonic crystalloid).
   Rationale: Replace ECF. Diarrhoea and post-gastric losses/alkaline ions.
5. **Action:** Ringer's solution (isotonic crystalloid).
   Rationale: Replace ECF; gastric losses from vomiting.
6. **Action:** Haemaccel/Gelofusine (isotonic colloids).
   Rationale: Expand plasma volume; moderate to severe fluid loss and blood loss where no blood products are available.
7. **Action:** Plasma (blood product – isotonic).
   Rationale: Replace plasma proteins; expand plasma volume as above; clotting defects.
8. **Action:** Whole blood (isotonic).
   Rationale: Replace blood loss; meet any ongoing or anticipated blood loss; anaemia; circulatory insufficiency.

Procedure: Oral fluid therapy

Indications. Animal willing to drink, not vomiting, absence of intestinal obstruction.
   Fluid choice. Hypotonic electrolyte solution or water.
1. **Action:** Select equipment – dosing syringe with catheter tip, towel, fluid. Ask for assistance.
   Rationale: A dosing syringe is the most suitable method of accurate administration. It is important to select all equipment prior to the procedure to ensure efficient administration.

2. **Action:** Measure correct volume of fluid in syringe.
   Rationale: Important to measure fluid replacement accurately to avoid excess or insufficient fluid.

3. **Action:** Request assistance holding patient (see Chapter 1).
   Rationale: Ensure that the patient is kept at ease and feels safe.

4. **Action:** Support patient's nose and mouth with left hand in normal position.
   Rationale: Firm but sympathetic handling will ensure fluid is delivered safely and effectively. Head must be in normal position to prevent aspiration pneumonia.

5. **Action:** Introduce the catheter tip syringe into the mouth between the upper and lower premolars above the tongue surface.
   Rationale: This area is the most suitable to administer fluid safely and accurately.

6. **Action:** Slowly introduce 5–10 ml of fluid into the mouth and allow the patient to swallow. Stroke the ventral aspect of the pharynx to encourage swallowing.
   Rationale: Avoid giving too much fluid at any one time as this may induce choking. Allow patient to swallow and breathe between administrations.

7. **Action:** Continue until required volume has been delivered or the patient becomes agitated.
   Rationale: Only continue if patient is taking fluid well and swallowing between doses. At any time, if the patient gets distressed or fails to swallow, stop the procedure immediately.

8. **Action:** Dry the patient's mouth and surrounding area and replace in prepared clean kennel.
   Rationale: Always dry the area to help prevent heat loss and make the patient comfortable.

9. **Action:** Record total fluid volume given and the frequency on the hospital record.
   Rationale: Ensure record keeping is accurate to prevent over- or under-administration.

10. **Action:** Dispose of equipment safely and appropriately.
    Rationale: It is essential to dispose of equipment correctly to avoid contamination and accidents.

Procedure: Subcutaneous fluid therapy

Indications. Mild dehydration with adequate peripheral circulation.

Fluid choice. Any crystalloid isotonic solution such as 0.9% NaCl, 0.18% NaCl + 4% dextrose or Hartmann's solution.

1. **Action:** Select and prepare equipment – prewarmed fluid, measured volume in sterile syringe with new sterile needle attached (maximum 10–20 ml/kg/site), clippers, surgical skin scrub, gloves, swabs (Fig. 4.2). Ask for assistance.
   Rationale: Fluid must be prewarmed to prevent shock and discomfort and aid absorption. Isotonic or hypotonic fluid is used to promote absorption. Ensure all equipment is prepared in advance to allow for efficient administration.

2. **Action:** Request assistant to restrain patient in lateral recumbency (see Chapter 1).
   Rationale: Firm, effective handling ensures that the patient remains comfortable throughout the procedure.

3. **Action:** Clip an area of approximately 3 × 3 cm on either side of the thorax over the ninth rib, midway between ventral and dorsal borders.
   Rationale: Area must be free of hair to reduce the risk of infection. This area allows effective movement and absorption of fluid.

4. **Action:** Prepare skin aseptically with surgical scrub solution. Wear gloves.
   Rationale: Skin must be cleaned aseptically to reduce risk of infection.

5. **Action:** Infiltrate local anaesthetic into the prepared site as per veterinary surgeon instructions. Drape the area.
   Rationale: Local anaesthetic will desensitize the area, preventing pain and discomfort. Draping the area will help to maintain asepsis.

6. **Action:** Tent the skin and introduce the needle, attached to the fluid-filled syringe, subcutaneously.
   Rationale: Administration must be subcutaneous, avoiding any puncture of thoracic cavity.

7. **Action:** Withdraw the plunger of the syringe and check for presence of blood.
   Rationale: To check that a vein has not been punctured by accident.

8. **Action:** Administer the volume of fluid slowly and withdraw the needle (maximum 10–20 ml/kg/site).
   Rationale: Fast infusion of fluid can cause considerable discomfort.

9. **Action:** Massage the area.
   Rationale: To ensure even and effective distribution.

10. **Action:** Repeat the procedure on the other side of the thorax.
    Rationale: To ensure equal distribution in the body.

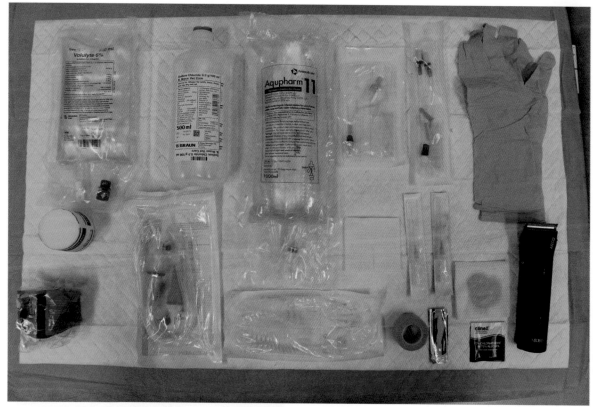

Fig. 4.2 Equipment used to provide intravenous fluid therapy.

11. **Action:** Remove the drapes and dry the area. Allow the patient to resume sternal recumbency and place back in the kennel.
    Rationale: Ensure patient is comfortable in kennel.
12. **Action:** Dispose of equipment safely and appropriately.
    Rationale: It is essential to dispose of equipment correctly to avoid contamination and accidents.

Procedure: Intraperitoneal fluid therapy

Indications. Mild dehydration where fluids cannot be administered orally; where larger volumes need to be infused rapidly; neonates and exotics.

Fluid choice. Any isotonic crystalloid fluid such as 0.9% NaCl, 0.18% NaCl + 4% dextrose, or Hartmann's solution.

1. **Action:** Select and prepare equipment – prewarmed fluid, measured volume in sterile syringe with sterile new needle attached, clippers, surgical skin scrub solution, swabs, gloves. Ask for assistance.

Rationale: Avoid shock and drop in body temperature by prewarming fluid. Prepare all equipment in advance of procedure to ensure efficient administration.

2. **Action:** Assistant to restrain patient in dorsal recumbency and reassure patient throughout procedure.
   Rationale: To present the correct area for administration and encourage the viscera to gravitate away from site, thereby avoiding puncture during procedure.
3. **Action:** Clip area surrounding umbilicus.
   Rationale: Reduce risk of infection by clipping hair, allowing a wide margin around umbilicus.
4. **Action:** Prepare skin aseptically and drape area.
   Rationale: To reduce risk of infection.
5. **Action:** Infiltrate local anaesthetic into prepared site – umbilicus region – as per veterinary surgeon instructions.

Rationale: To desensitize area prior to administration of fluid.

6. **Action:** Introduce sterile needle attached to fluid syringe through the skin and central line (linea alba) into the peritoneal cavity.
   Rationale: Ensure asepsis is maintained and introduction is efficient and smooth.

7. **Action:** Withdraw plunger of syringe.
   Rationale: To check that no organ or blood vessel has been penetrated by accident. If blood appears in hub of syringe, withdraw and start again. If urine or gut contents appear in the syringe, the bladder or intestine may have been punctured – withdraw and start again.

8. **Action:** Introduce prewarmed fluid into the peritoneal cavity.
   Rationale: If any resistance is felt, stop and restart procedure from point 6.

9. **Action:** Withdraw needle and syringe, putting gentle pressure over injection site.
   Rationale: Clean, swift removal of needle minimizes any discomfort. Applying pressure prevents leakage of body fluid.

10. **Action:** Remove drapes and dry the area. Allow patient to regain sternal recumbency, reassure and replace in kennel.
    Rationale: Resume normal position as soon as possible to restore equilibrium. It is important to ensure patient is comfortable before placing back in kennel.

11. **Action:** Record fluid administration details.
    Rationale: To ensure accurate monitoring.

12. **Action:** Dispose of equipment safely and appropriately.
    Rationale: It is essential to dispose of equipment correctly to avoid contamination and accidents.

Procedure: Preparation of equipment for intravenous fluid administration

1. **Action:** Wash hands and wear disposable gloves.
   Rationale: It is essential to maintain asepsis to avoid contamination and infection.

2. **Action:** Select correct equipment for intravenous fluid administration – clippers, surgical scrub solution, swabs, tapes, blade, intravenous catheter, heparinized saline, three-way tap or bung, fluid bag, infusion set, kick bowl, drip stand (Fig. 4.3).

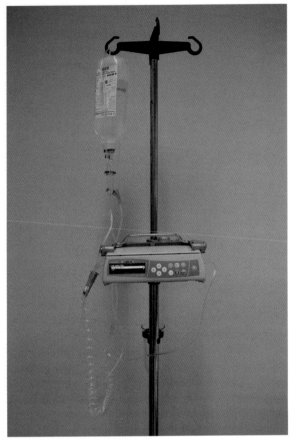

Fig. 4.3 Intravenous therapy set-up using a type of infusion pump

Rationale: All equipment must be selected prior to patient restraint to ensure that the procedure is performed efficiently and thoroughly.

3. **Action:** Check the expiry date on the fluid bag; look for any damage to the outside of the bag or for any artefacts within the fluid.
   Rationale: Any sign of damage, abnormality or passed expiry date indicates that sterility of the product cannot be guaranteed, rendering it unsafe to use.

4. **Action:** Remove the fluid bag from its outer covering and identify the correct outlet port. Prewarm fluid to body temperature and hang fluid bag on drip stand.
   Rationale: Careful handling to reduce risk of contamination. Use of a drip stand facilitates handling. Warming of fluid to just below body temperature will prevent shock.

5. **Action:** Remove infusion set from its outer coverings and switch off the flow control.
   Rationale: Switching off the flow control will prevent loss of fluid prior to connection to bag.
6. **Action:** Remove the cover from the infusion spike and introduce into the fluid bag carefully.
   Rationale: Careful handling will avoid puncture of fluid bag with the spike, thus avoiding contamination and fluid loss.
7. **Action:** Squeeze fluid chamber so that it fills by one-third.
   Rationale: To aid control of fluid during infusion and prevent air bubbles.
8. **Action:** Remove the cap from the end of infusion line, taking care not to touch a non-sterile surface.
   Rationale: It is important to maintain sterility at all times. If sterility is broken, you must use another sterile infusion set.
9. **Action:** Open flow control and allow fluid to travel down infusion set in a controlled manner, removing all air bubbles. Avoid excess fluid loss from the bag.
   Rationale: No air bubbles should enter the circulation. Excess fluid loss should be avoided from the fluid bag, as this affects the total volume being given.
10. **Action:** Switch off flow control and replace cap. Hang giving set on drip stand (Fig. 4.3).
    Rationale: To prevent leakage and maintain sterility.
11. **Action:** Dispose of equipment safely and appropriately.
    Rationale: It is essential to dispose of equipment correctly to avoid equipment clutter and reduce risk of contamination and accidents.

Procedure: Intravenous access to the cephalic vein and administration of fluid therapy

1. **Action:** Select equipment and prepare fluid infusion. Prewarm fluid to body temperature.
   Rationale: Prepare equipment in advance of restraining the patient. Maintain body temperature and minimize discomfort by prewarming the fluid.
2. **Action:** Assistant to restrain the patient in sternal recumbency, in the correct manner to allow access to the cephalic vein (see Chapter 1).
   Rationale: Firm handling will keep the patient at ease and reduce the risk of any accident.

3. **Action:** Wearing gloves, clip and prepare the site aseptically using surgical scrub or surgical spirit.
   Rationale: This will help to prevent infection.
4. **Action:** Ask the assistant to raise the vein (see Chapter 1).
   Rationale: This dilates the vein, making it easier to see.
5. **Action:** With gloved hands, insert the catheter tip into the vein. A cut-down technique with a scalpel blade may be employed for venous access. Once blood appears within the catheter, remove the needle and advance the catheter fully (Fig. 4.4).
   Rationale: The cut-down technique reduces risk of blunting the catheter tip. The needle is removed to prevent accidental puncture of vein further along the lumen.
6. **Action:** Ask the assistant to release the pressure over the vein. Place a bung or three-way tap to close the end of the catheter.
   Rationale: To avoid excess blood loss.
7. **Action:** Dry the area and secure the catheter to the leg with tapes.
   Rationale: It is important to dry the area to ensure that any tape adheres to the leg and holds the catheter in place, thus preventing movement and blood leakage.
8. **Action:** Flush the catheter with a small amount of heparinized saline.
   Rationale: This is to ensure patency of the catheter and prevent blood clot formation in the catheter.

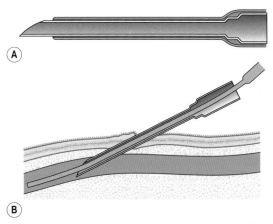

Fig. 4.4 Types of intravenous catheter. A, over-the-needle cannula; B, through-the-needle cannula.

9. **Action:** Remove the cap from the infusion set and attach the infusion tube to the intravenous catheter. Secure the infusion tube to the patient's leg with tapes. Bandage if necessary.

   Rationale: *To ensure that the fluid infusion tube remains in place if the patient moves. Movement could cause it to become dislodged, resulting in blood loss.*

10. **Action:** Open fluid flow control.

    Rationale: *To assess if the fluid is flowing freely. If the drip is not flowing, assess the reason and deal with it appropriately.*

11. **Action:** Adjust the fluid control to the drip rate required for the patient. Syringe drivers and infusion pumps may be used to facilitate the delivery of the calculated drip rate (Fig. 4.3).

    Rationale: *It is essential to control rate of delivery of the fluid replacement, to avoid over- or under-infusion.*

12. **Action:** Record fluid type and drip rate on hospital card (Fig. 4.5).

    Rationale: *This is to ensure accurate monitoring and clear communication between all veterinary personnel.*

13. **Action:** To prevent self-mutilation by the patient, bandage the area and apply an Elizabethan collar as necessary.

    Rationale: *If patient mutilates area, there is a risk of blood loss, sepsis and thrombosis.*

14. **Action:** Dispose of equipment safely and appropriately.

    Rationale: *It is essential that all items are disposed of correctly to avoid contamination and accidents.*

Procedure: Intravenous access to the saphenous vein and administration of fluid therapy

1. **Action:** Select equipment and prepared fluid infusion. Prewarm fluid to body temperature.

   Rationale: *Prepare all equipment in advance of restraining the patient. Maintain body temperature and minimize discomfort by prewarming fluids.*

2. **Action:** Ask the assistant to restrain the patient in lateral recumbency to allow intravenous access to the saphenous vein. Two assistants may be required to maintain patient in required position (see Chapter 1).

   Rationale: *Firm handling will keep the patient at ease and reduce the risk of any accident. As the*

patient will need to be in lateral recumbency, a second assistant is required to extend the hindlimb.

3. **Action:** Wearing gloves, clip and prepare site aseptically using surgical scrub or surgical spirit.

   Rationale: *This will help to prevent infection.*

4. **Action:** Ask the assistant to raise the vein (see Chapter 1).

   Rationale: *This dilates the vein, making it easier to see.*

5. **Action:** With gloved hands, insert the catheter tip into the vein. Once blood appears in the catheter, remove the needle and advance catheter fully.

   Rationale: *The needle is removed to prevent accidental puncture of the vein further along its lumen.*

6. **Action:** Ask the assistant to release the pressure on the vein. Place a bung or three-way tap to close the end of the catheter.

   Rationale: *To avoid excess blood loss and minimize the risk of infection entering the vein.*

7. **Action:** Dry the area and secure the catheter to the leg with tapes.

   Rationale: *It is important to dry the area to ensure any tape adheres to the leg and holds the catheter in place. Tapes are used to secure the catheter, preventing movement and blood leakage.*

8. **Action:** Flush the catheter with a small amount of heparinized saline.

   Rationale: *This is to ensure patency of the catheter and prevent blood clot formation in the catheter.*

9. **Action:** Remove the cap from the infusion set and attach the infusion tube to the intravenous catheter. Secure the infusion tube to the patient's leg with tapes. Bandage if necessary.

   Rationale: *To ensure that the fluid infusion tube remains in place if the patient moves. Movement could cause it to become dislodged, resulting in blood loss.*

10. **Action:** Open fluid flow control.

    Rationale: *To assess if the fluid is flowing freely. If the drip is not flowing, assess the reason and deal with it appropriately.*

11. **Action:** Adjust the fluid control to the drip rate required for the patient. Syringe drivers and infusion pumps may be used to facilitate the delivery of the calculated drip rate (Fig. 4.3).

Rationale: It is essential to control the rate of delivery of the fluid replacement to avoid over- or under-infusion.

12. **Action:** Record fluid type and drip rate on the hospital card (Fig. 4.5).
Rationale: This is to ensure accurate monitoring.

13. **Action:** To prevent self-mutilation by the patient, bandage the area and apply an Elizabethan collar as necessary.
Rationale: If the patient mutilates the area, there is a risk of blood loss, sepsis and thrombosis.

14. **Action:** Dispose of equipment safely and appropriately.
Rationale: It is essential that all items are disposed of correctly to avoid contamination and accidents.

Procedure: Intravenous access to the jugular vein and administration of fluid therapy

1. **Action:** Select equipment and prepared fluid infusion. Prewarm fluid to body temperature.
Rationale: Prepare all equipment in advance of restraining the patient. Maintain body temperature and minimize discomfort by prewarming fluid.

2. **Action:** Ask the assistant to restrain the patient in the correct manner to provide access to the jugular vein (see Chapter 1). Two assistants may be required to maintain the patient in the required position.
Rationale: Firm handling will keep the patient at ease and reduce any risk of accident.

3. **Action:** Wearing gloves, clip and prepare site aseptically using surgical scrub or surgical spirit.
Rationale: This will help prevent infection.

4. **Action:** The vein will be raised by the operator by applying pressure at the base of the neck (see Chapter 1).
Rationale: This dilates the vein, making it easier to see.

5. **Action:** With gloved hands, insert the catheter tip into the vein. Once blood appears in the catheter, remove the needle and advance the catheter fully.
Rationale: The needle is removed to prevent accidental puncture of the vein further along its lumen.

6. **Action:** Ask the assistant to release the pressure on the vein. Place a bung or three-way tap to close the end of the catheter.

Rationale: To avoid excess blood loss and risk of infection.

7. **Action:** Dry the area and secure the catheter to the skin with the aid of adhesive tapes and bandage, or suture in place.
Rationale: It is important to dry the area to ensure that any tape adheres to the skin holding the catheter in place. Accidental movement or displacement of the catheter must be avoided from the jugular vein, as blood loss could be considerable.

8. **Action:** Flush the catheter with a small amount of heparinized saline.
Rationale: This maintains the patency of the catheter and prevents blood clot formation in the catheter.

9. **Action:** Remove the cap from the infusion set and attach the infusion tube to the intravenous catheter. Secure the infusion tube to the neck region. Bandage if necessary.
Rationale: To ensure fluid infusion remains in place if patient moves, thereby preventing dislodgement and blood loss.

10. **Action:** Open fluid flow control.
Rationale: To assess if the fluid is flowing freely. If the drip is not flowing, assess the reason and deal with it appropriately.

11. **Action:** Adjust the fluid control to the drip rate required for the patient. Syringe drivers and infusion pumps may be used to facilitate the delivery of the calculated drip rate (Fig. 4.3).
Rationale: It is essential to control the delivery of the fluid replacement rate to avoid over- or under-infusion.

12. **Action:** Record fluid type and drip rate on the hospital card (Fig. 4.5).
Rationale: This is to ensure accurate monitoring and clear communication between all veterinary personnel.

13. **Action:** To prevent self-mutilation by the patient, bandage the area and apply an Elizabethan collar as necessary.
Rationale: If the patient mutilates the area, there is a risk of blood loss, sepsis and thrombosis.

14. **Action:** Dispose of equipment safely and appropriately.
Rationale: It is essential that all items are disposed of correctly to avoid contamination and accidents.

Procedure: Calculation of fluid deficit and maintenance requirements

Example. A 20 kg dog that has been off food and water for 3 days and has been vomiting four times a day for the last 2 days.

Fluid choice. Colloid to replace or expand plasma volume, e.g. Haemaccel or Gelofusine, followed by a crystalloid to replace remainder of deficit, e.g. 0.9% NaCl or Hartmann's solution, and crystalloid to meet maintenance requirements, e.g. 0.18% NaCl + 4% dextrose.

1. **Action:** Calculate insensible losses × 3 days (25 ml/kg/24 h × 20 kg) = 1500 ml.
   Rationale: Insensible losses (respiratory, cutaneous, faecal) will initially continue in spite of the lack of fluid intake.
2. **Action:** Calculate sensible losses × 3 days (25 ml/kg/24 h × 20 kg × 1) = 500 ml.
   Rationale: Sensible losses (urine) will be reduced by the lack of fluid intake, therefore the calculation is based on 1 day instead of 3 days.
3. **Action:** Calculate loss from vomiting four times a day for 2 days (4 ml/kg/vomit × 20 × 4 × 2) = 640 ml.
   Rationale: Fluid loss from vomit can only be estimated but does need to be taken into account when calculating the total deficit.
4. **Action:** Calculate total fluid deficit = all of the above factors added together = 2640 ml, of which ECF deficit is 880 ml and 220 ml represents plasma volume.
   Rationale: This amount has been calculated by adding all of the above factors and represents the deficit only.
5. **Action:** This volume should be replaced over 24 hours, with half of the replacement being administered over 6–8 hours.
   Rationale: One-twelfth of the total deficit should be replaced with a plasma substitute, as one-twelfth of the body fluid represents plasma volume (Fig. 4.1).
6. **Action:** Meet ongoing losses/maintenance requirements at 50 ml/kg/24 h × 20 kg = 1000 ml/24 h.
   Rationale: Whilst the deficit needs to be replaced, water loss will continue due to body metabolism, so it is essential to meet the ongoing maintenance requirements until the patient has recovered.
7. **Action:** Alternatively, calculate deficit from packed cell volume (PCV)/haematocrit measurement (see Chapter 11): for every 1% rise in PCV, allow for fluid deficit of 10 ml/kg.
   Rationale: This can only be assessed if compared with PCV reading for normal, healthy patient.

Procedure: Calculation of drip rate

Example. Daily maintenance for 25 kg dog to be administered over an 8-hour period.

1. **Action:** Calculate the daily maintenance fluid requirements for a 25 kg dog at 50 ml/kg body-weight/24 h = 1250 ml/24 h.
   Rationale: Daily fluid requirement is a total of 50 ml/kg to allow for 25 ml/kg/24 h sensible losses and 25 ml/kg/24 h insensible losses. The weight of the patient is multiplied by the millilitres of fluid for a 24-hour period.
2. **Action:** The above fluid is to be given over 8 hours. Calculate the volume of fluid to be given per hour = 156 ml/h.
   Rationale: The calculation in step 1 is based on a 24-hour period. This is to be administered over an 8-hour period. Divide 1250 ml by 8.
3. **Action:** Calculate the volume of fluid to be given per minute = 2.60 ml/min.
   Rationale: The hourly rate is 156 ml. There are 60 minutes in 1 hour, therefore divide 156 by 60.
4. **Action:** The infusion set delivers 20 drops/ml. Calculate the drips per minute = 52 drops per minute.
   Rationale: The volume in millilitres per minute is 2.60, and the infusion set delivers 20 drops/ml; therefore multiply 2.6 by 20.
5. **Action:** Calculate the drops per second = 0.8 drop per second, or approximately 1 drop per second.
   Rationale: 52 drops are to be delivered over 1 minute; there are 60 seconds in 1 minute, therefore divide 52 by 60 = 0.8.
6. **Action:** Once the drip rate is calculated, an infusion pump or syringe driver may be employed.
   Rationale: An infusion pump or syringe driver accurately delivers the calculated fluid rate, and an alarm will sound if problems arise.

Procedure: Maintenance of intravenous fluid therapy – general maintenance

1. **Action:** Ensure the infusion site is kept clean. Avoid touching the barrel of the catheter or the site of insertion.
   Rationale: It is essential that the area is kept clean to avoid infection. Bandage the area where possible.

2. **Action:** Replace dressings if they become soiled.

   Rationale: *Any soiled dressings near to the infusion site dressing could introduce infection, so the dressings must be checked and changed regularly. Antibiotic or antiseptic cream can be applied to the site of catheter insertion to reduce risk of infection.*

3. **Action:** Check catheter placement for any abnormalities such as redness, heat or swelling of the area.

   Rationale: *The signs of infection include perivascular leakage and thrombus. A new catheter may have to be placed.*

4. **Action:** Take the patient's temperature 3–4 times daily.

   Rationale: *An increasing body temperature could indicate infection.*

5. **Action:** Flush the catheter at least twice daily with a small amount of heparinized saline.

   Rationale: *This is to ensure patency of the catheter. If resistance is experienced, assess the viability of the catheter and replace with a new catheter if necessary.*

6. **Action:** Check that fluid is kept warm and is flowing freely and at the correct drip rate.

   Rationale: *Warm fluids will prevent infusion shock. Failure of the fluid to flow could mean that the catheter has moved or become blocked, or that there are problems with the infusion set or pump – all of which require immediate attention. Flush the catheter and assess the patency of the infusion set. If patency is not achieved, replace faulty or damaged equipment as necessary.*

7. **Action:** Check the patient's demeanour.

   Rationale: *If the patient shows any change in its behaviour pattern and appears to be in discomfort, examine the infusion site for any problems. Stop infusion and consult the veterinary surgeon.*

8. **Action:** Allow the patient to urinate either by catheterization, taking a dog for walks, providing litter trays for cats and providing absorbent bedding.

   Rationale: *To ensure the patient remains comfortable, it must be allowed to urinate while receiving fluids. The method will depend on each individual case. Remember to measure urine voided.*

Procedure: Maintenance of fluid therapy – replacement or changing of intravenous fluid bags

1. **Action:** Select and prepare equipment – prewarm correct fluid, check expiry date, wash hands, wear gloves and apron.

   Rationale: *It is essential that all equipment is ready prior to the procedure to ensure efficient changing of fluid bags.*

2. **Action:** Remove the new fluid bag from its outer wrapping. Identify the correct fluid outlet port and remove the cover, maintaining asepsis. Hang the new fluid bag on patient's drip stand.

   Rationale: *It is essential to identify the correct site to insert the infusion set to prevent damage or contamination. Placing the fluid bag on the drip stand will facilitate easy and efficient handling.*

3. **Action:** Ask assistant to restrain the patient.

   Rationale: *This is essential to avoid movement of the patient and risk of removal or contamination of equipment.*

4. **Action:** Switch off flow control on infusion set connected to patient.

   Rationale: *The infusion must be switched off before changing the bags to prevent any air entering the infusion tube.*

5. **Action:** Holding the empty fluid bag at the base, carefully remove the infusion set and immediately insert spike into new fluid bag, taking care not to puncture the bag or contaminate the infusion.

   Rationale: *Removal and reintroduction of the infusion set to a new bag need to be swift to reduce the likelihood of contamination. Any contamination could result in infection entering the circulatory system.*

6. **Action:** Switch on flow control to ensure that the fluid is flowing freely and adjust to required drip rate.

   Rationale: *It may be necessary to flush the patient's catheter after a fluid change as some back flow of blood into catheter and infusion line may occur.*

7. **Action:** Record all details of fluid replacement.

   Rationale: *It is essential to keep accurate records to prevent under- or over-infusion of the patient.*

8. **Action:** Dispose of all equipment safely and appropriately and disinfect area.

   Rationale: *It is essential for all areas to remain hygienic and for equipment to be disposed of correctly to prevent infection and accidents.*

Procedure: Maintenance of fluid therapy – removal of intravenous fluid therapy equipment from patient

1. **Action:** Select and prepare equipment – assemble tapes, swab and scissors; wash hands; enlist the help of an assistant; wear gloves and apron.

Rationale: It is essential to ensure all equipment is ready prior to starting the procedure to ensure efficient and safe removal of the catheter from the vein.

2. **Action:** Ask assistant to restrain patient.
   Rationale: It is essential that the patient is made to feel safe and that any movement is minimized to prevent discomfort or unnecessary haemorrhage during the procedure.

3. **Action:** Remove all tapes and sutures and terminate flow by switching off flow control.
   Rationale: The infusion must be switched off before removal to prevent fluid leakage and contamination.

4. **Action:** Gently and quickly remove catheter while assistant applies pressure over the vein.
   Rationale: Removal of the catheter should be quick and efficient to ensure minimal discomfort to the patient.

5. **Action:** Maintain pressure on the site of catheter removal while placing a swab over the area. Secure with adhesive tape or bandage.
   Rationale: Pressure must be exerted to prevent haemorrhage and haematoma formation. It may be necessary to apply sutures if a cut-down technique has been used for jugular access.

6. **Action:** Dispose of all equipment safely and appropriately and disinfect area.
   Rationale: It is essential for all areas to remain hygienic and for equipment to be disposed of correctly to prevent infection.

Procedure: Monitoring of fluid therapy – general guidelines

1. **Action:** Baseline parameters, such as pulse rate, heart rate, capillary refill time and colour of mucous membranes, must be recorded prior to any fluid administration.
   Rationale: It is essential to know the results of baseline tests to compare and assess the effectiveness of fluid administration.

2. **Action:** Monitoring must be performed at regular intervals and recorded on a fluid administration chart (Fig. 4.5).
   Rationale: Regular results will indicate a trend, which is more useful than a one-off measurement. Accuracy and regularity are essential requirements for effective monitoring. Everything must be recorded in writing to avoid error.

3. **Action:** All deviations or abnormalities must be noted immediately.
   Rationale: It is essential that any abnormalities are reported immediately to the veterinary surgeon and acted upon to avoid further deterioration or complications to the patient.

Procedure: Monitoring of fluid therapy – essential parameters

Indications. All patients receiving fluids (Figs 4.5 and 4.6).

1. **Action:** Pulse rate, rhythm and quality, including core and peripheral pulses.
   Rationale: To check circulatory volume is adequate for tissue perfusion and to ensure circulation is the same throughout the body.

2. **Action:** Mucous membrane colour and feel.
   Rationale: Check oxygenation levels are adequate – membranes will change colour. Check level of hydration by feel – membranes may feel moist, tacky or dry. Excess moisture and lacrimation may indicate over-infusion – contact the veterinary surgeon.

3. **Action:** Capillary refill time.
   Rationale: To assess effectiveness of circulating fluid volume – should be 1–2 seconds.

4. **Action:** Chest auscultation/respiratory rate and depth.
   Rationale: Should be clear lung sounds. Laboured, rapid or noisy respiratory patterns may indicate over-infusion or cardiac problems.

5. **Action:** Peripheral oedema.
   Rationale: This could indicate over-infusion of fluid.

6. **Action:** Body temperature – core and peripheral.
   Rationale: To assess vasoconstriction/vasodilation, and to check if patient is suffering from a systemic infection.

7. **Action:** Urine output.
   Rationale: Minimum output = 1 ml/kg/h. To assess renal function and associated circulatory volume. Less than 1 ml/kg/h could indicate renal problems due to insufficient circulatory volume.

8. **Action:** Skin turgor.
   Rationale: To assess pliability of skin. Tenting can indicate dehydration.

9. **Action:** Bodyweight.
   Rationale: To assess any change over a period of hours/days. Marked increase could indicate over-infusion.

Patient I.D.				Clinical history								
Species and breed												
Age	Sex		Weight									
Veterinary surgeon												
Veterinary nurse												

Monitor and record every............................. daily

Date and time	T	P	R	MM CRT	Demeanour	Fluid type	Drip rate	Fluid input	Fluid/urine output	Weight	Medication	Comments

Fig. 4.5 Example of a chart for monitoring patients receiving fluid therapy.

10. **Action:** General demeanour/clinical observation.
    Rationale: Any sign of distress or discomfort could indicate a problem, e.g. infection, over-infusion, deterioration of medical condition.

Procedure: Blood collection for transfusion

Indication. Blood required for storage or by a recipient to replace acute or chronic haemorrhage, anaemia or clotting problems.

1. **Action:** Select an appropriate donor that is of the same species, healthy and fully grown. The owner must be aware of what is involved and give permission for blood to be collected.
   Rationale: Different species have different blood groups, and blood groups also differ within the species. There are 13 recognized blood groups in the dog and three in the cat. It may be necessary to check for compatibility by testing for a reaction between a prepared sample of donor red cells and the recipient plasma. Absence of haemolysis or agglutination demonstrates compatibility.

2. **Action:** Select equipment for blood collection – acid citrate/citrate dextrose blood collection bag, local anaesthetic, syringe, needle, clippers, surgical skin scrub solution, gloves, swabs. Ask for assistance.
   Rationale: Anticipation and preparation are essential for effective collection.

3. **Action:** An assistant is needed to restrain the patient in a suitable position allowing access to the jugular vein. The patient is reassured throughout the procedure (see Chapter 1).
   Rationale: Firm restraint is required to make the donor feel safe and comfortable.

Name _____

Case number _____

Date and time	Fluid offered	Fluid intake	IV fluid	Drip rate

Fig. 4.6 Example of a chart for monitoring fluid balance.

4. **Action:** Clip small area over jugular vein and prepare skin aseptically.

   Rationale: To reduce risk of infection.

5. **Action:** Local anaesthetic is infiltrated into the prepared site as per the veterinary surgeon's instructions. Massage the area.

   Rationale: Local anaesthetic desensitizes the area. The area is massaged to help absorption.

6. **Action:** The needle attached to the donor blood bag is introduced by the veterinary surgeon into the jugular vein. Once blood flows into the donor bag, the needle is advanced and held in place manually.

   Rationale: As collection is via a needle rather than a catheter, it needs to be held securely to prevent further puncture of the jugular vein, which could result in considerable blood loss.

7. **Action:** Hold blood bag below the patient and roll it continually and gently.

   Rationale: Blood is collected by the action of gravity. The bag is rolled to ensure mixing of the acid citrate/citrate dextrose anticoagulant, thus preventing clotting.

8. **Action:** Once the required volume of blood has been collected, the veterinary surgeon removes the needle and the assistant exerts pressure on the jugular puncture site.

   Rationale: To prevent further blood loss by providing back pressure, thereby arresting haemorrhage from venepuncture site.

9. **Action:** Fold over the blood collection tube to occlude it.

   Rationale: To avoid excess wastage within the tube.

10. **Action:** If the blood is not to be administered immediately, store at 4–8°C for a maximum of 3 weeks. Label bag clearly with the species and date of collection.

    Rationale: It is essential that blood products are stored correctly to avoid deterioration.

11. **Action:** Dispose of equipment safely and appropriately.

    Rationale: It is essential to dispose of equipment correctly to avoid contamination and accidents.

Procedure: Blood transfusion

Indications. Acute or chronic haemorrhage, acute or chronic anaemia, platelet and clotting problems.

1. **Action:** Select and prepare equipment (Fig. 4.7) – blood warmed to body temperature (if from storage), blood infusion set, adhesive tape, bandage. Patient with intravenous catheter in place.

   Rationale: Blood must be prewarmed prior to administration to maintain body temperature and cause minimal discomfort to the patient. All equipment must be prepared in advance of the procedure to ensure efficient administration.

2. **Action:** Remove the cover from the spike of the blood infusion set. Switch off flow control and insert the spike into the correct port of the blood bag, taking care not to puncture the bag.

   Rationale: Puncturing the blood bag would result in a waste of blood and contamination of the blood bag, making it unsafe to use for transfusion.

3. **Action:** Squeeze both chambers of blood infusion set to fill one-third of each chamber with blood.

   Rationale: The extra chamber within the blood infusion set contains a fibrin filter to collect any fibrin clots, preventing them entering the circulation.

4. **Action:** Remove cap from the end of the infusion line and hold over kick bowl, taking care not to contaminate the tip.

   Rationale: It is essential to keep all items sterile.

5. **Action:** Remove all air bubbles by turning on flow control switch to allow blood to travel down infusion line to the tip in a controlled manner.

   Rationale: To avoid risk of air embolism, all air bubbles must be removed from the infusion line prior to connection to the patient.

6. **Action:** Replace cap on infusion line and hang infusion on drip stand prior to connection to the patient.

   Rationale: Ensure equipment remains aseptic.

7. **Action:** Restrain patient and ensure the patency of the catheter by flushing with a small amount of heparinized saline.

   Rationale: It is essential to check the patency of the catheter before attachment to the blood infusion line to avoid unnecessary contamination or wastage of blood.

8. **Action:** Remove cap from infusion line and attach to the intravenous catheter. Switch on flow control to allow blood to flow into the patient.

   Rationale: Connect and access patency. If not flowing freely, check equipment and reflush.

9. **Action:** When flowing freely, adjust flow control to required rate of transfusion.

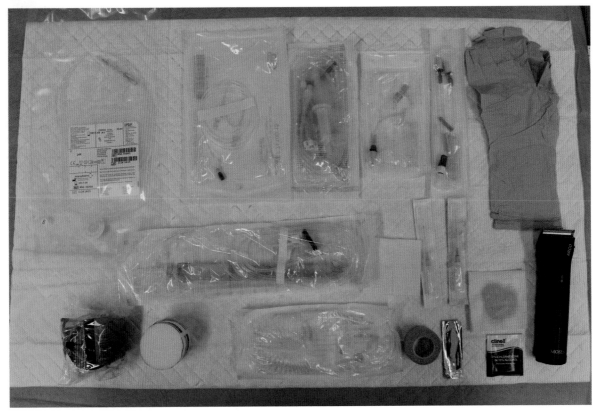

Fig. 4.7 Equipment required to collect and give whole blood.

Rationale: Rapid transfusion of blood should be avoided to prevent circulatory overload or reaction.

10. **Action:** Attach infusion line securely to the patient by means of tapes, bandages or sutures (depending on which intravenous route has been chosen).

    Rationale: It is essential that the infusion line is secure to avoid displacement or leakage.

11. **Action:** Monitor constantly for any signs of blood transfusion reaction and record details of transfusion rate and time.

    Rationale: It is essential to keep accurate records and monitor constantly as any reaction to a blood transfusion is undesirable and requires immediate attention.

12. **Action:** Dispose of equipment safely and appropriately.

    Rationale: It is essential to dispose of all equipment correctly to avoid contamination and accidents.

Procedure: Monitoring for blood transfusion reactions

Indications. All patients receiving blood transfusions.

1. **Action:** Assess baseline parameters prior to transfusion – temperature, pulse, respiration, mucous membrane colour, PCV.

    Rationale: It is essential to obtain baseline parameters to notice any deviations from normal during the transfusion.

2. **Action:** Continue to monitor patient parameters as above and record results.

    Rationale: Immediate action is required if any signs of a reaction become apparent.

3. **Action:** Monitor the patient for any of the following signs: pyrexia, salivation, vomiting, diarrhoea, tachycardia, muscle tremors, facial oedema.

    Rationale: Any of these signs could indicate a transfusion reaction due to incompatibility or over-administration and requires immediate attention.

4. **Action:** If any of the above signs are apparent, stop the infusion and inform the veterinary surgeon immediately.

   Rationale: *It is essential to stop the infusion if these signs are apparent, to prevent further deterioration.*

5. **Action:** Reassure the patient and make it comfortable.

   Rationale: *Patients can become disoriented and confused during a blood transfusion reaction and require reassurance to avoid undue stress.*

REFERENCES AND FURTHER READING

Aspinall, V., 2011. The Complete Textbook of Veterinary Nursing, second ed. Elsevier, Oxford.

Ackerman, N., 2012. Aspinall's Complete Textbook of Veterinary Nursing, third ed. Elsevier, Oxford.

Cooper, B., Mullineaux, E., Turner, L., 2011. Textbook of Veterinary Nursing, fifth ed. BSAVA, Gloucester.

Houlton, J.E.F., Taylor, P.M., 1987. Trauma Management. Wright, Bristol.

Lane, D., Cooper, B., 2003. Veterinary Nursing. Butterworth-Heineman, Oxford.

Masters, J., Bowden, C., 2003. Quick Reference Guide to Veterinary Medical Kits. Butterworth-Heinemann, Oxford.

Taylor, R.A., McGehee, R., 1995. Manual of Small Animal Postoperative Care. Williams and Wilkins, Baltimore.

REFERENCES AND FURTHER READING

5

Provision of nutritional support

Nicola Ackerman

CHAPTER CONTENTS

INTRODUCTION

All animals must receive a balanced diet to maintain optimum levels of health. When an animal is ill, it may not want to eat or may not be able to eat, leading to deficiencies of certain vital nutrients and energy. During certain life stages and periods of illness, there may be an increased requirement for certain nutrients above the 'norm' and, if not provided, a deficiency will seriously slow down the rate of recovery and impair the healing process. Failure to consider some method of nutritional support may compromise the patient's chances of recovery.

When nursing any animal, consideration must be given to certain factors regarding nutrition. These will differ depending on lifestyle, life stage and clinical health:

1. Energy requirement – animals need energy for basic metabolism and for activity. A sick animal will use much less energy in exercise, but disease and stress have the potential to increase the normal energy requirements. Energy calculations provide a starting point but are just guidelines; a full nutritional assessment is required to establish if these quantities are correct for that individual.

2. Type of food – anorexia (a lack or loss of appetite for food) and/or dysorexia (a diminished, disordered or unnatural appetite, usually linked to emotional or psychological response) are often seen in sick animals, and you must find a diet that they find palatable. Palatability can be affected by the food (taste, texture and smell), the animal (is the animal able to taste or smell?) and the environment (type of bowl, external stressors in the area). If a disease process requires a specific type of food (e.g. low sodium required in renal disease), there may be a limited range of available foods which must still be able to satisfy the basic nutrient requirements.

3. Route of administration – nutritional support can be given by the enteral route – making use of the

gastrointestinal tract – or by the parenteral route – providing nutrients intravenously.

4. Digestibility, absorption and utilization – even when the animal consumes the food or is given it via a feeding tube, it is important to assess whether the animal can then digest the food, absorb the nutrients and utilize them. The choice of diet plays a part, e.g. semi-elemental diets provide peptides (rather than whole proteins), simple sugars and medium-chain triglycerides to facilitate digestion. Digestive supplements such as pancreatic enzymes may be given to facilitate absorption of fats in cases where they are reduced or absent.

Energy Calculations

The **basal energy requirement (BER)** is the amount of energy expended while asleep, 12–18 hours after feeding, in a thermoneutral environment. The **resting energy requirement (RER)** differs from the BER as it includes the energy expended in recovery from physical activity and feeding. However, in many texts, the BER and RER are considered to be interchangeable, and in this chapter, we will simply refer to the RER.

The **maintenance energy requirement (MER)** is the amount of energy required by a moderately active animal in its daily search for and utilization of food. It does not include the energy required for growth, repair, pregnancy, lactation or work, which is known as the **daily energy requirement (DER)** (Table 5.1).

- Most of the energy used by the body is given off as heat through radiation and convection from the body surface. Energy expenditure is related to body surface area. Small animals have a larger body surface area related to body weight, and therefore have a greater heat loss and so a greater RER; larger animals have a smaller surface area in relation to their body weight, and consequently have a relatively smaller RER.

- The MER in dogs is approximately 2 × RER.
- The MER in cats is approximately 1.4 × RER. RER may be calculated thus:

$$RER\,(kcal/day) = 70\,(BW_{kg})^{0.75}$$
$$\text{(if body weight (BW) is less than 2 kg).}$$

Or $30\,(BW_{kg}) + 70$ (if BW is between 2 and 45 kg).

- In sickness, the energy requirement varies considerably. Pets are often less active, sleep more and lie in a warm environment. The RER can sometimes be lower, but if the animal has suffered from trauma, surgery or sepsis, the RER rises sharply. The precise rise or fall depends upon:
- the disease process
- the animal's response
- environmental factors such as external temperatures.
- Illness factors are no longer used to calculate the DERs for patients because of these varying requirements. These calculations should only be used as a starting calorific guideline and using adjusted nutritional assessment. During pregnancy, lactation, growth and obesity control, the energy needs also vary (Table 5.1).

Once the calorific requirements for the animal have been calculated, we can then ascertain how much food is required to provide this, depending on the **energy density** of the food. The energy density of a food, or its energy content, is highest in highly digestible foods and lowest in poorly digestible foods, such as foods with poor quality ingredients. All of these calculations are purely based on energy and do not take into consideration how much of a specific nutrient, e.g. protein or carbohydrate, is required by the individual. The gross energy of nutrients varies, but only a proportion are able to be digested – this is the **metabolizable energy (ME)**. Energy density is based on the ME of protein, fat and carbohydrates (Table 5.2).

TABLE 5.1 Daily energy requirements for cats and dogs

One full day's work	1.5 × maintenance energy requirement (MER)
Three weeks post gestation	1.3 × MER
Peak lactation	2–4 × MER
Birth to 3 months	2.0 × MER
Sub-freezing temperatures	1.7 × MER
Tropical heat	2.5 × MER
Resting	0.8 × MER
Obesity	0.6 × MER

TABLE 5.2 Metabolizable energy content of nutrients

Nutrient	kcal/g
Protein	3.5
Fat	8.7
Carbohydrate	3.5

ENTERAL FEEDING

This may be defined as the administration of nutritional support using the gastrointestinal tract. The gastrointestinal tract should always be used, if possible, as this is the function for which it is most effective.

Procedure: Calculate the energy needs of the patient

1. **Action:** Calculate the RER for any animal over 2 kg BW.
   Formula: RER = $(30 \times BW_{kg}) + 70$ kcal.
   For example, to find the RER for a 10 kg dog:
   RER = $(30 \times 10) + 70$
   $= 300 + 70$
   $= 370$ kcal/day
   Calculate RER for an 800 g puppy:
   Formula: $70\,(BW_{kg})^{0.75}$
   RER = $70 \times (0.8)^{0.75}$
   $= 70 \times 0.856$
   $= 59$ kcal/day
   Rationale: *Animals under 2 kg have a faster metabolic rate than larger animals, so require more energy per BW_{kg} than do animals over 2 kg. This also applies to neonates, where the metabolic rate is greater than that of adults.*

2. **Action:** Calculate the MER for a 10 kg dog.
   MER in dogs is approximately $2 \times$ RER.
   MER in cats is approximately $1.4 \times$ RER.
   MER = RER $\times$ 2
   $= ((30 \times 10) + 70) \times 2$
   $= 370 \times 2$
   $= 740$ kcal/day
   Rationale: *MER is the amount of energy required by a moderately active animal.*

3. **Action:** Calculate DER.
   DER depends on the life stage of the animal.
   For example, using Table 5.1, a 10 kg obese dog requires 444 kcal/day.
   $= 0.6 \times$ MER
   $= 0.6 \times 740$
   $= 444$ kcal/day

Procedure: Calculation of the amount of food to be given to the patient

1. **Action:** Calculate the energy density or ME of the food; this may be available from the food labelling or the manufacturing company.

Find the amount of protein, fat, and carbohydrates in the diet. The carbohydrate content may not be stated on the label but can be calculated by subtracting the total amount of all other nutrients from 100. The water content may not be given for all dry diets. Assume a figure of 10% if none is stated.
Rationale: *It is essential to know the amount of energy that is available to the patient.*

2. **Action:** Multiply the percentage of each nutrient in the diet by the ME of each nutrient (Table 5.2).
   For example, if the diet had 10% protein, 10% fat, 20% carbohydrate and 50% water:
   Protein = $10 \times 3.5 = 35$ kcal
   Carbohydrate = $20 \times 3.5 = 70$ kcal
   Fat = $10 \times 8.7 = 87$ kcal
   Add these together, $35 + 70 + 87 = 192$ kcal per 100g of the diet.
   Rationale: *This is based on assumption that the digestibility of the diet allows this amount of metabolizable energy in this individual. In this example, the food has over 14% moisture, and therefore is required to be recorded on the label.*

3. **Action:** Calculate the quantity of food in ml or grams to be fed to a 10 kg dog based on its RER. Food value: 2 kcal/ml.
   For example, the dog requires 444 kcal/day:
   $= 444 / 2 = 222$ ml/day

4. **Action:** Divide quantity in ml into equal feeds to be administered throughout the day:
   222 ml / 6 meals per day = 37 ml per meal
   Rationale: *Always divide the food quantity into equal workable amounts depending on the method of artificial feeding. Consider the time available for feeding and each patient's needs. Avoid excessive quantities in single feeds to prevent discomfort, regurgitation or vomiting. Gastric capacities of 5–10 ml/kg for cats and dogs have often been quoted when reintroducing feeding and can be a good guide for calculating the number of meals.*

Procedure: Force feeding, including syringe feeding

These procedures are deemed not suitable in cats and dogs. Force feeding an animal, whether by placing food in the mouth or syringe feeding, has the potential to cause food aversions. Feeding by these methods will not achieve reaching the calorific requirements for the animal. In these cases, a feeding tube should be placed.

Procedure: Micro-enteral nutrition

The gastrointestinal system derives a large portion of its nutrient and energy requirements from the gut lumen, not the blood stream. In times where it is not clinically recommended to enterally feed the patient, though these are uncommon, micro-enteral or semi-elemental nutrition, i.e. diets that supply basic nutrients in smaller more easily digested molecules (e.g. protein as peptides, polysaccharides as simple sugars, etc.) should be used, and these can be taken voluntarily or administered via a feeding tube.

1. **Action:** Provide a 10 kg dog with micro-enteral nutrition. Administer 0.25–0.5 ml/kg/h orally, increasing by 50% every 8–12 hours, or until the animal is able to be fed enterally.

   $10 \times 0.25 = 2.5$–5 ml hourly.

   Rationale: Nutrient requirement by the gastrointestinal system is met via micro-enteral nutrition and will aid in maintaining gastro-mucosal integrity, thus reducing the risk of bacterial translocation and sepsis.

Procedure: Naso-oesophageal tube placement

Indications. Generally short-term tube feeding where there is failure to stimulate voluntary eating or a physical inability to eat, and there is a contraindication for anaesthesia. Contraindications include any animals with nasal pathology or oesophageal disease, poor gag reflex, protracted vomiting or with a reduced mentation or head trauma.

1. **Action:** Select and prepare equipment – naso-oesophageal tube of the appropriate size, topical local anaesthetic agent, water-soluble lubricant, adhesive tape, gloves, tissue glue or suture equipment, swabs, syringe and water.

   Rationale: It is essential to prepare equipment prior to beginning the procedure to ensure efficient administration.

2. **Action:** Request an assistant to restrain the patient, supporting its head in a normal position.

   Rationale: Firm handling makes the patient feel safe and facilitates the procedure. General anaesthesia is not normally used for placement of these tubes because if the patient can be

anaesthetized, it is better to place an oesophageal feeding tube.

3. **Action:** Measure the distance from the external nares to the seventh rib space (Fig. 5.1). Mark position on the tube with a biro.

   Rationale: It is important to measure the distance prior to the procedure to check placement is correct later on.

4. **Action:** Local anaesthetic gel or spray can be applied to the internal aspect of nares.

   Rationale: Local anaesthetic agents desensitize the nasal mucous membrane, reducing any discomfort.

5. **Action:** Lubricate the tip of the tube with water-soluble lubricant (avoid the use of petroleum jelly on silicone tubes).

   Rationale: This will allow for easy passage of the tube and minimize discomfort for the patient. Petroleum jelly reacts with silicone.

6. **Action:** The tube is introduced into the nasal cavity and advanced down the pharynx and oesophagus until the biro mark is at the external nares.

   Rationale: At this point you know that the tip of the tube is in the oesophagus at the level of the seventh rib. Nasogastric, i.e. into the stomach, tube placement is preferred in some cases. The placement is more caudal than that of a naso-oesophageal tube. Nasogastric tubes can also be used to remove excess fluid or air from the stomach.

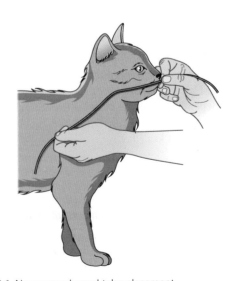

Fig. 5.1 Naso-oesophageal tube placement.

7. **Action:** Check for correct positioning by observing any coughing and by the introduction of up to 5 ml of water followed by auscultation for borborygmi. Once in place, occlude end of tube with a suitable bung. Better still is to use an end-tidal carbon dioxide monitor or capnography, as a trace will indicate that the tube is in the trachea rather than the oesophagus.

   Rationale: It is essential to ensure that the tube is placed correctly, to prevent inhalation of food. Coughing and lack of borborygmi could indicate that the tube is in the trachea, in which case the tube should be repositioned. The end of the tube must be occluded once in place to prevent excessive air being swallowed.

8. **Action:** Secure the exterior part of the tube to the patient's head with the aid of tissue glue or sutures over the nose and between the eyes (Fig 5.2).

   Rationale: The remainder of the tube must be secured to prevent displacement.

9. **Action:** Food may now be administered to the conscious patient (Fig 5.3). If feeding is not to take place immediately, occlude the end of the tube with a bung and apply an Elizabethan collar.

   Rationale: It is essential to prevent patient interference, tube displacement and swallowing of air if the patient is not to be fed immediately.

10. **Action:** Measure the correct volume of prewarmed food into a syringe, as calculated previously. If the animal has been without food for more than

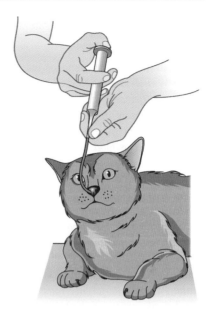

Fig. 5.3 Naso-oesophageal tube feeding.

48 hours, then food should be re-introduced slowly. The total calorific requirement should be slowly increased over 3 days to prevent refeeding syndrome.

   Rationale: It is important that the food quantity/ energy requirements are calculated prior to the procedure, facilitating easy measurement at this point. Prewarming food to at least room temperature helps to reduce the likelihood of vomiting.

   Refeeding syndrome *is associated with calorific depletion in starved cats and is characterized by the development of severe hypophosphataemia following the introduction of enteral or parenteral nutrition. Typically, it may occur with 2–5 days of restarting feeding, but signs may develop within 10 hours.*

11. **Action:** Remove bung from the feeding tube and flush the tube with 3–10 ml of water. Carbonated water may be used in cases where food and mucus may be blocking the tube.

   Rationale: Flushing the tube will ensure it is patent. If resistance is experienced, repeat the procedure. The bubbles in carbonated water are thought to help the blockage.

12. **Action:** Administer the food slowly, constantly monitoring for any changes in respiration, coughing, sneezing or vomiting.

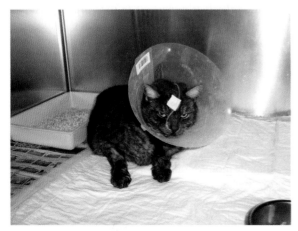

Fig. 5.2 Naso-oesophageal feeding tube and Elizabethan collar to prevent interference. (Courtesy Ackerman, own photo)

Rationale: Rapid administration can lead to discomfort, regurgitation and vomiting, and should therefore be avoided.

13. **Action:** Flush tube with a further 5–10 ml water.

    Rationale: Water must be flushed after the food to ensure tube is clear of any particles.

14. **Action:** Replace bung in feeding tube.

    Rationale: The bung must be replaced to prevent any leakage of fluid or food and to prevent air being ingested.

15. **Action:** Clean around tube site.

    Rationale: It is essential to keep the tube insertion site clean. An antibiotic or antiseptic cream may be applied to the area to help moisturize and to prevent infection.

16. **Action:** Apply an Elizabethan collar to the patient and return patient to the kennel.

    Rationale: Patient interference must be avoided to prevent displacement of the tube.

17. **Action:** Follow same feeding regime for repeat feeds. Record all administration details on the hospital chart (Fig. 5.9).

    Rationale: It is essential to keep accurate records to avoid any error in administration.

18. **Action:** Store any remaining food according to the manufacturer's instructions and dispose of all other equipment safely and appropriately.

    Rationale: It is essential that any food is stored hygienically and equipment is disposed of correctly to avoid contamination.

Procedure: Oesophagostomy tube placement

Indications. Can be used to provide at-home nutritional support for weeks or months for patients that are unable to meet their calorific or water requirements voluntarily.

1. **Action:** Select and prepare equipment (Fig. 5.4) – feeding tube of appropriate size and diameter, clippers, surgical skin scrub solution, forceps, gloves, minor surgical kit and suture equipment, swabs, syringe and water.

    Rationale: It is essential to prepare equipment prior to beginning the procedure to ensure efficient administration.

2. **Action:** The patient will be anaesthetized, as this is a painful surgical procedure. Position the patient in right lateral recumbency.

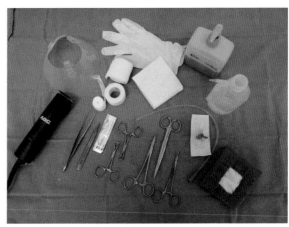

Fig. 5.4 Oesophagostomy tube placement kit. (Reproduced, with permission, from Textbook of Veterinary Medical Nursing, Masters and Bowden (2003), Butterworth-Heinemann.)

Rationale: Correct positioning is essential in aiding correct placement of the tube. Endotracheal intubation of the patient may potentially lead to mispositioning of the feeding tube.

3. **Action:** The surgical area is clipped and prepared. This area is from the mandibular ramus to the thoracic inlet and extends to both the dorsal and ventral midlines. Drape the area.

    Rationale: It is essential to provide asepsis for the surgical procedure.

4. **Action:** The feeding tube is measured from the mid-cervical oesophagus caudal to the larynx to the seventh or eighth intercostal space.

    Rationale: It is important to measure the distance prior to the procedure to check that the placement is correct. The distal end of the tube needs to lie in the distal oesophagus.

5. **Action:** The veterinary surgeon then places the pre-measured feeding tube surgically.

    Rationale: This ensures that the patient suffers minimal discomfort.

6. **Action:** Correct positioning of the tube is checked by radiography or the use of an end-tidal carbon-dioxide monitor or capnograph. Careful monitoring of the anaesthesia throughout the procedure is required.

    Rationale: It is essential to ensure that the tube is placed correctly to prevent inhalation of food.

7. **Action:** The tube is then sutured to the skin at the insertion site. Remove drapes and cover the tube with sterile dressing and light bandage or specialized feeding tube cover, e.g. Kit-E-Collar (Figs 5.5 and 5.6).

   Rationale: *To prevent the tube from being displaced, to prevent patient interference and to prevent the risk of infection.*

8. **Action:** The end of the tube must be occluded once in place.

   Rationale: *To prevent excessive air travelling down tube.*

9. **Action:** Water and fluids should only be introduced once the veterinary surgeon is satisfied that the tube is correctly placed.

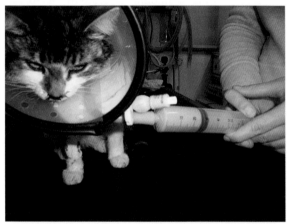

Fig. 5.5 Cat with a fractured jaw being fed through an oesophagostomy tube. (Taken from The Complete Textbook of Veterinary Nursing, Aspinall, V., (2011), Elsevier, p. 260, Fig. 15.10a.)

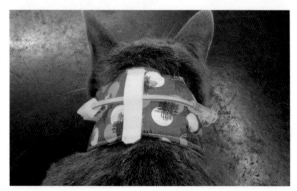

Fig. 5.6 Use of specialized oesophageal feeding tube protective covering.

Rationale: *To prevent material being administered into the respiratory system.*

10. **Action:** Label the feeding tube.

    Rationale: *If a central venous line has also been placed, it is vital that the tubes do not become mixed up. All lines (tubes) should be labelled.*

11. **Action:** As placement is performed under general anaesthetic, do not administer food until the patient has regained consciousness.

    Rationale: *Food must not be administered in the unconscious patient due to the absence of or reduced swallow and cough reflexes.*

12. **Action:** Measure the correct volume of prewarmed food into a syringe, as calculated previously. If the animal has been without food for more than 48 hours, then food should be re-introduced slowly. The total calorific requirement should be slowly increased over 3 days to prevent refeeding syndrome.

    Rationale: *It is important that the food quantity/energy requirements are calculated prior to the procedure, facilitating easy measurement at this point. Prewarming food to at least room temperature helps to reduce the likelihood of vomiting.* **Refeeding syndrome** *is associated with calorific depletion in starved cats and is characterized by the development of severe hypophosphataemia following the introduction of enteral or parenteral nutrition. Typically, it may occur with 2–5 days of restarting feeding, but signs may develop within 10 hours.*

13. **Action:** Remove the bung from the feeding tube and flush tube with 3–10 ml of water.

    Rationale: *Flushing the tube will ensure it is patent. If resistance is experienced, repeat procedure. Carbonated water may be used in cases where food and mucus may be blocking the tube – the bubbles are thought to help clear the blockage.*

14. **Action:** Administer the food slowly, constantly monitoring for any changes in respiration, sneezing, coughing or vomiting.

    Rationale: *Rapid administration can lead to discomfort, regurgitation and vomiting, and should therefore be avoided.*

15. **Action:** Flush tube with a further 5–10 ml of water.

    Rationale: *Water must be flushed after the food to ensure tube is clear of any particles.*

16. **Action:** Replace bung in feeding tube.

    Rationale: To prevent any leakage of fluid or food and to prevent air being ingested.

17. **Action:** Clean around tube site.

    Rationale: It is essential to keep the tube insertion site clean. An antibiotic or antiseptic cream may be applied to the area to help moisturize and prevent infection, as directed by the veterinary surgeon (Fig 5.7).

18. **Action:** Repeat the procedure as required and record all food administration details.

    Rationale: It is essential to record accurately to prevent an error in administration.

19. **Action:** Store any remaining food according to the manufacturer's instructions and dispose of all other equipment safely and appropriately.

    Rationale: It is essential that any food is stored hygienically and equipment is disposed of correctly to avoid contamination.

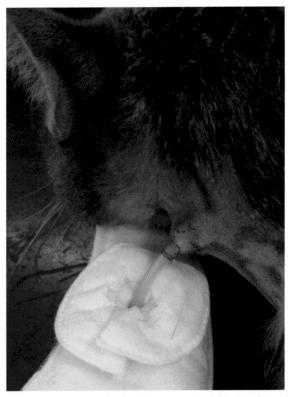

Fig. 5.7 Example of dressing around an oesophageal feeding tube.

Procedure: Gastrostomy tube placement

Indications. For longer-term feeding, underlying disease, surgery or trauma to the oesophagus. The tube can be left in place for several months; only use liquidized foods.

1. **Action:** Select equipment (Fig. 5.8) – gastrostomy (mushroom-tipped) catheter, stylet and introducing equipment, clippers, surgical skin scrub solution, forceps, gloves, minor surgical kit and suture equipment, swabs.

   Rationale: It is essential to prepare equipment prior to beginning the procedure to ensure efficient administration.

2. **Action:** The patient will be anaesthetized. Position in right lateral recumbency. The tube may also be placed during a midline laparotomy; if so, the patient will be in dorsal recumbency.

   Rationale: As the placement of this tube requires surgical intervention, a general anaesthetic is required. Correct positioning of the patient is essential to facilitate efficient preparation and tube placement.

3. **Action:** Surgically prepare the left flank in an area from the costal arch to the mid-abdomen in a cranial to caudal direction, and from the transverse processes of the lumbar vertebrae to the level of the ventral end of the last rib in a dorso-ventral direction. Prepare skin aseptically and drape area.

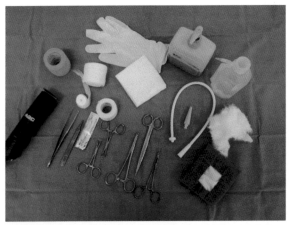

Fig. 5.8 Gastrostomy tube placement kit. (Reproduced, with permission, from Textbook of Veterinary Medical Nursing, Masters and Bowden (2003), Butterworth-Heinemann.)

Rationale: It is essential to provide asepsis for surgical procedures to reduce the risk of infection.

4. **Action:** The veterinary surgeon places the gastrostomy tube surgically. This can be facilitated by a specially designed introducer or with the aid of an endoscope (percutaneous endoscopic gastrostomy – PEG).

   Rationale: This allows for easy passage of the tube and minimizes discomfort for the patient.

5. **Action:** Correct placing of the tube is checked by the introduction of 2–3 ml of water. Gastric sounds are monitored. Once confirmed, occlude the end of tube.

   Rationale: It is essential to ensure that the tube is placed correctly in the stomach and not between the visceral and parietal layers of the peritoneum. The end of the tube must be occluded once in place to prevent excessive air being ingested.

6. **Action:** The exterior part of the tube is secured to the patient's body wall by means of a suture or tissue glue.

   Rationale: The remainder of the tube must be secured to prevent displacement by movement or patient interference.

7. **Action:** As placement is performed under general anaesthetic, it is not advisable to administer food until the patient has regained consciousness. Apply a dressing and an abdominal bandage to cover the tube until food is administered.

   Rationale: Food must not be administered in the unconscious patient due to an inability to swallow or cough if gastric reflux occurs. Covering the end of the tube protects against ingestion of air.

8. **Action:** When ready to feed the patient, measure the correct volume of prewarmed food into a syringe, as calculated previously. If the animal has been without food for more than 48 hours, then food should be re-introduced slowly. The total calorific requirement should be slowly increased over 3 days to prevent refeeding syndrome.

   *Rationale: It is important that the food quantity/ energy requirements are calculated prior to the procedure, facilitating easy measurement at this point. Prewarming food to at least room temperature helps to reduce the likelihood of vomiting. **Refeeding syndrome** is associated with calorific depletion in starved cats and is characterized by the development of severe hypophosphataemia following the introduction of enteral or parenteral nutrition. Typically,*

it may occur with 2–5 days of restarting feeding, but signs may develop within 10 hours.

9. **Action:** Remove bung from the feeding tube and flush the tube with 3–10 ml of water (the volume will depend on the size of the tube).

   Rationale: Flushing the tube will ensure it is patent. If resistance is experienced, repeat the procedure. Carbonated water may be used in cases where food and mucus may be blocking the tube – the bubbles help remove the blockage.

10. **Action:** Slowly administer the food amount calculated previously. Larger quantities of food can be administered by this route – do not exceed 50 ml/ kg/feed.

    Rationale: Rapid administration can lead to discomfort and vomiting and should therefore be avoided.

11. **Action:** Flush tube with a further 5–10 ml water.

    Rationale: To ensure tube is clear of any particles.

12. **Action:** Replace bung in feeding tube.

    Rationale: To prevent any leakage of fluid or food and to prevent air being ingested.

13. **Action:** Clean around tube site.

    Rationale: It is essential to keep the tube insertion site clean. An antibiotic or antiseptic cream may be applied to the area to help moisturize and to prevent infection, as directed by the veterinary surgeon.

14. **Action:** Apply a dressing and an abdominal bandage to the area. Also put on an Elizabethan collar.

    Rationale: Patient interference must be avoided to prevent displacement of the tube.

15. **Action:** Repeat feeding regime as required, and record administration details.

    Rationale: It is essential to record feeding accurately to prevent any error in administration on the hospital chart (Fig. 5.9).

16. **Action:** Store any remaining food according to the manufacturer's instructions and dispose of all other equipment safely and appropriately.

    Rationale: It is essential that any food is stored hygienically and equipment is disposed of correctly to avoid contamination.

Procedure: Maintenance of feeding tubes

1. **Action:** Ensure tube and insertion site are clean and dry at all times.

   Rationale: As the food being administered contains the ideal constituents for the growth of microorganisms, it is essential to remove any food leakage from the tube and the surrounding area and to keep the area dry, to prevent infection. Antiseptic and antibiotic creams may be applied to the skin at the tube insertion site under the direction of the veterinary surgeon. Dried-on food particles could attract flies and, in the very worst scenario, result in fly strike.

2. **Action:** Check the position and condition of the tubes at each feed.
   Rationale: It is important to check tube position and check for signs of movement or displacement. The tubes should also be checked for cracks or damage. Administration of food into the wrong area could cause infection and even death.

3. **Action:** Flush tube before and after administration of fluids.
   Rationale: Always flush the tube with water prior to the administration of food to ensure that the tube is not blocked. Always listen for any coughing or lack of borborygmi, indicating that the tube has moved. If in doubt, do not continue, and inform the veterinary surgeon. Always flush after feeding to ensure no food particles remain within the tube and cause a blockage later.

4. **Action:** Ensure tube remains occluded when not in use.
   Rationale: It is essential to occlude the tube when not in use to prevent unnecessary ingestion of air leading to discomfort and distension of the abdomen.

5. **Action:** Keep tube area covered and free from patient interference.
   Rationale: It is essential to prevent patient interference, which may cause tube displacement. In the case of oesphagostomy and gastrostomy tubes, it is advisable to cover with dressings and bandages, or with specialized coverings.

6. **Action:** When tube is to be removed, remove all tapes and sutures. Pull the tube out gently but quickly while an assistant exerts pressure on the exit site. Sutures may be placed if necessary.
   Rationale: Tube removal is indicated if there are problems or if the animal begins to eat sufficient food voluntarily. Gastrostomy tubes should be left in place for at least 5 days to ensure adhesion of the stomach to the body wall. The procedure needs to be quick and efficient to produce minimal discomfort and reduce risk of aspiration of air or stomach contents.

7. **Action:** Dispose of all equipment and disinfect the area.
   Rationale: It is essential to maintain a clean environment at all times, thereby reducing the risk of infection.

Procedure: Monitoring techniques for enteral feeding

1. **Action:** Baseline parameters such as body temperature, respiratory rate and pulse must be recorded prior to any enteral feeding.
   Rationale: It is essential to know the results of baseline tests in order to assess the effectiveness of enteral feeding. Electrolyte imbalances can occur in cases of refeeding syndrome, and careful monitoring is required.

2. **Action:** Nutritional assessment of BW, body condition score (BCS) and muscle condition score (MCS) should occur at each consultation. Weigh hospitalized patients once or twice daily. Record all results in the clinical history (Fig 5.9).
   Rationale: Regular results will indicate a trend, which is more useful than a one-off measurement. Accuracy and regularity are essential requirements for effective monitoring.

3. **Action:** All deviations or abnormalities must be noted immediately and reported to the veterinary surgeon.
   Rationale: It is essential that any abnormalities are reported so that steps can be taken to prevent further deterioration or development of complications in the patient.

Procedure: Monitoring enteral feeding – essential parameters

Indications. All patients receiving enteral nutrition (Fig. 5.9).

1. **Action:** Temperature, pulse and respiration.
   Rationale: To identify infection or inflammation.

2. **Action:** Measure body weight once or twice daily.
   Rationale: To identify any large fluctuations that may indicate fluid imbalance and to ensure that the required amount of calories is being supplied.

3. **Action:** Plasma glucose concentration – dependent on situation (once/twice daily/hourly) until stable.
   *Rationale: Metabolic abnormalities, especially those associated with blood glucose levels, may indicate sepsis and refeeding syndrome. **Refeeding***

syndrome is associated with calorific depletion in starved cats and is characterized by the development of severe hypophosphataemia following the introduction of enteral or parenteral nutrition. Typically, it may occur with 2–5 days of restarting feeding, but signs may develop within 10 hours.

4. **Action:** Urine output and concentration (specific gravity).

   Rationale: *Minimum output per hour = 1 ml/kg, once any dehydration has been addressed and sufficient fluids are being taken on board. The concentration of the urine will indicate the renal function.*

5. **Action:** Observe the general demeanour/clinical observation and pain score.

   Rationale: *Any sign of distress or discomfort could indicate a problem.*

6. **Action:** Check tube insertion site for any signs of heat, redness or swelling.

   Rationale: *It is essential to monitor the insertion site to check for any signs of discomfort or infection.*

7. **Action:** Continue to feed until the patient eats 2/3 to 3/4 of its nutritional requirements voluntarily.

   Rationale: *This would indicate that the patient is making progress towards recovery, and that there may be a need to reduce or cease tube feeding.*

8. **Action:** Record all results accurately on the hospital chart (Fig 5.9).

   Rationale: *It is essential to record all results accurately to measure the patient's progress or deterioration. All of this is an integral part of the nursing care plan for the patient.*

Patient I.D.						Clinical history							
Species and breed													
Age		Sex		Weight									
Veterinary surgeon													
Veterinary nurse													

Monitor and record every ———————— intervals daily

Date and time	T	P	R	MM CRT	Demeanour	Food administration	Type and rate	Food input	Fluid/urine output	Weight	Medication	Comments

Ⓐ

Fig. 5.9 A, B Examples of charts used for monitoring patients undergoing enteral feeding.

(Continued)

Small animal nutrition sheet		

Client name

Patient name

Sex

Admission date

Age

Weight

Veterinary surgeon

Veterinary nurse

Condition

emaciated ☐

underweight ☐

correct for breed ☐

overweight ☐

grossly obese ☐

....

....

Medical/surgical problems

1.   3.

2.   4.

Dietary recommendations

Protein ☐   Fat ☐

Fibre ☐   Other ☐

Selected food ....

Calorific density ....

Amount to feed daily = $\dfrac{\text{RER}}{\text{Calorific density}}$ OR

Amount =	ml/day
Amount =	g/day

Food dosage and route

DAY 1

DAY 2

DAY 3

Plan

Continue diet for:	2 weeks	Post surgery
	2–4 weeks	Trauma
	4–12 weeks	Head trauma/burns
	months	Chronic disease/neoplasia

Continue ....diet   for .... weeks

Ⓑ

Fig. 5.9, Cont'd

PARENTERAL FEEDING

Parenteral nutrition (PN) is the administration of nutritional support via a number of intravenous routes in dogs and cats. These include central venous catheters (mainly the jugular vein), peripheral venous catheters (the cephalic and saphenous veins) and also peripherally inserted central catheters accessing the caudal vena cava via the femoral vein. Generally, high osmolarity solutions should be administered by a central venous catheter.

PN is associated with higher catheter complication rates, including thrombotic events, catheter-related infections and sepsis. PN should only be used when the gastrointestinal system is not functioning as required. When PN is being used, micro-enteral nutrition should still be utilized.

PN can be divided into two types:

- **Total parenteral nutrition (TPN)**, which is designed to meet 100% of the patient's total energy needs. Solutions such as intravenous dextrose should be used as the sole source of energy for no more than 2–3 days because of potential complications and only be administered through a central line.
- **Partial parenteral nutrition (PPN)**, which is designed to meet 40–70% of the patient's total energy needs. The solutions are diluted, decreasing the protein and calorific density but allowing them to be administered through a peripheral vein.

Calculating PN requirements is based on RER, the clinical requirements of the animal and how the veterinary surgeon would like the calories to be provided, i.e. by fat, protein or sugars. Illness factors are not utilized in the calculation of energy requirements for PN. The nutrient requirements should be made by the veterinary surgeon and then programmed into an automated PN compounder, within a sterile environment. '3-in-1' bags of PN can be utilized but are less ideal.

Once the patient is taking in enough of its energy requirement voluntarily, PN can be discontinued. PPN can be stopped abruptly, but TPN should be stopped gradually over a 6- to 12-hour period. All patients must continue to be monitored. The catheter site must be cleaned and checked for signs of infection. Record all signs on the hospital chart (Fig. 5.9).

Nutritional Assessment

It is important that all animals undergo a nutritional assessment every time they are seen in practice, whether they are to be admitted for critical treatment or simply sent home on a diet. Nutritional assessment can be based on visual observations, such as Body Condition Score (BCS) and Muscle Condition Score (MCS), and specific measurements, such as weight and plasma protein measurements.

1. **BCS** – this is based on a 5- or 9-point scale. Some leaner breeds such as whippets and greyhounds, even if in good condition, do not suit some aspects of the BCS index. They have limited fat cover, so the MCS should be utilized alongside the BCS. To perform a BCS for an overweight dog, palpate the animal all over, following through the BCS chart (Fig 5.10) and making a note of any bony prominences you can feel (sometimes this is quite difficult!). By estimating a BCS you are putting the animal's body weight into perspective, and this will help you to set a goal of the ideal weight for that animal.

2. **MCS** – the MCS differs from the BCS in that it estimates muscle mass (Fig 5.10) rather than fat. Evaluation of muscle mass includes visual examination and palpation over the temporal bones, scapulae, lumbar vertebrae and pelvic bones. Assessing muscle condition is important, as muscle loss is greater in patients with most acute and chronic diseases, i.e. stressed starvation, compared to healthy animals deprived of food when primarily fat is lost, i.e. simple starvation. Muscle loss adversely affects strength, immune function and wound healing, and is independently associated with mortality in humans. It is especially important to use the MCS when initiating a weight loss diet, as dramatic losses could be due to a drop in lean muscle mass, which should be prevented.

A condition known as 'overcoat syndrome' occurs when an MCS of 1 or 2 (Fig. 5.10) is present but the animal is still carrying excessive amounts of weight. The large fat deposits mask the muscle wastage that is occurring. This can easily occur in animals that suffer from a dramatic decrease in food consumption, e.g. acute anorexia. Other aspects of physical examination of the patient should be taken into consideration. These aspects include hair/coat quality and skin condition, evidence of peripheral oedema or ascites (which may

Body condition score (5 point scale, can use 1/2 points for 9 point scale)

1	Very thin	Ribs, spine and pelvis: • Visible (especially shorthair cats/dogs) • Pronounced, very easy to palpate • No fat covering Marked abdominal tuck Loss of body muscle	
2	Thin	Ribs, spine and pelvis: • Easily palpated • Very little fat covering Tops of lumbar vertebrae visible Obvious waist behind ribs	
3	Normal	Ribs and spine: • Palpable but not visible • Slight (but not excess) fat covering Waist and abdominal tuck present Minimal abdominal fat pad	
4	Over-weight	Ribs and spine: • Not easy to palpate • Moderate fat covering Little or no waist present Rounding of abdomen	
5	Obese	Ribs and spine: • Hard to palpate • Marked fat cover Fat over other body areas No waist, marked abdominal fat Marked inguinal fat pad	

Muscle condition score

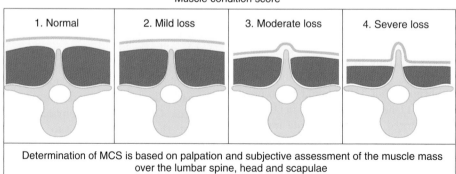

| 1. Normal | 2. Mild loss | 3. Moderate loss | 4. Severe loss |

Determination of MCS is based on palpation and subjective assessment of the muscle mass over the lumbar spine, head and scapulae

Fig. 5.10 Body and muscle condition scores as shown in the cat and in the dog.

No muscle wasting Normal muscle mass	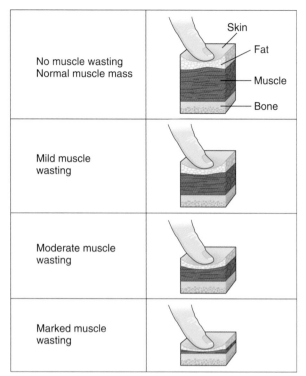
Mild muscle wasting	
Moderate muscle wasting	
Marked muscle wasting	

Fig. 5.11 Relative proportions of muscle to body fat used in body condition scoring and muscle condition scoring.

indicate hypoproteinaemia) and clinical signs that indicate certain deficiencies in micronutrients, e.g. neck ventroflexion or tetany.

REFERENCES AND FURTHER READING

Agar, S., 2001. Small Animal Nutrition. Butterworth-Heinemann, Oxford.

Ackerman, N., 2016. Aspinall's Complete Textbook of Veterinary Nursing, third ed. Elsevier, Oxford.

Cooper, B., Mullineaux, E., Turner, L., 2011. Textbook of Veterinary Nursing, fifth ed. BSAVA, Gloucester.

Lewis, L.D., Morris, M., Hand, M.S., 2000. Small Animal Clinical Nutrition, fourth ed. Morris Marks, Topeka, Kansas.

6

Anaesthetic procedures

Denise Prisk

CHAPTER CONTENTS

INTRODUCTION

Anaesthesia may be defined as the production of a controlled, reversible state of unconsciousness. By using certain drugs designed to have an effect on the nervous system, anaesthesia may be described as being general, i.e. the animal is unconscious and the entire nervous system is rendered insensitive to stimuli, or local, whereby a specific area is rendered insensitive to stimuli. Anaesthesia is used for welfare reasons as it is obviously unpleasant (and illegal) for painful procedures to be performed on a fully conscious animal. It may also be used as a means of restraint; for example, when performing radiography or to examine an aggressive animal.

Local anaesthesia is used in small animal practice either to perform superficial surgery, such as suturing a small skin wound; for nerve blocks, such as those performed prior to dental procedures; or as an adjunct to other anaesthetic protocols, including sedation and general anaesthesia.

General anaesthesia can be achieved with the use of injectable agents alone or with inhalant agents. In small animal practice, it is frequently the veterinary nurse who is responsible for setting up and maintaining anaesthetic equipment, as well as monitoring the depth of anaesthesia in the patient. It is vital that the veterinary nurse has a thorough understanding of the anaesthetic process if the patient is to survive the procedure and make a good recovery.

This chapter describes the procedures involved in preparing the anaesthetic equipment and in caring for the patient perioperatively (before, during and after the procedure). It also describes the different types of anaesthetic breathing systems in common veterinary usage.

THE ANAESTHETIC MACHINE

Anaesthetic machines are designed to deliver accurate amounts of carrier gases and volatile liquids in a vapour form to the patient to produce anaesthesia (Figs 6.1 and 6.2). Table 6.1 describes the parts of the anaesthetic machine.

Procedure: Checking the anaesthetic machine before use

1. **Action:** Turn on the *spare* oxygen cylinder and check that it is full.
   Rationale: The contents of the spare cylinder must be noted to ensure a constant supply of oxygen is available throughout the anaesthetic.
2. **Action:** Turn the cylinder off and label it as full.
   Rationale: If the in-use cylinder and the spare cylinder are both open, they will empty at the same time.
3. **Action:** Turn on the *in-use* cylinder or piped oxygen supply, check the contents and replace if necessary. Label the cylinder as in-use.
   Rationale: If the pressure reading is in the red area of the gauge, the cylinder should be changed.
4. **Action:** Repeat the process for the nitrous oxide cylinders or piped supply.
5. **Action:** Open and close the oxygen flowmeter valve.
   Rationale: This confirms that the ball or bobbin can move and rotate freely in its column of gas.
6. **Action:** Check the low oxygen alarm by turning the oxygen cylinder off and pressing the oxygen flush valve. Turn the oxygen back on.
   Rationale: The alarm should sound as the oxygen pressure falls to a dangerously low level. The flow of fresh gas through the oxygen flush valve is also confirmed.
7. **Action:** Check that the correct vaporizer is properly fitted and that it is full.

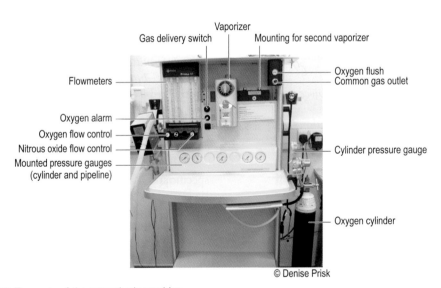

© Denise Prisk

Fig. 6.1 The parts of the anaesthetic machine.

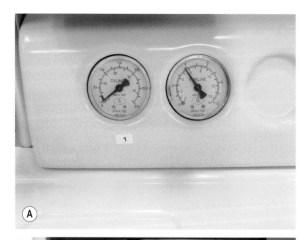

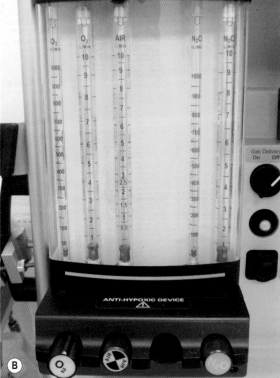

Fig. 6.2 A, Pressure gauges set into the front panel of an anaesthetic machine. B, Flowmeters calibrated in ml/min and l/min.

Rationale: The dial should move freely and the vaporizer should contain sufficient agent to avoid having to fill it during anaesthesia.

8. **Action:** Connect the correct breathing system, having checked it carefully for faults.

Rationale: Leaks may result from disconnected inner tubes in coaxial circuits or from leaking reservoir bags.

9. **Action:** Connect the scavenging system. Switch active systems on.

Rationale: It is a legal requirement that waste gases are scavenged to avoid pollution of the environment.

Procedure: Shutting down the anaesthetic machine

1. **Action:** Check contents of gas cylinders and replace as necessary.

Rationale: This ensures the machine is ready for the next use.

2. **Action:** Turn the oxygen cylinder off and press the oxygen flush valve until no pressure reads on the pressure gauge. Turn the piped gas supply off.

Rationale: All oxygen must be flushed from the pipes. Oxidizing gases are a fire hazard.

3. **Action:** Wipe the anaesthetic machine with disinfectant.

Rationale: This minimizes the risk of contamination.

PATIENT PREPARATION

Procedure: Pre-anaesthetic instructions

1. **Action:** Food should be withheld for the required period of time, as necessary, depending on species, age and condition. For routine procedures in healthy adult dogs and cats, food is generally withheld for 6–12 hours. Water should be available up until the time of premedication.

Rationale: If food is present in the stomach of animals that are able to vomit, regurgitation or vomiting may occur. This may lead to fatal aspiration, as the swallowing reflex is reduced or lost during anaesthesia. However, it has been shown that feeding a small amount of wet food to dogs 3 hours before anaesthesia increases the pH of gastric content but does not increase the chances of regurgitation. If regurgitation does occur, acidic damage is less likely.

2. **Action:** Cats should be kept inside overnight with a litter tray until ready to be taken to the practice the following morning.

Rationale: This prevents the cat from disappearing and possibly missing its scheduled procedure.

3. **Action:** Dogs should be walked prior to admittance.

Rationale: This allows the patient to urinate and defecate before admission.

TABLE 6.1 Parts of the anaesthetic machine (Figs 6.1, 6.2A and B)

Component	Description	Function
Gas supply	In the UK, medical gas cylinders are identified by the colour of the shoulder (top part). Oxygen cylinders are black with a white shoulder or all white. Nitrous oxide cylinders are blue. Cylinders may either be attached to the anaesthetic machine (sizes E and F) or kept remotely and gas piped to the machine (size J)	Supplies fresh oxygen and nitrous oxide to the patient
Pressure-reducing valve or regulator	Placed between the cylinder/pipe and the flowmeter. Often not visible, as may be incorporated into the yoke or positioned underneath the machine	Reduces the pressure of the gas, leaving the cylinder at a safe working pressure
Pressure gauges	Colour-coded for different gases, these may be attached to the anaesthetic machine near the gas supply (cylinder or pipe) or incorporated into the front panel of the machine (Fig. 6.2A). As the pressure in the cylinder of non-liquid gases falls, so does the pressure reading, indicating the amount of gas remaining in the cylinder. The pressure gauge of piped gases shows the pressure in the pipelines only, not in the cylinder. A separate gauge is attached to large cylinders. The gauge of nitrous oxide cylinders always reads full until the cylinder is empty, as it shows the pressure of the vapour above the liquid. Therefore, the pressure gauge cannot be used to assess the amount of nitrous oxide remaining in a cylinder – it must be weighed	For non-liquid gases, such as oxygen, the volume of gas remaining in the cylinder is proportional to the pressure reading on the gauge
Flowmeters (or rotameters)	Consist of a tapered glass or plastic tube, calibrated and colour-coded for different gases. A bobbin (oblong) or ball (round) should rotate freely within the tube, providing an accurate reading of the flow rate. The reading is taken from the top of a bobbin or the middle of a ball. The dot in the centre of the bobbin helps assess whether it is spinning in the gas	Control and measure the flow of gas. Calibrations are in l/min. Some machines also have flowmeters that are calibrated in 100 ml/min increments up to 1.0 l, in addition to those that are calibrated in l/min increments (Fig. 6.2B)
Vaporizers	Modern vaporizers, such as the TEC and Penlon type, are designed to remain accurate in output despite temperature and gas flow changes. They are agent-specific	Deliver a known concentration of anaesthetic vapour to the patient
Back bar	Flowmeters and vaporizers can be attached to the back bar. This allows more than one volatile agent to be available	Supports the flowmeters and vaporizers
Common gas outlet	Location varies between anaesthetic machines	Enables connection to anaesthetic breathing systems and ventilators
Oxygen flush valve	A button or valve that allows pure oxygen to be released at high pressure and high flow, bypassing the vaporizer. The valve should never be activated when a patient is attached to the system, as barotrauma to the lungs is likely	Provides oxygen in emergency situations and purges anaesthetic gases from the system, to minimize pollution
Low-oxygen alarm	An alarm sounds when oxygen levels become low. In modern anaesthetic machines, the delivery of nitrous oxide stops when the oxygen alarm sounds, also activating the nitrous oxide alarm	Warns the anaesthetist of low oxygen levels

4. **Action:** Cats must be brought to the surgery in a secure cage or basket. Dogs must wear a secure collar and be on a lead.
   Rationale: This minimizes the risk of escape.
5. **Action:** The client is given a time to arrive at the surgery.
   Rationale: This enables the nursing team to plan the surgery list and allow time for each patient to be admitted.

Procedure: Admitting the patient

1. **Action:** Check that the patient is included on the day's list and confirm the procedure.
   Rationale: A consent form should have been prepared in advance. The owner must be fully aware of what the procedure entails to give informed consent.
2. **Action:** Take the client and pet into a consulting room.
   Rationale: This is more professional than dealing with the client in a busy waiting room.
3. **Action:** Weigh the patient.
   Rationale: The exact weight is essential for accurate administration of all anaesthetic and analgesic drugs.
4. **Action:** Obtain a complete history (Table 6.2).
   Rationale: An accurate history is vital to evaluate the patient's anaesthetic risk.
5. **Action:** For small mammals and exotic species, it is especially important to find out the animal's normal routine, including its usual diet and preferred drinking method.
   Rationale: This ensures the post-operative period is as stress-free as possible and that a diet likely to be eaten is offered. It is preferable for clients to bring the usual food with them to minimize the risk of post-operative anorexia.
6. **Action:** Check the sex of patients admitted for neutering procedures.
   Rationale: It is far better to discover a mistake prior to surgery.
7. **Action:** Identify a cryptorchid patient prior to castration.
   Rationale: The owner must give consent for any additional surgery and can also be informed of an increased fee.
8. **Action:** Obtain a contact telephone number for the duration of the patient's stay.

TABLE 6.2   Questions to ask when obtaining a history

Question	Significance
1. How old is the animal?	The animal's age should be on the client records, but should be checked: old and very young patients may pose a higher anaesthetic risk
2. When did the animal last eat?	If food has been recently consumed, there may be an increased risk of vomiting or regurgitation during anaesthesia
3. Has the animal had any previous illnesses, and, if so, what treatment was given?	Client records should supplement this information. Any condition involving the major body systems may increase the anaesthetic risk
4. Have there been any signs of illness in the past 24 hours? If so, what were the symptoms and has the animal recovered?	Anaesthetic risk might be increased due to dehydration, fever or electrolyte imbalance. Pathogens may also be introduced to the environment
5. How well does the animal tolerate exercise?	Poor exercise tolerance may indicate cardiovascular or respiratory problems
6. Is the patient on any medication? If so, has it been administered today?	Some drugs can alter the effects of anaesthetic agents
7. Is there any history of allergies or drug reactions?	Prolonged recovery from a previous anaesthetic or anaphylactic reactions to any medication should be noted
8. Is the patient entire, or has it been neutered? If an entire female, is she in season or pregnant?	If ovariohysterectomy is to be performed on a pregnant female, surgery time may be prolonged, and there might be an increased risk of haemorrhage

Rationale: It is vital to be able to contact the owner or an agent of the owner in the event of an emergency.

9. **Action:** Check the owner understands all the details, then obtain a signature on the consent form.

   Rationale: The owner or agent must read, understand and sign the consent form. The owner or agent must be over 18 if agreeing to pay veterinary fees.

10. **Action:** Transfer the patient to a kennel, making sure it cannot escape on the way.

    Rationale: It is best to ask the owner to leave before the dog is taken away as it is more likely to leave its owner willingly. Cats should be transferred in a secure basket.

Procedure: Pre-anaesthetic check

Assessment should be carried out before anaesthesia and surgery. This is usually performed by the veterinary surgeon.

1. **Action:** Assess the function of the cardiovascular system by auscultation of the heart and palpation of the pulse. (For normal values, see Table 2.1.)

   Rationale: The cardiovascular system is affected by anaesthesia. Note the heart rate and rhythm, abnormal heart or lung sounds, pulse rate and presence of a pulse deficit.

2. **Action:** Assess the function of the respiratory system.

   Rationale: This is also affected by anaesthesia. Note the respiratory rate and any abnormalities.

3. **Action:** Palpate the abdomen.

Rationale: This may detect the presence of an enlarged liver or abnormally small kidneys, either of which may lead to inefficient excretion of anaesthetic agents.

4. **Action:** Palpate superficial lymph nodes.

   Rationale: Enlarged lymph nodes may indicate the presence of infection, allergy or neoplasia.

5. **Action:** Take the patient's temperature.

   Rationale: Note any temperature outside the normal range. Premedicant and anaesthetic agents decrease body temperature.

6. **Action:** Assess pain, if relevant, prior to the administration of a premedicant.

   Rationale: Most premedicants contain an analgesic, which may mask signs of pain in conditions such as lameness, rendering further physical examination useless.

7. **Action:** Take a blood sample to perform a pre-anaesthetic blood screen, if required.

   Rationale: Pre-existing conditions may be evaluated, along with the patient's hydration status and function of the liver and kidneys.

8. **Action:** Administer a premedicant.

   Rationale: Premedication is performed to sedate the patient, to relieve anxiety, to enable reduced doses of anaesthetic drugs to be used and to allow a smooth recovery. In addition, analgesia is provided with the inclusion of analgesic drugs. The patient should be kept warm after premedication as many drugs used for sedation cause a drop in body temperature. Common premedicant agents are shown in Table 6.3.

TABLE 6.3	**Common premedicant drugs**		
Drug	**Type/group**	**Use**	**Warnings**
Acepromazine	Sedative/ataractic: phenothiazine	Calms the patient prior to induction and allows the use of lower doses of induction agent Used with opioid analgesics to produce neuroleptanalgesia	May reduce the seizure threshold, although this theory is controversial and not supported with data. Its use may be avoided in known epileptic patients Boxers are very sensitive to the effects of acepromazine, and it is used with caution at low dose rates in this breed

TABLE 6.3 Common premedicant drugs—cont'd			
Drug	**Type/group**	**Use**	**Warnings**
Diazepam and midazolam	Sedative/ataractic: benzodiazepine	Calms the patient prior to induction and allows the use of lower doses of induction agent Used as a premedicant for sick patients and those prone to seizures	Usually only produces sedation in very young or very sick patients
Medetomidine and dexmedetomidine	Sedative: alpha-2 agonist	Used as a premedicant or in combination with other drugs to produce sedation for minor procedures. It can reduce the dose of induction agent by up to 80%. These agents also have analgesic properties. The sedative and analgesic effects are antagonized with atipamezole	Alpha-2 agonist agents cause cardiovascular and respiratory depression. They should only be used in healthy patients. Spontaneous arousal is possible, and care should be exercised when using in aggressive animals
Morphine, methadone, pethidine	Analgesic: full opioid agonist	Produce pain relief. Given prior to surgery to provide pre-emptive (also referred to as preventive) analgesia, which leads to decreased requirements in the post-operative period	Full opioid agonist agents may cause respiratory depression, although this is rarely a problem in veterinary medicine. Morphine causes vomiting in healthy dogs
Buprenorphine	Analgesic: partial opioid agonist	As above	Butorphanol is also a partial opioid agonist but it is used for its sedative effects as it only produces weak and short-acting analgesia
Carprofen, meloxicam	Analgesic: non-steroidal anti-inflammatory drug (NSAID)	May be given at premedication, after induction or during recovery, to provide multimodal analgesia	Renal toxicity and gastric irritation

GENERAL ANAESTHESIA

In modern practice, stages and planes of general anaesthesia are no longer referred to, as surgical anaesthesia can be attained with the use of several different drugs working together (a process known as synergy). This means that patients do not need to be at a great depth of anaesthesia for painful surgical procedures to be performed. The time of greatest risk to the patient is said to be at induction and during recovery, and close monitoring at all times is essential.

Induction. During the induction period the patient passes from consciousness to unconsciousness. Induction is usually performed by intravenous injection, using one of the induction agents described in Table 6.4. Other methods are also possible, and the advantages and disadvantages of each method are discussed in Table 6.5.

Maintenance. During this period the state of unconsciousness is usually maintained with the use of an inhalant agent, delivered by means of an endotracheal tube connected to an anaesthetic breathing system and machine. In some cases, an anaesthetic mask may be necessary; for example, if intubation is not possible. Total intravenous anaesthesia (TIVA) is a method of maintaining anaesthesia with the constant infusion of a suitable intravenous agent or by giving incremental doses of the agent. It is preferable that patients undergoing TIVA are intubated to ensure the airway is maintained and protected. This also allows the administration of oxygen. The common inhalant agents are described in Table 6.6.

TABLE 6.4　Common induction agents

Agent	Effects	Warnings
Propofol	A propyl phenol agent Rapidly metabolized in the dog by the liver, lungs and muscles. Its effects are therefore not cumulative in dogs. Anaesthesia in the dog can be maintained by giving incremental doses or by constant rate infusion – a technique known as total intravenous anaesthesia (TIVA). It is cumulative in cats, causing prolonged recovery, and should not be topped up or infused continuously	Muscle twitches are sometimes seen at induction or during recovery A brief period of apnoea and a fall in blood pressure may be seen on induction, especially if administered quickly Two preparations are currently available: preservative-free, which should be discarded 6 hours after opening; and preserved with benzyl alcohol, giving a broached shelf-life of 28 days
Alfaxalone	A neurosteroid anaesthetic agent Non-cumulative in both dogs and cats, so can be used for TIVA without prolonging recovery time	Post-induction apnoea is sometimes seen. Its occurrence can be minimized by administering the dose slowly, over 1 minute. Induction time may therefore be prolonged
Ketamine	A dissociative agent Produces anaesthesia and profound analgesia Combined with alpha-2 agonists, opioid analgesics and benzodiazepines to produce anaesthesia in cats, dogs, rabbits, small rodents, birds and reptiles	Cannot be used alone, as it causes muscle rigidity and central nervous system stimulation Hallucinations and emergence phenomena are often seen during recovery in the cat

TABLE 6.5　Methods of induction

Method	Advantages	Disadvantages
Mask induction A tightly fitting clear plastic mask with a diaphragm is placed over the animal's face. 100% oxygen is administered for several minutes; this maximizes tissue perfusion and allows the patient to adjust to the mask. The anaesthetic concentration is then gradually introduced	Used to administer oxygen and inhalant agents when endotracheal intubation is not possible Useful for small mammals and birds	May be very distressing for the patient The airway is not protected, and obstruction can occur Masks increase mechanical dead space Atmospheric pollution is a significant hazard
Chamber induction The conscious patient is placed inside an anaesthetic induction chamber, which should be large enough for the animal to lie with its neck extended. Oxygen and the inhalant agent are delivered via a gas inlet. Waste gases are scavenged via an appropriate outlet. The patient is removed when it loses the ability to stand	Induction chambers are useful for small mammals and uncooperative patients	Only suitable for small patients Risk of vomiting Cardiopulmonary function cannot be monitored Atmospheric pollution occurs when the chamber is opened
Intravenous The induction agent is injected into a peripheral vein over the recommended period of time, depending on the agent being used	Smooth and usually rapid induction Induction agents can be given to effect, so minimal quantities are used	Patients must be restrained well Perivascular injection can be avoided by placing an intravenous catheter before induction
Intramuscular This method can only be used for certain drugs such as those used in combination mixtures	Technically easier than intravenous injection Useful in fractious patients when intravenous access is not possible	Dosage is according to weight; it is therefore not easy or possible to dose to effect Slower onset of anaesthesia

TABLE 6.6 Common inhalant agents

Agent	Properties	Effects	Warnings
Isoflurane	Low solubility, so quick onset of action	Rapid induction and recovery Good muscle relaxation	Little effect on cardiac output Respiratory depression Hypotension Approximately 0.2% is metabolized by the liver; the rest is exhaled unchanged
Sevoflurane	Very insoluble, so less potent than isoflurane with very quick onset of action	Rapid and smooth induction and recovery Less odour than other inhalant agents, so useful for mask and chamber inductions	Dose-dependent decrease in cardiac output Respiratory depression and hypotension as for isoflurane Decomposes in the presence of soda lime – higher than normal fresh gas flows may be needed (unless using soda lime formulated for low-flow usage)
Desflurane	The least soluble of all inhalant agents	Extremely rapid onset of action and recovery	Similar cardiovascular depression as seen with other agents Pungent and irritant to airways, so not suitable for induction by inhalation

ENDOTRACHEAL TUBES

After induction, an endotracheal tube should be placed in the patient's airway (tracheal intubation). This tube conducts anaesthetic gases and oxygen from the anaesthetic machine to the lungs, bypassing the nasal passages and pharynx. Tubes come in a variety of sizes, may be made of rubber or silicone and may be cuffed or uncuffed.

Procedure: Intubation of a patient

The patient must be sufficiently anaesthetized to carry out intubation. This is indicated by the following signs:

- The jaw is relaxed
- The tongue can be held with no resistance
- There is no gagging or swallowing reflex on introduction of the tube.

  Equipment required. Selection of suitably sized endotracheal tubes, lubricant to facilitate intubation, laryngoscope, local anaesthetic spray to prevent laryngeal spasm in cats, syringe or cuff inflator, stylet if necessary, suitable tie to secure the tube in place.

1. **Action:** Select several endotracheal tubes of varying sizes and measure the required length against the patient's head and neck.

   Rationale: This will enable selection of the most suitable tube for the patient. The largest diameter tube possible should be used, as long as tracheal damage

does not occur. This avoids resistance to ventilation, which occurs when tubes which are too small are used; it also decreases mechanical dead space.

2. **Action:** Inflate the cuff of cuffed tubes and leave for several minutes; inspect for excessive wear and check the patency of the tube.

   Rationale: Rubber tubing can perish over time, causing malfunction of the cuff. If the cuff does not remain inflated, anaesthetic gases may leak around it during anaesthesia, and fluid and debris may be inhaled. Patency is essential for adequate patient ventilation and for the delivery of oxygen and anaesthetic gases.

3. **Action:** Lubricate the tube with water-soluble lubricant.

   Rationale: This allows smooth, atraumatic introduction of the tube; it also enhances the seal produced by the cuff.

4. **Action:** The patient is restrained in sternal recumbency. An assistant extends the neck and holds the head so the nose is pointing upwards (Fig. 6.3).

   Rationale: Intubation in sternal recumbency reduces the risk of regurgitation and aspiration.

5. **Action:** The upper jaw is held still whilst the tongue is pulled out and down so that it lies between the lower canines. Pull the lower jaw downwards by pulling the tongue down until the epiglottis can be clearly seen.

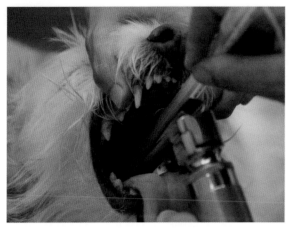

Fig. 6.3 Position of an animal for intubation.

Rationale: In this position, visibility of the anatomy of the pharynx is maximized (Figs 6.4 and 6.5).

6. **Action:** Gently push the epiglottis down with the tip of the tube and insert it through the glottis into the trachea (Figs 6.6 and 6.7).

   Rationale: The tube should pass smoothly between the arytenoid cartilages and enter the trachea and not the oesophagus.

7. **Action:** When intubating a cat, topical local anaesthetic (lidocaine) is first sprayed on to the larynx before introducing the tube during inhalation, at which point the vocal folds are open.

   Rationale: The larynx of a cat is very sensitive, so local anaesthetic is used to desensitize it, preventing laryngospasm. One spray is sufficient. A short period of time – around 30–60 seconds – should elapse between desensitizing the larynx and attempting intubation.

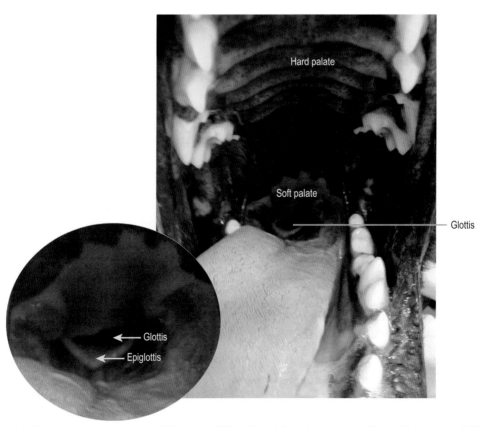

Fig. 6.4 How to place an endotracheal tube. Inset: When the epiglottis is depressed, the glottis is exposed. The endotracheal tube is advanced through the glottis.

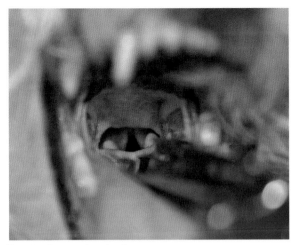

Fig. 6.5 A normal canine larynx.

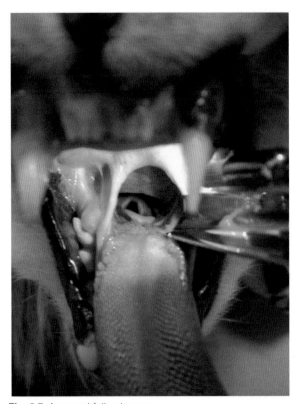

Fig. 6.7 A normal feline larynx.

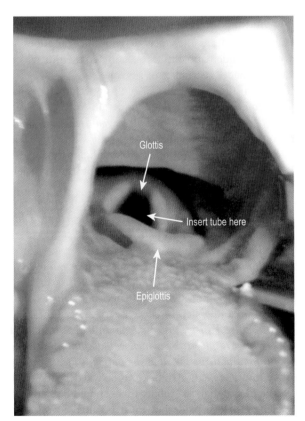

Fig. 6.6 Anatomy landmarks for feline intubation.

8. **Action:** A laryngoscope is very useful in assisting intubation.
   Rationale: *The smooth blade enables the operator to depress the epiglottis, and the light source illuminates the larynx.*
9. **Action:** The tube must not be introduced too far or endobronchial intubation may occur (Fig 6.8).
   Rationale: *This results in ventilation of one lung only.*
10. **Action:** Once the tube is inserted, confirm correct placement in the trachea (rather than the oesophagus). This can be performed in a number of ways, including using a capnograph to determine the presence of end-tidal carbon dioxide, visual checking with a laryngoscope and watching the breathing system bag for movements that coincide with breathing/chest movements.
    Rationale: *Oesophageal intubation results in oxygen and anaesthetic gas being delivered to the stomach rather than the lungs.*

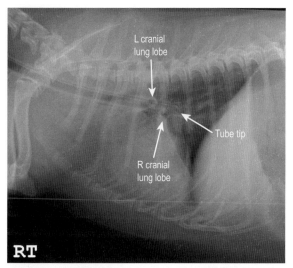

L cranial
lung lobe

Tube tip

R cranial
lung lobe

RT

Fig. 6.8 Radiograph showing incorrect (endobronchial) placement of an endotracheal tube in a dog.

11. **Action:** If a cuffed tube has been used, the minimum occluding volume technique, whereby the cuff is inflated just enough to prevent gas escaping, should be used.

    Rationale: Over-inflation can damage the tracheal mucosa or cause occlusion of the tube. Under-inflation enables the patient to breathe around the tube, and foreign material may pass into the trachea. Pollution of the environment will also occur.

12. **Action:** To avoid accidental extubation, secure the tube in place using a suitable tie. This is ideally tied around the end of the tube over the plastic connector and secured behind the ears with a quick-release bow. Alternatively, it may be tied to the mandible or maxilla.

    Rationale: The plastic connector will support the tube, preventing it from collapse when the tie is pulled tight. A quick-release fastening is used for easy removal in an emergency.

Procedure: Extubation (removal of the endotracheal tube) of a patient

1. **Action:** Release the tie holding the endotracheal tube in place.

    Rationale: This is usually untied before signs of arousal are seen so the tube can be removed quickly at the appropriate time.

2. **Action:** Deflate the cuff after the cough reflex has returned in dogs, and before it returns in cats.

    Rationale: Deflation of the cuff is essential as an inflated cuff can easily damage the tracheal mucosa. After oral surgery, the cuff may be left partially inflated to dislodge debris and fluid in the proximal trachea as the tube is withdrawn slowly.

3. **Action:** Withdraw the tube in a slight downward arc as the animal exhales.

    Rationale: This will help to avoid damage to the laryngeal structures.

4. **Action:** In dogs, the tube is left in place until the swallowing or gag reflex returns.

    Rationale: The swallowing reflex helps protect against aspiration in the event of regurgitation or vomiting.

5. **Action:** Cats should be extubated before the swallowing reflex returns. Signs of impending arousal include tail, limb or head movements or an active palpebral reflex.

    Rationale: Delayed extubation may lead to laryngospasm.

Procedure: Care of endotracheal tubes

The care and maintenance of endotracheal tubes is partly dependent on the type of material from which they are made, i.e. rubber or silicone.

1. **Action:** Rinse the tubes in running water.

    Rationale: Any debris and fluid that would otherwise deactivate a detergent will be removed.

2. **Action:** Soak in a suitable detergent solution.

    Rationale: This will soften any residual debris.

3. **Action:** Scrub the tubes inside and out using specialist brushes.

    Rationale: All debris and mucus will be removed. It is imperative that the lumen is cleaned thoroughly and that it remains patent.

4. **Action:** Thorough rinsing is essential.

    Rationale: All traces of detergent must be removed to prevent chemical or ischaemic tracheitis.

5. **Action:** Dry thoroughly and check for patency, cuff inflation and general wear. Discard faulty tubes.

    Rationale: This ensures that no animal is intubated with a faulty tube, which could compromise the anaesthetic or threaten the patient's life.

6. **Action:** The method of sterilization will depend on the type of material: red rubber tubes should be sterilized using ethylene oxide but must be aired for at least 48 hours before use; silicone tubes can be autoclaved.

Rationale: Heat will damage rubber tubes, so they should not be autoclaved. Airing after sterilization with ethylene oxide is essential to avoid chemical tracheitis.

7. **Action:** Store the tubes in a dry, cool environment away from direct sunlight.
   Rationale: Correct care and storage of endotracheal tubes will prolong their life.

ANAESTHETIC MASKS

There may be some instances where an anaesthetic mask is required. Masks come in a range of sizes and are made of either clear plastic or malleable black rubber. They can be used to:

- Supply oxygen, either in a first aid situation or as a means of pre-oxygenating a patient, as long as it does not cause stress
- Provide gases for maintenance of anaesthesia in short procedures if for some reason intubation is not possible
- Supply gases to induce anaesthesia in neonates for which intravenous access cannot be gained
- Provide oxygen during procedures where the patient has been sedated.

Gas flow rates have to be higher than those used with an endotracheal tube due to increased dead space. The risk of atmospheric pollution is therefore increased. The use of a plastic mask with a rubber diaphragm is preferred as a closer fit is possible. Unfortunately, intermittent positive pressure ventilation (IPPV) cannot be carried out effectively using a mask.

ANAESTHETIC BREATHING SYSTEMS

The anaesthetic breathing system connects the patient to the anaesthetic machine. The most common systems fall into two categories: rebreathing and non-rebreathing. All systems have advantages and disadvantages, depending on the clinical situation, so a practice should have a range of systems available for use. Rebreathing systems are those where carbon dioxide is removed from the system and the same gas is recirculated and rebreathed. Non-rebreathing systems rely on fresh gas flow (FGF) to flush out exhaled gases and prevent rebreathing of carbon dioxide.

The common components of a breathing system are an inspiratory limb (takes fresh gas from the machine to the patient), expiratory limb (removes waste gas and carbon dioxide from the patient and conveys it to the scavenge system), reservoir or rebreathing bag (available in various sizes) and an adjustable pressure-limiting (APL) valve (also called pop-off or exhaust valve). Rebreathing systems have a soda lime canister.

Functions of the anaesthetic breathing system are to:

- Supply oxygen to the patient
- Supply anaesthetic gases to the patient
- Remove carbon dioxide and waste gases from the patient
- Enable IPPV.

Whether a system is suitable for performing IPPV or not will depend on the position of the bag. Not all systems can be used to provide long-term IPPV. In general, if the bag is on the expiratory limb, IPPV can be performed. If it is on the inspiratory limb, IPPV should not be performed for long periods of time, as rebreathing of carbon dioxide will occur.

Jackson Rees modified Ayre's T-piece (non-rebreathing) (Fig. 6.9)

This consists of a long, narrow inspiratory limb and a short, wide expiratory limb to which a 0.5-litre bag is attached. (An open-ended bag is the true modification, with no valve; however, the system with a closed bag and low-pressure APL valve is also marketed under the same name.)

Advantages
- Can be used for long-term IPPV
- Minimal apparatus dead space and resistance
- Suitable for small patients.

Disadvantages
- High gas flow rates are required
- Scavenging is difficult when an open-ended bag is used.

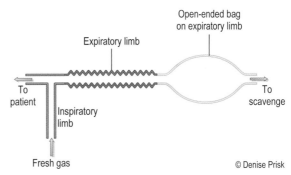

Fig. 6.9 Jackson Rees modified Ayre's T-piece anaesthetic breathing system.

Suitable for. Small dogs (less than 8–10 kg ideal weight), cats, neonates, birds and exotic species.

Flow rates. 2.5–3.0 × minute volume.

Lack and mini Lack (non-rebreathing) (Fig. 6.10)

The parallel Lack, which is the most common type of Lack, consists of an inspiratory limb to which the reservoir bag is attached, an expiratory limb and an APL valve. A coaxial version exists, where the expiratory limb is a tube inside the outer, inspiratory limb. The bag is found on the inspiratory limb. The coaxial Lack is rarely seen.

Advantages
- Low gas flow rates are required.

Disadvantages
- Cannot be used for prolonged IPPV because rebreathing will occur, causing hypercapnia
- The coaxial tubing may become disconnected, causing rebreathing.

Suitable for. Patients weighing more than 8 kg (ideal weight).

Flow rates. 0.8 × minute volume.

The mini Lack system is similar to the parallel Lack but consists of smooth, narrow-bore tubing, a low-resistance valve and a 0.5-litre bag. It works in the same way as the parallel Lack and is suitable for animals weighing 1–10 kg (ideal weight).

Magill (non-rebreathing) (Fig. 6.11)

This consists of one wide corrugated tube only, a valve at the patient end, a reservoir bag and two T-connectors. The Magill is not commonly in use in modern practice as it is thought to be less efficient than the Lack.

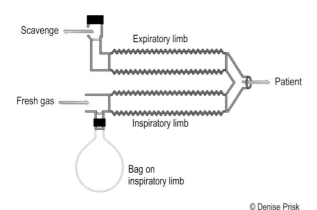

Fig. 6.10 Parallel Lack anaesthetic breathing system.

© Denise Prisk

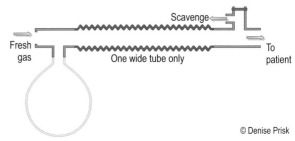

© Denise Prisk

Fig. 6.11 Magill anaesthetic breathing system.

Advantages
- Low gas flow rates are required.

Disadvantages
- The tube must hold a volume greater than the patient's tidal volume to prevent rebreathing
- Cannot be used for prolonged IPPV
- The location of the valve is inconvenient for scavenging and for surgery involving the head and neck.

Suitable for. Patients weighing more than 8–10 kg (ideal weight).

Flow rates. 0.8 × minute volume.

Modified Bain (non-rebreathing) (Fig. 6.12)

The Bain consists of coaxial tubing: the inner tube is the inspiratory limb, and the outer tube is the expiratory limb. The bag is attached to the expiratory limb. An APL valve is located on the expiratory limb.

Advantages
- Can be used for long-term IPPV
- Expired gas passing through the outer tubing warms the inspired gas, thereby conserving patient temperature.

Disadvantages
- Inner tube disconnection increases dead space and will cause rebreathing. This can be checked using a recommended technique
- High gas flow rates are required.

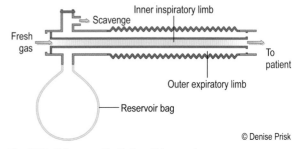

© Denise Prisk

Fig. 6.12 Bain anaesthetic breathing system.

Suitable for. Patients weighing more than 8–10 kg (ideal weight).

Flow rates. 2.5–3.0 × minute volume.

Circle system (rebreathing) (Fig. 6.13)

Circle systems can vary in configuration and appearance but they generally consist of an inspiratory and an expiratory limb with unidirectional valves, a Y-connector, a rebreathing bag of suitable size, a soda lime canister and a valve. As gas is literally recirculated in the system, the term 'circuit' is only really correct for this type of breathing system.

Advantages
- Warmed, humidified gas is circulated so heat and moisture are conserved with less risk of hypothermia
- Economical due to low flow rates
- Less environmental pollution
- IPPV can be carried out (as long as the bag is on the expiratory limb).

Disadvantages
- Increased resistance
- Soda lime is required
- Nitrous oxide should only be used if the patient's oxygenation status is monitored

- Changes in anaesthetic gas concentration occur slowly at low flow rates, and the inhaled gas concentration is not the same as that dialled on the vaporizer.

Suitable for. Patients weighing more than 8–10 kg (ideal weight). Note: the Cyclo-Flo circle is suitable for patients weighing 7 kg or more. Paediatric circle systems are also available for patients weighing less than 10 kg.

Flow rates. The gas requirement in circle systems is related to minute oxygen consumption and not to minute volume, so there is no circuit factor. FGF need only supply sufficient oxygen to satisfy metabolic requirements – around 5–10 ml/kg/min. However, in practice, higher flow rates are used to allow for deficiencies in the performance of vaporizers at low gas flows and variable specific patient requirements. To achieve a stable state of anaesthesia and to allow denitrogenation of the lungs and the circuit, 100 ml/kg/min is used for the first 5–10 minutes and also at the end of anaesthesia, to lighten the plane of anaesthesia quickly and to purge gas from the system. Once a suitable depth of anaesthesia has been achieved, the FGF can be reduced to 0.5–1.0 l/min (or according to capnography), with the valve partly closed.

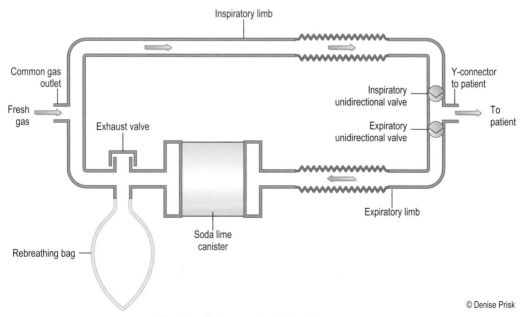

© Denise Prisk

Fig. 6.13 Circle anaesthetic breathing system.

Humphrey ADE system (hybrid system: rebreathing and non-rebreathing) (Fig. 6.14)

This versatile system consists of a special four-phase exhaust valve, smooth-bore tubing with less resistance to gas flow and suitable-sized rebreathing bag. It can be used with (rebreathing – more than 8–10 kg ideal weight) or without (non-rebreathing – less than 8–10 kg ideal weight) the Humphrey low-volume soda lime canister.

Advantages

- The valve supplies positive end expiratory pressure (PEEP), which keeps the alveoli open and prevents their collapse at the end of expiration
- The valve conserves dead space gas with no increase in airway resistance; this means that gases are warmed and humidified
- Very low flow rates are required, so it is economical to use
- IPPV can be performed in any mode; there is no evidence of rebreathing, even when used as a Lack
- One system is suitable for use on any size animal
- Can be used with a ventilator attached – the position of the lever determines whether or not the bag or ventilator is in circuit. The lever must be in the correct position for the patient to be able to breathe.

Disadvantage

- Expensive.

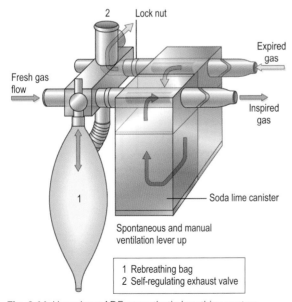

Fig. 6.14 Humphrey ADE anaesthetic breathing system.

Labels on figure:
2 Lock nut
Expired gas
Fresh gas flow
Inspired gas
Soda lime canister
1
Spontaneous and manual ventilation lever up
1 Rebreathing bag
2 Self-regulating exhaust valve

Procedure: Replacing soda lime

Soda lime is used to absorb carbon dioxide from rebreathing systems. It consists of granules consisting of:

- Approximately 90% calcium hydroxide
- Approximately 5% or less of sodium hydroxide
- Silicates – make granules less likely to disintegrate into powder
- pH indicator – this causes the soda lime to change colour as it becomes exhausted. Common colour changes in the UK are pink to white and white to violet. A type of soda lime that is marketed specifically for use with low gas flows (LoFloSorb) is green when fresh and changes to violet when exhausted.

1. **Action:** Put on protective clothing, including gloves, apron, mask and goggles.
   Rationale: Soda lime is caustic and must be handled with care. The dust is irritant if inhaled.

2. **Action:** Follow the manufacturer's instructions when filling the soda lime canister.
   Rationale: The canisters of most standard circle systems should be filled almost completely but not tightly packed as a small gap decreases circuit resistance and increases efficiency of carbon dioxide absorption.

Note: the Humphrey canister must be filled completely with no gap.

CONTROL OF POLLUTION – SCAVENGING

Anaesthetic gases must be scavenged from the breathing system to avoid atmospheric pollution and potential damage to personnel. Hazards arise from short- or long-term exposure. Disorders such as neoplasia, organ damage, abortion and infertility have been linked to exposure to anaesthetic gases. Under the Control of Substances Hazardous to Health (COSHH) regulations, employers must assess the risk of exposure and take appropriate action to protect their employees.

Scavenging can be achieved in two ways – active scavenging and passive scavenging. In both cases, a scavenge tube is connected to the exhaust valve of the breathing system to conduct waste gases away from the system and environment to a safe site. (With an open-ended bag on a modified Ayre's T-piece, an attachment is needed to connect the scavenge tube to the open end of the bag.)

1. **Active scavenging** – gas is drawn along the scavenge tube by negative pressure generated by a vacuum pump or extractor fan. An atmospheric equalizer

prevents air being sucked from the circuit, which would otherwise cause the bag to collapse. All gases can be scavenged by this method.

2. **Passive scavenging** – passive systems either direct the gas into an activated charcoal adsorber unit or pass it straight to the outside through a duct in the wall. These systems rely on the combined effects of gas flowing into the anaesthetic circuit and expiratory effort. The scavenge tube must travel downwards and not be excessively long or it will offer too much resistance to expiration and could lead to rebreathing. All gases can be scavenged by being ducted to the outside. Activated charcoal units do not scavenge nitrous oxide. These are sealed units which are depleted at a certain weight – usually 200 g heavier than when new. They must be weighed regularly and disposed of correctly when exhausted.

CALCULATING ANAESTHETIC GAS FLOW RATES

When using a non-rebreathing system, an accurate flow rate should be calculated for each patient to prevent hypoxia (reduced oxygen concentration in the tissues) and hypercapnia (increased carbon dioxide levels in the blood). Several factors must be taken into account when calculating flow rates, including the patient's tidal volume and respiratory rate and the circuit being used. Note: if a capnograph is used, the flow rate is set according to the inspiratory value of carbon dioxide, which should be 0 mmHg or 0%. It is therefore not necessary to calculate the flow rate, and, as a rule, much lower flow rates can be achieved than those calculated.

Respiratory rate. The number of breaths taken per minute during normal, resting respiration.

Tidal volume. The amount of air passing into and out of the lungs in each respiratory cycle. It is estimated as follows:

- Cats/small dogs weighing less than 10 kg: 15 ml/kg
- Dogs weighing more than 10 kg: 10 ml/kg.

Minute volume. The amount of air passing into and out of the lungs in one minute. This is calculated from the tidal volume and respiratory rate of the patient:

- Minute volume (ml/kg) = tidal volume × respiratory rate.

Note: as a rough estimate, if accurate calculation is not possible, the minute volume of dogs is approximately 200 ml/kg, using an average tidal volume of 10 ml/kg

TABLE 6.7 Circuit factors for non-rebreathing systems

Anaesthetic breathing system	Circuit factor
Jackson Rees modified Ayre's T-piece	2.5–3.0 × minute volume
Bain	2.5–3.0 × minute volume
Lack and mini Lack	0.8 × minute volume
Magill	0.8 × minute volume

and an average respiratory rate of 20 breaths/min. This figure is higher for small dogs, cats and small mammals, and lower for large dogs.

Circuit factor. This relates to non-rebreathing systems only. It is the factor by which the minute volume must be multiplied to prevent rebreathing (unless capnography is used). Circuit factors for individual systems are shown in Table 6.7.

Calculating the fresh gas flow of anaesthetic gas to the patient

The formula is:

$$\text{Bodyweight (kg)} \times \text{tidal volume (ml)} \times \text{respiratory rate} \times \text{circuit factor} = \text{FGF (ml/min, then converted to litres/min)}$$

Example. The FGF for a 12 kg spaniel with a respiratory rate of 15 breaths/min on a Bain circuit would be calculated as follows:

First, calculate the patient's tidal volume (body weight × 10 ml):

$$12 \text{ kg} \times 10 \text{ ml} = 120 \text{ ml}$$

Then calculate the minute volume (tidal volume × respiratory rate):

$$120 \times 15 = 1800 \text{ ml}$$

Finally, multiply the minute volume by the circuit factor:

$$1800 \times 2.5 - 3 = 4500 - 5400 \text{ ml/min} (4.5 - 5.4 \text{ litres/min})$$

Combining gases

When nitrous oxide (an effective analgesic agent) is used, the amount of oxygen delivered to the patient is governed by the fact that, to prevent hypoxia, i.e. low oxygen levels, oxygen levels must not drop below 33% of the total inspired gas. When calculating flow rates, the maximum ratio of nitrous oxide to oxygen is 2:1 (i.e. two-thirds or 66% of the total gas flow is nitrous oxide, and one-third or 33% of the total gas flow is oxygen). The minimum effective ratio of nitrous oxide to oxygen is 1:1 (50% of each gas).

Example. A 4 kg cat with a respiratory rate of 20 breaths/min is connected to an Ayre's T-piece. Nitrous oxide is to be used. The flow rate would be calculated as follows:

$$\begin{aligned} \text{Bodyweight(kg)} \times \text{tidal volume (ml)} \times \\ \text{respiratory rate} \times \text{circuit factor} = \\ \text{FGF(ml/min)} \end{aligned}$$

First, calculate the patient's tidal volume (body weight × 15 ml):

$$4\,kg \times 15ml = 60\,ml$$

Then calculate the minute volume (tidal volume × respiratory rate):

$$60 \times 20 = 1200\,ml$$

Finally, multiply the minute volume by the circuit factor:

$$1200 \times 2.5 - 3 = 3000 - 3600\,ml/min$$
$$(3.0 - 3.6\,litres/min)$$

To split this into a ratio of 2:1, divide the total gas flow by 3:

$$3000 \div 3 = 1000; \ 3600 \div 3 = 1200$$

One-third of the gas flow is 1000 ml or 1200 ml. Two-thirds of the total gas flow is therefore 2000 ml or 2400 ml. The safest maximum gas flow of nitrous oxide to the patient is 2000–2400 ml/min (2.0–2.4 l/min),

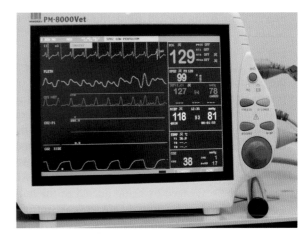

Fig. 6.15 A type of multiparameter monitor.

and the safest minimum gas flow of oxygen is 1000–1200 ml/min (1.0–1.2 l/min).

MONITORING ANAESTHESIA

It is vital that the status of the central nervous, cardio-vascular and cardiopulmonary systems is monitored continuously throughout anaesthesia and data recorded on a chart at 5-minute intervals. To minimize cardio-pulmonary depression, the patient should be maintained at a depth of anaesthesia that just prevents a response to surgery. Multiparameter monitors, which monitor and display a variety of parameters continuously (Fig. 6.15), are becoming popular in veterinary practice. However, machines should not be relied upon, and the undivided attention of the person monitoring the anaes-thetic is crucial. The range of techniques and equipment that is available for monitoring is listed in Table 6.8,

TABLE 6.8 **Methods of monitoring the patient during anaesthesia**		
Method	**Parameter measured**	**Description**
Palpation of peripheral and central pulses	Pulse rate and rhythm Pulse quality	Central pulses can be palpated at the femoral and brachial arteries. Peripheral pulses can be assessed by palpation of the dorsal metatarsal, digital, lingual, facial and coccygeal arteries. Palpation of peripheral pulses is recommended as they are more sensitive to changes and can provide early indication of developing hypotension

TABLE 6.8 Methods of monitoring the patient during anaesthesia—cont'd

Method	Parameter measured	Description
Palpation of the heart	Heart rate and rhythm	Used in small mammals or when peripheral pulses are not palpable due to hypotension
Thoracic auscultation	Heart rate and rhythm Valve action Lung sounds	Oesophageal stethoscopes are recommended because they remain in place throughout anaesthesia and provide continuous monitoring of breathing and heart sounds
Electrocardiography (ECG)	Electrical activity of the heart	Heart rhythm can be seen and the rate ascertained Electrolyte imbalances can alter the ECG and arrhythmias can be detected The ECG gives no indication of cardiac output
Pulse oximetry	Percentage of haemoglobin molecules that are saturated with oxygen. Pulse rate is also shown	Various types of sensors are available. The most common type clips on to the tongue but can also be used on the toe web, pinna or lip. Oxygen saturation of arterial blood is measured
Blood pressure monitors	Blood pressure	Non-invasive blood pressure monitoring can be performed using Doppler or an oscillometric method. Both methods involve placing an inflatable cuff of suitable size around a limb or the base of the tail, proximal to a distal artery. On inflation, the cuff occludes arterial blood flow. As the cuff is deflated, returning blood flow is detected Taping the Doppler transducer in place provides audible monitoring of peripheral pulse
Capnography	End-tidal carbon dioxide levels to assess ventilation	The concentration of carbon dioxide at the end of expiration is analyzed using sidestream or mainstream capnography. This reflects the concentration in arterial blood
Examination of mucous membranes	Peripheral perfusion Hydration status	Mucous membrane colour should be salmon pink and can be assessed by looking at the gingiva, conjunctiva, anus, vulva or prepuce
Capillary refill time (CRT)	Peripheral perfusion Hydration status	A mucous membrane is blanched and the time taken to return to normal is the CRT
Respiratory and apnoea alert monitors	Respiratory rate ± tidal volume Apnoea	Respirometers measure tidal volume. Adequate ventilation (exchange of gases) is not assessed in this way An alarm is triggered after a period of apnoea. The trigger period can be set by the operator
Thermometer or thermistor	Body temperature	Multiparameter monitors have oesophageal and rectal probes that are left in situ to provide continuous monitoring and display the core temperature. Alternatively, the rectal temperature can be periodically taken using a thermometer
Pedal reflex	Depth of anaesthesia	This reflex is tested by pinching in between the digits. Reaction indicates a light plane of anaesthesia in dogs and cats. Rabbits retain the forelimb pedal reflex until a very deep plane of anaesthesia is reached, so a hindlimb should be used. The ear pinch reflex can also be tested in rabbits

Continued

TABLE 6.8   Methods of monitoring the patient during anaesthesia—cont'd

Method	Parameter measured	Description
Palpebral reflex	Depth of anaesthesia	The eyelids will blink when the medial canthus is lightly touched. Reaction indicates a light plane of anaesthesia
Jaw tone	Depth of anaesthesia	The jaws are opened, and the amount of resistance gauged. As the depth of anaesthesia increases, the jaw becomes more relaxed. Little or no resistance indicates an excessively deep plane of anaesthesia
Blood loss	Hypovolaemia	The contents of a suction bottle should be measured. Blood loss can be estimated by weighing blood-soaked swabs and subtracting their dry weight: 1 ml blood weighs approximately 1 g
Urine output	Hydration status Renal function	Placement of a urinary catheter with a closed collection system allows measurement of urine. Urine production should be at least 1 ml/kg/h

TABLE 6.9   Changes in respiration seen during anaesthesia

Term	Definition	Cause	Action
Bradypnoea	Respiratory rate slower than normal	Effects of anaesthetic drugs Anaesthesia too deep Hypothermia	Lighten anaesthesia Increase body temperature – active warming and prevention of heat loss. Use of a heat and moisture exchanger (HME) between the endotracheal tube and breathing system can help preserve warmth
Tachypnoea	Respiratory rate faster than normal	Light plane of anaesthesia Pain	Deepen anaesthesia Administer analgesics
Dyspnoea	Difficulty breathing	Obstruction in the airway, endotracheal tube or anaesthetic breathing system	Check airway is patent Suction pharynx and/or endotracheal tube if necessary Extubate and reintubate with a different tube
Apnoea	Absence of respiration	Effects of some induction agents such as propofol and alfaxalone Respiratory arrest	Check airway is patent Check tube positioning and patency Perform intermittent positive pressure ventilation with 100% oxygen

and the clinical signs that may change during anaesthesia are described in Tables 6.9–6.11.

PATIENT RECOVERY

Once surgery has been completed, the vaporizer is switched off. Pure (100%) oxygen should be given for at least 5 minutes after turning off nitrous oxide to avoid diffusion hypoxia. The system should be flushed with oxygen from the flowmeter, not the oxygen flush valve, before final disconnection to avoid atmospheric pollution.

It is essential to monitor the patient closely throughout the recovery period – post-operative mortality occurs when attention relaxes. The patient should be placed in a warm, quiet, accessible kennel with

TABLE 6.10 Changes in heart rate seen during anaesthesia

Term	Definition	Cause	Action
Bradycardia	Heart rate slower than normal	Effects of drugs such as alpha-2 agonists and acepromazine Increasing depth of anaesthesia Hypothermia Pre-existing condition	Administer atipamezole if necessary to antagonize alpha-2 agonist agents Lighten anaesthesia if too deep Active warming and prevention of heat loss Maintain normal blood pressure (intravenous fluid therapy) Prepare anticholinergic drugs such as atropine
Tachycardia	Heart rate faster than normal	Effects of drugs such as atropine, glycopyrrolate and ketamine Light or decreasing plane of anaesthesia pain	Deepen anaesthesia if necessary Administer analgesics
Cardiac arrest	Total absence of heart beat	Many reasons, including drug overdose, hypoxia, hypercapnia, severe hypotension, hypothermia, vagal stimulation, electrolyte imbalances and cardiac disease	Start cardiac massage Intermittent positive pressure ventilation with 100% oxygen Abdominal compressions or abdominal wrap to increase intrathoracic pressure and improve venous return

TABLE 6.11 Changes in the colour of mucous membranes seen during anaesthesia

Colour	Cause	Action
Pale	Hypovolaemic shock Haemorrhage Hypotension Anaemia	Administer suitable fluid therapy Lighten plane of anaesthesia if appropriate
Cyanotic	Hypoxaemia Cardiac failure	Check airway is patent Suction pharynx and/or endotracheal tube Administer 100% oxygen ± intermittent positive pressure ventilation Cardiac massage
Icteric (yellow)	Hepatic abnormalities	Inform veterinary surgeon Monitor closely
Brick red	Toxaemia	Septic patients often require lower than normal concentrations of inhalant agent to maintain anaesthesia Monitor closely

emergency equipment close to hand. The length of time taken to recover depends on various factors, including:

- Anaesthetic agents used
- Duration of the anaesthetic
- Body temperature
- Environmental temperature
- Health of the patient.

Procedure: Care of the patient during recovery

1. **Action:** Monitor vital signs.
   Rationale: A change can be detected swiftly and acted upon immediately.
2. **Action:** Keep the patient calm.
   Rationale: Excitement on recovery causes increased blood pressure, which may dislodge clots and

cause haemorrhage. Injury to the patient is also possible.

3. **Action:** Keep the patient warm.
   Rationale: Hypothermia will delay recovery.
4. **Action:** Keep surgical sites covered if possible.
   Rationale: This minimizes the risk of contamination.
5. **Action:** Administer post-operative medication and assess the patient for signs of discomfort.
   Rationale: If there are any signs of pain, such as vocalization, panting, abnormal posture or tachycardia, inform the veterinary surgeon immediately. Analgesia should be maintained to prevent breakthrough pain.
6. **Action:** Prevent patient interference with wounds.
   Rationale: Apply dressings, bandages or an Elizabethan collar as necessary.
7. **Action:** Monitor fluid and nutritional intake.
   Rationale: If the patient is on intravenous fluids, maintain at the given rate. Allow access to water and a small amount of suitable food, unless contraindicated.
8. **Action:** Allow the patient the opportunity to urinate and defecate.
   Rationale: Patient comfort is improved. Urinary catheterization may be indicated if prolonged recovery is expected or if the patient is unable to walk.

Procedure: Discharging the patient

1. **Action:** Make sure all drugs, instructions and invoices are prepared in advance.
   Rationale: The reception staff can take payment and make follow-up appointments while the owner is waiting to speak to a veterinary nurse or veterinary surgeon.
2. **Action:** Take the client into a consulting room.
   Rationale: This ensures privacy and minimal distraction.
3. **Action:** Give instructions regarding feeding, exercise, medication, care of dressings, care of wounds, follow-up appointments, suture removal and possible complications.
   Rationale: Instructions should be given verbally and supported with written information to which the owner can later refer.
4. **Action:** Return the patient to the owner, making sure wounds are clean and intravenous catheters have been removed.

Rationale: This should be the last step because the client will be unlikely to take in any information once reunited with the pet.

ANAESTHETIC EMERGENCIES

An anaesthetic emergency is any anaesthesia-related incident that poses a threat to the patient's life. Constant monitoring is essential to detect the early warning signs of a potential emergency, such as a gradual decrease in respiratory rate prior to respiratory arrest.

The outcome of an emergency depends on:
- Correct preparation of an emergency kit
- Early observation of warning signs
- Correct assessment of the problem
- Prompt action.

Table 6.12 describes the contents of an anaesthetic emergency box, which should be regularly checked for out-of-date drugs and restocked as necessary. It is usually kept near the theatre and should always be readily available. Table 6.13 illustrates possible emergencies and the actions to be taken.

Intermittent positive pressure ventilation

IPPV is carried out for a number of reasons:
- To control ventilation (manually or with a ventilator)
- To ensure oxygenation of the patient
- To maintain anaesthesia in a patient that is not breathing spontaneously
- To maintain normocapnia (normal carbon dioxide levels) in a patient whose levels are either too high or too low
- To reduce the risk of acidosis in a bradypnoeic patient (one with a slow respiratory rate).

IPPV does, however, have some disadvantages, including:
- Reduced venous return (blood flow returning to the heart via the vena cava)
- Reduced cardiac output (blood leaving the heart)
- Trauma to the lungs from pressure or volume (barotrauma or volutrauma).

Procedure: Performing IPPV

A suitable breathing system must be used, i.e. circle, Bain, T-piece or Humphrey.

1. **Action:** Partly close the APL valve, squeeze the rebreathing bag and release. It may be necessary to increase the flow rate to fill the bag.

TABLE 6.12 Contents of an anaesthetic emergency box

Contents	Reason for use	Indication
Adrenaline	Increases the force of cardiac contractions (cardiac contractility) and stimulates sinus rhythm	Cardiac arrest Severe bradycardia that is unresponsive to atropine or glycopyrrolate
Atropine and glycopyrrolate	Increases the heart rate	Bradycardia Atrioventricular block
Dobutamine	Increases the force of cardiac contractions and cardiac output	Myocardial depression Cardiogenic shock Cardiac failure Hypotension
Dopamine	Increases renal blood flow and organ perfusion (low dose) Increases cardiac contractility and blood pressure (high dose)	Decreased urine output Decreased cardiac output Hypotension – but high doses cause reduced renal blood flow
Doxapram	Respiratory stimulant	Stimulates respiration, especially in neonates after birth by caesarean Note: the use of doxapram in hypoxaemic patients is contraindicated as it decreases cerebral perfusion with a subsequent increase in oxygen demand
Lidocaine	Treats ventricular arrhythmias and fibrillation	Ventricular premature contractions Ventricular tachycardia Atrial or ventricular fibrillation Note: lidocaine does not convert ventricular fibrillation to sinus rhythm
Naloxone	Opioid antagonist	Antagonizes the effects of opioid drugs
Sodium bicarbonate	Alkalotic agent	Metabolic acidosis
Tracheostomy tubes	Emergency tracheostomy	Laryngeal/pharyngeal obstruction
Long dog urinary catheter	Intratracheal/endobronchial drug administration	Some drugs may be given in this way, e.g. adrenaline and atropine. The catheter is inserted down the endotracheal tube and the drug diluted with saline before administration, followed by a flush with 1–5 ml saline to ensure the drug reaches the alveoli. An increased dose of the drug is usually used
Miscellaneous sundries such as syringes and needles, intravenous catheters, three-way taps, bungs, scissors, tape, emergency drug dosage chart		

Rationale: This will oxygenate the patient's lungs and remove waste gases from the patient and circuit via the scavenge system. The patient must be allowed to exhale fully.

2. **Action:** Allow an expiratory pause.

Rationale: During this time the bag refills with gas, and waste gases are purged. It also allows venous return.

3. **Action:** Continue at a rate of around 10–12 breaths/min.

TABLE 6.13 Anaesthetic emergencies

Emergency	Signs	Action
Airway obstruction	Dyspnoea Exaggerated respiratory effort Inspiratory or expiratory snoring Cyanosis Respiratory arrest	Remove any obvious obstruction Check patency of airway and ET tube – reintubate if necessary IPPV with 100% oxygen Tracheostomy may be necessary
Apnoea	Absence of breathing Irregular gasping can signify impending apnoea Cyanosis No movement of reservoir bag	IPPV with 100% oxygen
Cardiac arrest	Absence of heart beat and pulses Agonal or Cheyne–Stokes breathing Grey, white or cyanotic mucous membranes Eye fixed and central with dilated pupils	Turn off vaporizer and start cardiopulmonary resuscitation (reference should be made to the RECOVER guidelines)
Haemorrhage	Visible blood loss Pale mucous membranes Prolonged CRT Tachycardia Weak, thready pulse	Replace blood loss – whole blood transfusion, packed red blood cells IVFT – crystalloids ± colloids Decrease concentration of inhalant agent Prevent hypothermia
Hypotension	Low measured blood pressure Prolonged CRT Pale mucous membranes Weak peripheral pulses Tachycardia	Increase rate of crystalloid intravenous fluid administration or start IVFT Colloid administration Decrease concentration of inhalant agent Prevent hypothermia Drug therapy may be necessary
Hypothermia	Low body temperature Cold extremities Excessive depth of anaesthesia Bradycardia Pale mucous membranes Cardiac arrest	Decrease concentration of inhalant agent Provide active warming and prevent further heat loss – bubble wrap extremities and cover with bubble wrap, use circulating warm air blanket, insulate table top, administer warm intravenous fluids, use warm lavage fluids, increase environmental temperature, use a heat and moisture exchanger, recalculate and reduce fresh gas flow rates accordingly for non-rebreathing systems Minimize anaesthesia time

ET, endotracheal tube; IPPV, intermittent positive pressure ventilation; CRT, capillary refill time; IVFT, intravenous fluid therapy; RECOVER, Reassessment Campaign on Veterinary Resuscitation.

Rationale: *This mimics the average respiratory rate of the anaesthetized patient, thus enabling adequate oxygenation, removal of carbon dioxide and provision of anaesthetic gas (if relevant).*

4. **Action:** At the end of anaesthesia, reduce the ventilation rate gradually.
   Rationale: *Carbon dioxide levels will rise and stimulate spontaneous respiration.*

Note: When performing manual IPPV with a Humphrey system, the lever must be in the *up* position. The valve can be closed by placing a finger on the central orange valve stem. The bag is squeezed with the other hand, then the valve stem and the bag are both released simultaneously to allow exhalation. This method is also employed when using an IPPV button valve attached between the APL valve and the scavenge system of any circuit. Depressing the button effectively closes the valve so there is no need to partially close the APL valve.

SPECIALIZED TECHNIQUES

Local anaesthesia

Local anaesthetic agents may be used for a variety of reasons, including:

- To perform superficial surgery in a conscious or sedated patient
- Before or during surgery to reduce the depth of general anaesthesia
- To cause topical desensitization, e.g. in the eye, on the skin and on the larynx
- To enhance multimodal analgesia, by infusing lidocaine alongside analgesic drugs as a constant rate infusion (CRI)
- Lidocaine may be used in an emergency situation to treat cardiac arrhythmias.

Local anaesthetic agents work by blocking nerve conduction, thus preventing the transmission of toxic information from peripheral tissues to the central nervous system. They therefore block pain perception. The most common injectable local anaesthetic agents used in small animal practice include lidocaine, bupivacaine and ropivacaine. Table 6.14 describes the local anaesthetic techniques in common use.

TABLE 6.14 **Local anaesthetic techniques**		
Technique	**Description**	**Use**
Surface	Drops, creams, gels and sprays are available to be applied to the skin or mucous membranes	Drops can be applied to the eye to facilitate ocular examination Cream can be applied to the skin prior to intravenous catheterization Gel can be applied to urinary catheters to facilitate placement Spray can be applied to the larynx of cats to prevent laryngeal spasm during endotracheal intubation
Infiltration	Injection of local anaesthetic along the line of surgical incision	Facilitates suturing of skin wounds
Regional: perineural	Local anaesthetic is injected around nerve trunks to produce loss of sensation	Intercostal block during and after thoracotomy Maxillary and mandibular nerve blocks prior to dental extractions or facial surgery
Regional: intravenous	A tourniquet is placed around a limb and local anaesthetic is injected intravenously distal to the tourniquet. Analgesia of the distal limb is provided, which lasts until the tourniquet is removed	Rarely used in small animal veterinary practice
Extradural (epidural)	Local anaesthetic is injected into the epidural space to block nerves from the spinal cord. Preservative-free morphine may be included to provide additional analgesia	Used to provide muscle relaxation and analgesia during pelvic limb orthopaedic procedures, and for surgery of the abdomen and perineum
Others	Intrapleural and intra-articular blocks	Local anaesthetic agent is administered via a chest tube to provide intrapleural analgesia and into a joint to provide intra-articular analgesia

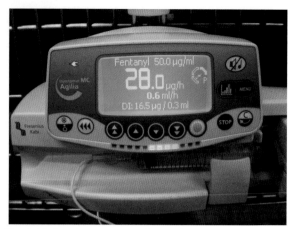

Fig. 6.16 A syringe pump can be used to deliver low volumes of fluid.

Constant rate infusion

CRI is the continuous administration of an agent or agents to a patient to provide constant and uniform levels and avoid the peaks and troughs in concentration of the drug that are seen with intermittent dosing. CRI may be administered to maintain anaesthesia, as in TIVA, or as a means of providing analgesia. When used intraoperatively for analgesic purposes, it significantly reduces the concentration of inhalant agent needed and therefore reduces its undesirable side-effects. To achieve therapeutic levels, a loading dose is given before starting the infusion. As only low volumes are infused, it is preferable to use a syringe pump for administration (Fig. 6.16). Drugs which are commonly infused as a CRI to provide analgesia include morphine, fentanyl, ketamine, lidocaine and medetomidine/dexmedetomidine.

REFERENCES AND FURTHER READING

Aspinall, V., 2011. The Complete Textbook of Veterinary Nursing, second ed. Elsevier, Oxford.

Ackerman, N., 2016. Aspinall's Complete Textbook of Veterinary Nursing, third ed. Elsevier, Oxford.

Bryant, S. (Ed.), 2010. Anesthesia for Veterinary Technicians. Wiley-Blackwell, Iowa.

Cooper, B., Mullineaux, E., Turner, L. (Eds.), 2011. Textbook of Veterinary Nursing. fifth ed. BSAVA, Gloucester.

Dugdale, A., 2010. Veterinary Anaesthesia: Principles to Practice. Wiley-Blackwell, Oxford.

Duke-Novakovski, T., de Vries, M., Seymour, C. (Eds.), 2016. Manual of Canine and Feline Anaesthesia and Analgesia. third ed. BSAVA, Gloucester.

Grimm, K.A., Lamont, L.A., Tranquilli, W.J., Greene, S.A., Robertson, S.A. (Eds.), 2015. Veterinary Anesthesia and Analgesia, The Fifth Edition of Lumb and Jones. fifth ed. Wiley-Blackwell, Iowa.

Savvas, I., Rallis, T., Raptopoulos, D., 2009. The effect of pre-anaesthetic fasting time and type of food on gastric content volume and acidity in dogs. Vet Anaesth Analg 36 (6), 539–546.

7

Theatre practice

Jo Hobbs and Suzanne Wildman

CHAPTER CONTENTS

INTRODUCTION

The management and maintenance of the theatre environment are of prime importance in a situation where patients, already weakened by their existing condition, are further subjected to procedures that may be painful, bewildering and traumatic.

The main focus in running an efficient operating theatre is on maintaining a good aseptic technique. This must be applied not only to the more obvious care of instruments, preparation of the surgical site and scrubbing-up techniques, but also to the daily routine of maintaining the hygiene of the theatre and associated preparation areas and to the personal hygiene of all who work in the area. It takes very little upset in any of the procedures to compromise asepsis and introduce infection, which could in turn lead to wound breakdown, systemic infection, reduced surgical success rate and, inevitably, an effect on the reputation of the practice.

It is usually the responsibility of the veterinary nurse to organize all matters concerned with the operating theatre and its efficient function, and it is to the nurse and his or her management routines that the veterinary surgeon will turn if things go wrong.

STERILIZATION

Sterilization can be defined as the process by which instruments and drapes are rendered aseptic (or sterile) by the destruction or removal of all microorganisms, including spores. This can be achieved by various methods, including:

- Heat sterilization: hot-air oven, autoclave
- Cold sterilization: ethylene oxide, radiation.

Boiling cannot be considered a method of sterilization because it does not reach a high enough temperature to destroy bacterial spores.

Chemical solutions based on chlorhexidine or glutaraldehyde will kill bacteria if items are soaked in them, but should only be considered as a method of disinfection.

Hot-Air Oven

Hot-air ovens produce a dry heat. Microorganisms are more resistant to dry heat, so high working temperatures are required for a long period of time (Table 7.1). Long cooling periods are also required, and the very high temperatures may damage metal items. A safety device should be fitted to the door to prevent accidental

TABLE 7.1 Hot-air ovens: working temperature and time requirements

Item	Temperature (°C)	Time (min)
Glassware and non-cutting instruments	180	60
Powders and oils	160	120
Sharp cutting instruments	150	180

opening before the oven is cool. Care should be taken not to overload the oven, as air will be unable to circulate freely.

Use of the hot-air oven is limited due to the long period of time required for sterilization and cooling. However, hot-air ovens are useful for items damaged by moist heat such as glassware, powders, oils and sharp cutting instruments.

Autoclave

This is the most common method of sterilization used in veterinary practice. In normal circumstances, water cannot reach temperatures greater than 100°C (boiling point) before producing steam. If water is boiled under pressure, the boiling point is raised, so the temperature of the steam is greater. This steam penetrates to the innermost layer of the packs being sterilized. Care should be taken to avoid overloading or blocking the inlet and outlet valves of the autoclave. Items to be sterilized should be free from grease and protein to achieve effective penetration of the steam.

The majority of autoclaves designed for modern veterinary practice incorporate a drying cycle. Steam is exhausted and replaced by filtered air, which dries the packs (Table 7.2).

Autoclaves are used for sterilizing instruments, drapes, gowns and swabs.

TABLE 7.2 Autoclaves: working temperature, time and pressure requirements

Pressure (kg/cm²)	Pressure (psi)	Temperature (°C)	Time (min)
1.2	15	121	12
1.4	20	126	10
2	30	134	3.5

Ethylene Oxide

Ethylene oxide gas sterilizes by inactivating DNA in the cells of the pathogen, thus rendering them inactive and preventing their replication. It is, however, toxic, irritant to tissues and inflammable. To comply with Control of Substances Hazardous to Health (COSHH) regulations, the manufacturer's instructions must be followed.

The ethylene oxide unit contains a ventilation system and should be located in a well-ventilated area. Room temperature must be kept at a minimum of 20°C during the sterilization cycle.

Procedure: Use of the ethylene oxide sterilizer

1. **Action:** Place individually packed items into a polythene liner bag (refer to the manufacturer's instructions).
   Rationale: Specific liner bags allow the diffusion of gas through their membrane.
2. **Action:** Place a scored ampoule containing ethylene oxide liquid inside the liner bag and seal the bag with a tie.
   Rationale: The bag must be sealed to keep the gas circulating around the contents.
3. **Action:** Put the liner bag into the sterilizer unit.
4. **Action:** Snap the ampoule from outside the bag to release the gas.
   Rationale: To minimize exposure to gas.
5. **Action:** Close and lock the door to the sterilizer unit and turn the ventilator on.
   Rationale: Accidental opening of the unit can be prevented if the unit is locked.
6. **Action:** In some units, the pump may need to be turned on manually after 12 hours.
   Rationale: This aerates the unit to make it safe for the operator to open.
7. **Action:** Two hours after aerating, remove sterilized items.
   Rationale: This will ensure that any toxic gas has been removed.

Sterilization by ethylene oxide is suitable for anaesthetic tubing, endotracheal tubes, endoscopic equipment, optical instruments, plastic items, laparoscopic surgical equipment and high-speed and battery-operated drills.

Everyday items such as instruments, gowns and drapes may also be sterilized in this manner.

Radiation

Sterilization is achieved using gamma irradiation. It can only be carried out under controlled conditions within an industrial context. Many prepackaged items used in practice, such as needles, syringes and catheters, are sterilized in this way.

Monitoring the efficacy of sterilization

It is essential that the effectiveness of any sterilization method is constantly monitored to ensure that all microorganisms, including bacterial spores, are destroyed. Different sterilization methods require different working conditions in terms of time and temperature. It is also important to choose the correct method of monitoring the efficacy of sterilization (Table 7.3).

Packing materials for sterilization

There are several types of packaging materials available for the preparation of items to be sterilized. Selection will depend largely on the method of sterilization but factors such as cost and personal preference may also be taken into account (Table 7.4).

Procedure: Packing surgical items for sterilization

1. **Action:** Select the appropriate packaging material for the chosen method of sterilization.
   Rationale: A packing material that is non-permeable to steam would not be suitable for an autoclave.
2. **Action:** Select the correct size of packaging for the item or surgical kit.
   Rationale: This will reduce cost.
3. **Action:** Label the pack with the contents.
   Rationale: This will save opening incorrect packs, which would then require re-sterilization.
4. **Action:** Write the date of sterilization on the pack.
   Rationale: Sterilized items should be repackaged and sterilized again if not used within 3 months.
5. **Action:** The initials of the person preparing the pack should be included.
   Rationale: This allows any problems with the packing to be traced.
6. **Action:** Ensure that the tips of sharp instruments are adequately protected.
   Rationale: To prevent the piercing of packaging material.

TABLE 7.3 Methods of monitoring the efficacy of sterilization

Method	Description	Use
Chemical indicator strips	Paper strips which change colour when the correct temperature and time have been reached. They are placed in the centre of the pack prior to sterilization.	Autoclave – select the correct strip for the cycle Ethylene oxide
Browne's tubes	Small glass tubes filled with an orange liquid which turns green when the correct temperature is reached and maintained for the correct time.	Autoclave Hot-air oven
Bowie-Dick indicator tape	A beige tape impregnated with chemical stripes that change to black when the correct temperature has been reached (121°C). It does not indicate that the pack has been exposed for the correct time; therefore, it is not a reliable method.	Autoclave
Ethylene oxide tape	As above, only the tape is green with lines that change to red on exposure to ethylene oxide.	Ethylene oxide
Spore strips	Strips of paper impregnated with spores (usually *Bacillus stearothermophilius*) are placed in the load. After sterilization, they are cultured for 72 hours. Provided that sterilization has been achieved, no growth will be visible. This is an accurate method, although the delay in obtaining the results is a major disadvantage.	Autoclave Ethylene oxide Hot-air oven
Thermocouples	Electrical leads with temperature-sensitive tips that are placed in the autoclave with the leads passed out and attached to a recording device. The temperature is checked throughout the cycle, and the results are recorded.	Autoclave

TABLE 7.4 Packing materials for sterilization

Packing material	Advantage	Disadvantage	Method of sterilization
Self-seal pouches	Easy to pack Clear front to view contents Paper back with sterilization indicator Ideal for individual instruments	Can be punctured by heavy or sharp instruments (double packing will prevent puncturing but increase the cost)	Autoclave Ethylene oxide
Nylon film	Cheap May be reused Sealed with Bowie-Dick tape	Repeated use leads to brittleness and can cause tiny holes, which can go unnoticed	Autoclave
Polythene bags supplied by ethylene oxide manufacturers	Easy to pack Strong	Overpacking can lead to poor gas circulation	Ethylene oxide
Linen drapes	Conforming Used to pack surgical equipment Strong Reusable	Permeable to moisture Require laundering Liable to wear	Autoclave (with a drying cycle) Ethylene oxide (if not too tightly packed)
Paper drapes	Water-repellent Disposable Used to pack surgical equipment	Non-conforming Can tear easily	Autoclave (with a drying cycle) Ethylene oxide (if not too tightly packed)

TABLE 7.4   Packing materials for sterilization—cont'd

Packing material	Advantage	Disadvantage	Method of sterilization
Metal tins	Long-lasting Useful for gowns, drapes, swabs, instruments Cannot be punctured	Expensive to buy Require a large autoclave Often multi-use, which may lead to contamination of contents	Autoclave (with a drying cycle) Hot-air oven
Cardboard cartons	Reusable Cannot be punctured easily Sturdy Useful for specialized kits	Expensive to buy Bulky to store	Autoclave (with a drying cycle)

Packing drapes for sterilization

When preparing a drape for sterilization, the aim is to ensure that all parts are sterilized evenly, and that when the drape is handled by the surgical team, it will unfold easily. This can be achieved by either folding the drape in a concertina fashion widthways or lengthways. Both methods are illustrated in Fig. 7.1.

When folding a fenestrated drape, it is important to use a similar method to that for a plain drape but the fenestration should end up on top of the drape so it can be clearly identified in the sterilization packaging.

MAINTAINING THE THEATRE ENVIRONMENT

It is vital to have a strict cleaning regime in the operating theatre and preparation room to maintain a high standard of asepsis. Both daily and weekly cleaning procedures are essential. In addition to this, there are some general rules for maintaining asepsis in the theatre (Table 7.5).

Procedure: Daily cleaning routine

1. **Action:** Damp-dust all surfaces and equipment using disinfectant.
   Rationale: Using a dry cloth would merely move dust around the room.
2. **Action:** Wipe the table and surfaces with disinfectant in between patients. Clean the floor if it is soiled.
   Rationale: This prevents cross-contamination from one patient to the next.
3. **Action:** Remove used instruments and drapes after each procedure.
   Rationale: To avoid contaminating the next surgical site.

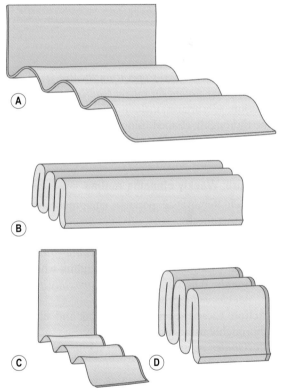

Fig. 7.1 Folding surgical drapes. A, Concertina cloth widthways. B, Pack cloths in autoclave bags. C, Concertina lengthways. D, Pack cloths in autoclave bags. (Redrawn from Cooper, Mullineaux and Turner (2011), BSAVA.)

4. **Action:** At the end of the day, vacuum to remove debris and hair.
   Rationale: Fine particles will be collected more efficiently using a vacuum.
5. **Action:** All waste material and soiled equipment must be removed.

TABLE 7.5 Maintaining an aseptic theatre

Action	Rationale
1. The least number of people should be present and movement kept to a minimum	1. Any movement will increase the risk of wound contamination by airborne particles
2. Personnel must wear the correct theatre attire at all times	2. This will avoid contamination from clothing, skin and hair
3. Clip and disinfect the patient away from the theatre	3. Hair and debris would contaminate the theatre
4. Use a new set of instruments for each surgical procedure	4. Cross-contamination between patients must be avoided
5. Carry out 'clean' operations before contaminated procedures	5. Contamination from high-risk procedures should then not occur
6. Discard any instrument that becomes contaminated	6. The remaining surgical instruments must remain aseptic
7. If asepsis is broken by any member of the surgical team, it must be rectified	7. Further contamination can then be avoided

Rationale: The warm operating theatre is an ideal breeding ground for microorganisms.

6. **Action:** All surfaces, including lights and sinks, must be thoroughly cleaned using disinfectant.
   Rationale: Contaminated dust particles will settle on all surfaces and must be removed.

Procedure: Weekly cleaning routine

1. **Action:** Remove all portable equipment from the operating theatre.
   Rationale: Dirt and debris quickly build up in less accessible areas such as those behind equipment.
2. **Action:** Clean the equipment, including wheels.
   Rationale: Wheels soon fail to run smoothly if they are not cleaned regularly.
3. **Action:** Clean the ceiling, walls, floor and all fixtures thoroughly using disinfectant.
   Rationale: Disinfecting will ensure a cleaner environment.
4. **Action:** Use separate cleaning equipment for the operating theatre.
   Rationale: This will minimize cross-contamination from other areas of the veterinary practice.

HAND CLEANING

A general hand-washing procedure following the WHO guidelines (Fig 7.2) should be carried out at the beginning of the day and then repeated at intervals throughout the day.

Prior to the first surgical procedure of the day, a full surgical scrub lasting up to 10 minutes is carried out,

then a shorter scrub may be carried out in between subsequent procedures, provided there has been no major contamination of the hands.

Before beginning any hand-washing procedure, all jewellery and watches must be removed. Nails should be short and free from varnish. If you wear a wedding ring, it is acceptable to wash thoroughly around and under it – the ring must be easily movable to do this. If the ring is too tight to move, you should remove it entirely. All other rings must be removed.

Procedure: Surgical scrub (Fig. 7.3)

The surgical scrub is performed to reduce the levels of both resident and transient microbes on the hands, as it is not possible to sterilize the skin.

The correct equipment should be prepared in advance so the complete process from scrubbing to gowning and gloving can be carried out in an aseptic manner.

The equipment required:
* Sink with elbow, knee or foot controls
* Liquid soap
* Skin disinfectant solution
* Disposable orange stick for cleaning under fingernails
* Sterile scrubbing brush (these may be prepackaged with scrub solution)
* Sterile material for drying hands
1. **Action:** Turn on the tap to produce a gentle stream of water.
   Rationale: A gentle stream will minimize splashing.

Duration of entire procedure: 20–30 seconds

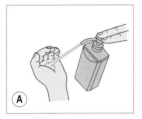

A

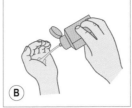

B

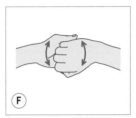

C

Apply a palmful of the product in a cupped hand, covering all surfaces

Rub hands palm to palm

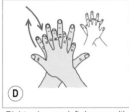

D

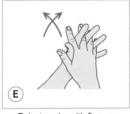

E

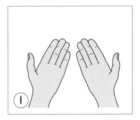

F

Right palm over left dorsum with interlaced fingers and vice versa

Palm to palm with fingers interlaced

Backs of fingers to opposing palms with fingers interlocked

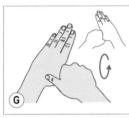

G

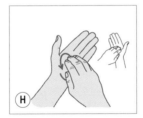

H

I

Rotational rubbing of left thumb clasped in right palm and vice versa

Rotational rubbing, backwards and forwards with clasped fingers of right hand in left palm and vice versa

Once dry, your hands are safe

Fig. 7.2 Hand hygiene technique with alcohol-based formulation. (Reproduced with permission from the World Health Organization (2009).)

2. **Action:** Keeping forearms higher than the elbows at all times, wet the arms and hands and apply liquid soap to all surfaces.
   Rationale: *It is important to keep the hands above the elbows to avoid recontamination.*

3. **Action:** Work the soap into a lather and spread over the hands and arms to 5 cm above the elbow.
   Rationale: *Any surface dirt and grease will be removed.*

4. **Action:** With the fingers under the stream of water, clean the nails with an orange stick.
   Rationale: *To ensure the area under the nails is as clean as possible.*

5. **Action:** Repeat step 3 using a surgical scrub solution.

6. **Action:** Take a sterile brush, moisten it under the stream of water and apply the surgical scrub solution.

7. **Action:** Scrub the nails using a straight stroke. Make sure the bristles of the brush clean under the nails.

8. **Action:** Starting with the little finger, scrub each of the four planes of each finger in straight strokes. Continue to scrub the palm of the hand using a circular motion.
   Rationale: *To ensure all skin surfaces are cleaned.*

9. **Action:** Wash the back of the hand and arm.

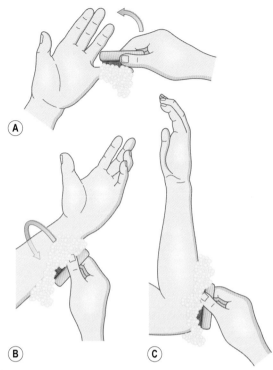

Fig. 7.3 The surgical scrub sequence. A, Starting with the little finger and working across to the thumb, scrub each surface of each digit. B, Scrub the forearm, again scrubbing the entire circumference. C, Scrub elbow area to 5 cm above the elbow, including all surfaces.

>   *Rationale: Care must be taken not to scrub these*
>   *areas, as the skin is more delicate, and therefore*
>   *susceptible to excoriation and infection.*

10. **Action:** If using two brushes, discard the first brush into the sink and take the second brush in the scrubbed hand. If not, rinse the brush and add scrub solution before transferring to the other hand.
    Rationale: Once one hand is scrubbed, it must not be re-contaminated, otherwise the procedure must be repeated.
11. **Action:** Repeat the process for the remaining hand and forearm.
    Rationale: Use the same method to ensure that no part of the skin is missed.
12. **Action:** Maintaining the hands above the elbows, rinse both hands thoroughly and allow the water to drain into the sink.
    Rationale: To prevent contamination.

13. **Action:** Repeat the above procedure, but this time do not include the elbows.
    Rationale: This ensures that the hands and arms are as clean as possible.
14. **Action:** Rinse hands, then dry them using a sterile towel.
    Rationale: Using a sterile towel will prevent contamination.
15. **Action:** Using separate quarters of the towel, dry each hand and arm.
    Rationale: By using a separate quarter for each hand and arm, a degree of asepsis is maintained.

Newer personnel surgical skin preparation regimes using products such as Sterillium are becoming popular in veterinary practices. Manufacturer instructions should be adhered to when using these products.

THEATRE ATTIRE

In order to achieve asepsis, specific theatre attire should be worn by the surgical team (Table 7.6).

Procedure: Folding a surgical gown for sterilization (Fig. 7.4)

1. **Action:** Lay the gown flat on a clean work surface with the inside of the gown face down.
    Rationale: In this position, all creases can be removed, ties identified and sleeves straightened. The outer surface of the gown will be folded in so that ungloved hands will not contaminate it when it is put on.
2. **Action:** Fold one side of the gown into the centre, tucking the ties in.
    Rationale: Ties must be tucked in to avoid accidental contamination when gowning.
3. **Action:** Fold the other side of the gown right across to the other side, also tucking ties in.
    Rationale: This enables the gown to be folded neatly into a sterile pack but still unfold easily when put on.
4. **Action:** Making sure that the inside collar of the gown is on top, concertina the rest of the gown lengthways until it is the size required to fit into the sterilizing pack.
    Rationale: This enables the gown to be picked up by the inside shoulders and allowed to unfold gently.

TABLE 7.6	**Theatre attire**
Item	**Description**
Scrub suits	A top and trousers worn only in the operating room. The top should be tucked into the trousers, and the trousers should either have cuffed legs or be tucked into surgical boots. They should be changed daily or more often if soiled. Sterilize periodically.
Footwear	Shoes or boots designed to be non-slip, antistatic, comfortable and easily cleanable. Not to be worn outside the theatre. Alternatively, shoe covers may be used.
Headwear	Hair can be a major source of contamination, so it should be completely covered in the operating room. There are various types of theatre hats available, some paper-based and designed to be single-use, and others lint-free and machine-washable.
Face masks	Face masks filter air from the nose and mouth but must be close-fitting to avoid bacteria entering the surgical environment through the sides of the mask. They should be changed between operations.
Surgical gowns	Surgical gowns are sterile and worn over the scrub suit. Ideally, they should be long-sleeved with cuffs. Both reusable and disposable gowns are available. Reusable gowns require the correct folding technique prior to sterilization in order for the veterinary surgeon to put the gown on in an aseptic manner.
Surgical gloves	Surgical gloves should be worn for all surgical procedures. They come prepacked in a variety of sizes and are sterile. Gloves without powder are recommended because the powder acts as a foreign body and may cause wound-healing problems.

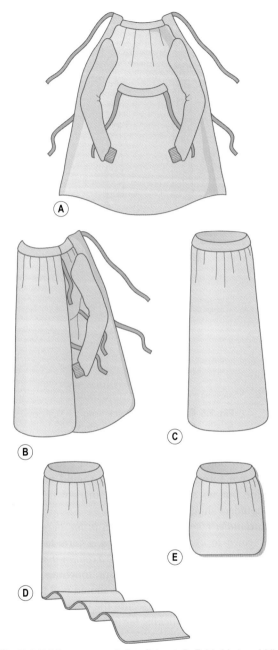

Fig. 7.4 Folding a gown. A, Lay flat out. B, Fold side to middle. C, Fold over other side of edge. D, Concertina lengthways. E, Pick up by inside of collar after autoclaving. (Redrawn from Cooper, Mullineaux and Turner (2011), BSAVA.)

Procedure: Putting on a back-tying surgical gown (Fig. 7.5A)

1. **Action:** Remove the sterile gown from its pack, hold it by the shoulders and allow it to unfold gently.

Rationale: Holding the gown correctly allows the sleeves to be clearly identified, and the act of unfolding it gently minimizes air movement and the risk of contaminating the gown.

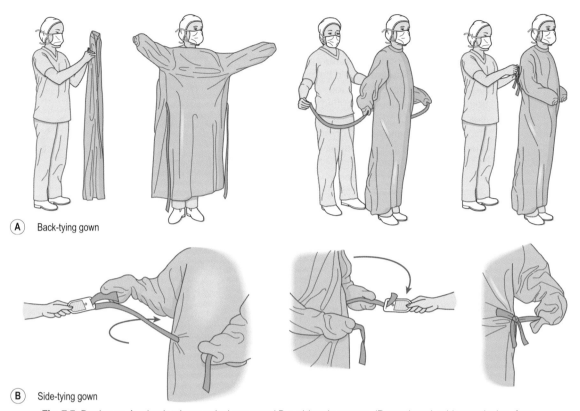

(A) Back-tying gown

(B) Side-tying gown

Fig. 7.5 Putting on A, a back-tying surgical gown and B, a side-tying gown. (Reproduced, with permission, from Martin and Masters (2007), Butterworth-Heinemann.)

2. **Action:** Slip one hand into each sleeve and push up to but not through the cuff. Arms should be opened wide but no attempt to adjust the gown over the shoulders should be made.
   Rationale: Hands should remain in the sleeves of the gown to avoid contamination. Efforts to pull the gown over the shoulders create a contamination risk.
3. **Action:** An unscrubbed assistant, touching only the inside of the back of the gown, should pull the gown over the shoulders and secure the ties at the back.
   Rationale: Only touching the inside of the gown maintains sterility.
4. **Action:** With hands still inside the gown sleeves, pick up the waist ties and hold them out to the sides. The assistant should grasp the ends and secure them at the back, taking care not to *touch any part of the gown.*
   Rationale: The back of the gown is now considered non-sterile and should not come into contact with any sterile equipment or drapes.

Procedure: Putting on a side-tying gown (Fig. 7.5B)

1. **Action:** Follow points 1–3 above.
2. **Action:** Keeping hands within the sleeves, pass the side tie (which is attached to a paper tape) to the assistant.
   Rationale: There is no risk of contamination if the hands are kept inside the sleeves.
3. **Action:** The assistant passes the tie around the gown. Take the tie back, leaving the assistant holding the paper tape, and secure the gown at the side.
   Rationale: The assistant has not contaminated the gown because he or she has only held the paper tape. The gown is now sterile all the way around, not just at the front, as with the previous method.

Procedure: Closed gloving (Fig. 7.6)

1. **Action:** Keeping the hands inside the sleeves of the gown, turn the glove packet so that the fingers face towards the body.

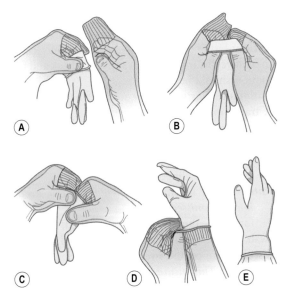

Fig. 7.6 Closed gloving technique. (Reproduced, with permission, from Martin and Masters (2007), Butterworth-Heinemann.)

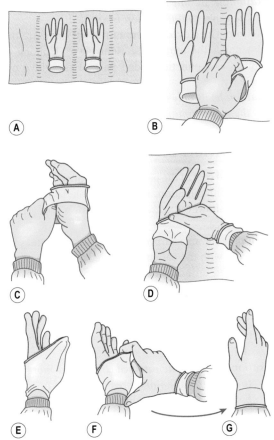

Fig. 7.7 Open gloving technique. (Reproduced, with permission, from Martin and Masters (2007), Butterworth-Heinemann.)

Rationale: The risk of contamination is minimized because the outsides of the gloves do not have the opportunity to come in contact with the skin.

2. **Action:** Pick up the right glove (which is on the left) by the rim of the cuff with the right hand.
   Rationale: By turning the glove packet round, the right glove is on the left and vice versa.

3. **Action:** Turn the hand over so that the palm is upwards, with the fingers of the glove facing towards the body.
   Rationale: The glove will be in the correct position to be pulled on.

4. **Action:** Using the left hand, grasp the other rim of the glove and pull it over the right hand until it covers the cuff of the gown.
   Rationale: Both hands remain within the sleeves of the gown to prevent contamination of the outer surface of the gloves.

5. **Action:** The left hand, within the sleeve of the gown, can adjust the fingers of the right glove until comfortable.
   Rationale: The glove must fit snugly but not too tightly.

6. **Action:** Pick up the left glove with the left hand and repeat the same process.
   Rationale: At no time will the hands come into contact with the outside of the gloves, thus preventing contamination.

Procedure: Open gloving (Fig. 7.7)

A disadvantage of using the open method of gloving is that the gloves may become contaminated by the skin.

1. **Action:** With the pack of gloves facing forward, pick up the right glove with the left hand, touching only the inner folded-down surface of the glove.
   Rationale: The inside of the glove may be touched freely because it will never come into contact with sterile items.

2. **Action:** Pull the glove on to the right hand, leaving the cuff folded back, and hook over the thumb.
   Rationale: This will avoid touching the contaminated inner surface with the gloved left hand when unfolding.

3. **Action:** Slide the gloved fingers of the right hand under the left cuff and pull onto the left hand.

Rationale: By only touching the sterile outer surface of the glove, contamination is avoided.

4. **Action:** The gloved fingers of the left hand are then slid under the fold of the right glove. Unhook the thumb and pull the folded part of the glove over the wrist.

   Rationale: By only touching the sterile outer surface of the glove, contamination is avoided.

PREPARATION OF THE SURGICAL SITE

The skin and coat of the patient are major sources of surgical site contamination. It is impossible to remove all pathogens; however, careful preparation will reduce their presence.

Clipping the area surrounding the surgical site is best carried out with the patient anaesthetized. If the patient is considered an anaesthetic risk, clipping the patient prior to induction can reduce anaesthetic time.

Procedure: Clipping

1. **Action:** Ensure the clippers are clean and in good working order.

   Rationale: Poorly maintained clippers are more likely to cause irritation and breaks in the skin surface, both of which can be contributing factors to surgical site infections.

2. **Action:** Initially clip in the same direction as hair growth, then clip in the opposite direction.

   Rationale: For a closer clip, cutting against the direction of the hair growth is most effective.

3. **Action:** Clip 10–20 cm beyond the line of the incision.

   Rationale: The surgeon will be able to safely extend the incision if necessary.

4. **Action:** If clipping around an open wound or near the eyes, apply an appropriate gel into/around the area.

   Rationale: Tiny hairs will act as foreign bodies in an open wound and are very difficult to remove. They cause intense irritation and are a source of contamination.

Procedure: Preparation of the skin

1. **Action:** Carry out steps 2–7 in the preparation area.

   Rationale: Contamination of the theatre is avoided.

2. **Action:** Put on examination gloves.

   Rationale: This will protect the patient's skin from being contaminated by the nurse's hands.

3. **Action:** Use a chlorhexidine or povidone-iodine solution.

Rationale: These both have antiseptic and detergent properties.

4. **Action:** Using lint-free swabs, clean the surgical site to remove dirt from the skin surface. A back and forth motion should be used.

   Rationale: This will ensure surface dirt is removed.

   A traditional method of surgical site preparation is described below.

5. **Action:** Starting at the incision site, clean the skin surface, working in a circular pattern out towards the edge of the clipped area.

   Rationale: By moving in a circular pattern, no area should be missed.

6. **Action:** Once the edge has been reached, discard the swab, select a fresh swab and repeat until there is no discoloration on the swab.

   Rationale: This ensures that dirt is not returned to the incision site.

7. **Action:** Wearing sterile gloves and using sterile swabs and scrub solution, repeat the scrub procedure described above.

   Rationale: Sterile equipment is used to create an environment that is as aseptic as possible.

8. **Action:** An alcohol solution of skin disinfectant is applied and left to dry on the skin.

   Rationale: The alcohol solution will provide residual bactericidal activity. Do not apply to open wounds or mucous membranes. Do not use diathermy if an alcohol solution has been applied.

Chlorhexidine gluconate and isopropyl alcohol preparations such as Chloraprep are starting to become widely used for preparing surgical sites. An initial scrub takes place (as in points 1–8 above), and the patient is then moved to theatre, where the solution is applied via an applicator in a back and forth motion for 30 seconds and allowed to dry.

DRAPING THE PATIENT

The patient is draped to maintain asepsis during surgery. A member of the surgical team who is gowned and gloved is responsible for draping the patient. See Table 7.7 for commonly used draping materials.

Procedure: Draping with four plain drapes (Fig. 7.8)

1. **Action:** Pick up the first drape and allow it to unfold away from any surfaces in the room.

   Rationale: The sterile drape must not be allowed to become contaminated by touching a non-sterile surface.

TABLE 7.7 Types of drape

Drape	Advantages	Disadvantages	Comments

Disposable	Water-resistant
	Prepacked and folded
	Presterilized
	Will prevent strike-through
	Lint-free
	Always in perfect condition
		Expensive
		Less conforming
		Large stock required
		Less accurate fenestration
		  size
			Can be used under or over a cloth drape
			Ideal for surgery where fluid is likely to be
			  present
			Can be secured with sterile spray or may
			  be self-adhesive

Reusable	Cheaper
	Conforming
	Required size fenestration
	  using four plain drapes
		Porous, which can lead to
		  strike-through
		Labour-intensive: washing and
		  drying
		Become poor-quality with
		  repeated use
		Require an autoclave with an
		  effective drying cycle
			Secured to the skin with towel clips: if the
			  tips puncture the cloth they are no longer
			  sterile and must be replaced

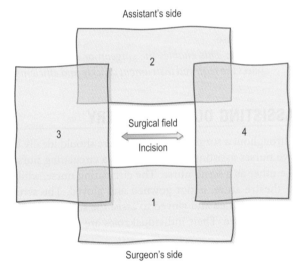

Fig. 7.8 Draping with four plain drapes. (Redrawn from Ackerman (2016), Elsevier.)

2. **Action:** Fold back the edge of the drape underneath itself. This folded edge will be used to line the edge of the incision.
   Rationale: This will produce a double layer at the edge of the draped area, protecting it from strike-through.
3. **Action:** Apply the first drape on the surgeon's side.
   Rationale: This prevents contamination when leaning over the patient to place the subsequent drapes.
4. **Action:** Walking around the patient, place the second drape on the opposite side to the first drape. The third and fourth drapes are placed at either end of the surgical site.
   Rationale: Following this method will reduce the risk of contamination.
5. **Action:** Apply further drapes to cover any remaining exposed areas of the patient or table.
   Rationale: Following this method will reduce the risk of contamination.
6. **Action:** If not using self-adhesive drapes, then towel clips can be used to secure the drape to the patient.
   Rationale: This prevents the drapes from moving.

Procedure: Draping a limb (Fig. 7.9)

1. **Action:** Cover the lower part of the limb with a bandage and hold it upright. It may either be held by an assistant or secured to a transfusion stand.
   Rationale: The lower part of the limb is a source of contamination. The limb is held upright to allow further drapes to be placed.
2. **Action:** Place a plain drape over the patient and the opposite limb.
   Rationale: This reduces the risk of contamination from the rest of the body.
3. **Action:** Place a smaller drape on top of the initial drape and lower the limb.
   Rationale: The limb should only be in contact with the second drape.
4. **Action:** Wrap the second drape around the limb and secure with a towel clip.
   Rationale: The limb is now covered, avoiding contamination of the surgical site.

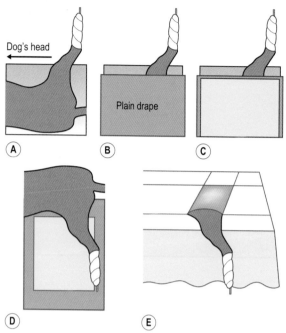

Dog's head

Plain drape

(A)   (B)   (C)

(D)   (E)

Fig. 7.9 Draping a limb for surgery. A, The lower limb is bandaged and attached by tape to a transfusion stand. B, A plain drape is laid over the body and the opposite limb of the patient. C, A smaller plain drape is laid on top of this. D, The tape is then cut and the limb lowered on to the inner drape. E, The drape is carefully wrapped around the limb and secured with a towel clip. Plain drapes or a fenestrated drape are then applied over the surgical site.

5. **Action:** Further drapes are placed around the surgical site.
   Rationale: The patient should now be fully draped, with only the surgical site visible.

Procedure: Draping with a fenestrated drape

1. **Action:** Pick up the drape and, holding it by the edge, allow it to unfold away from the trolley or table.
   Rationale: This prevents contact of the drape with non-sterile surfaces. If asepsis is broken, discard the drape and start again.
2. **Action:** Place the fenestration over the surgical site.
   Rationale: The 'window' cut into the drape allows visualization of and access to the surgical site.
3. **Action:** Secure the drape with towel clips at each corner.
   Rationale: This prevents the drape from moving.

INSTRUMENTATION

Preparation of the Instrument Trolley

The instrument trolley should be prepared immediately prior to use. If there is a delay in the start of surgery, the instruments must be covered with a sterile drape to minimize the risk of contamination from the environment.

The instrument trolley will not be sterile. It should be covered with a waterproof sterile drape, followed by a cloth drape, to prevent bacterial strike-through in the event that the trolley gets wet.

Procedure: Laying out an instrument trolley

1. **Action:** Identify the instruments and equipment required for the surgical procedure to be carried out.
   Rationale: Having all equipment prepared in advance can reduce surgical and anaesthetic time.
2. **Action:** Place the instruments on to the trolley in order of use.
   Rationale: This enables the surgeon or scrub nurse to select the required instrument quickly and efficiently.

ASSISTING DURING SURGERY

Throughout a surgical procedure there should ideally be two nurses assisting – one acting as a circulating nurse, the other as a scrub nurse. The circulating nurse, whilst in theatre attire, is not gowned and gloved. The scrub nurse is gowned and gloved to assist the surgeon during the procedure. Their individual roles are as follows:

The Circulating Nurse

- Assist in the preparation of the theatre, instruments and equipment.
- Adjust and tie the gowns of the surgical team.
- Position the patient on the operating table.
- Prepare the surgical site.
- Connect equipment such as diathermy and suction.
- Unwrap suture material and extra equipment required.
- Record suture material and swabs used.
- Assist the anaesthetist if required.
- Prepare and apply post-operative dressings when necessary.
- Maintain the cleanliness of the theatre in readiness for the next procedure.

The Scrub Nurse

- Prepare the instrument trolley.
- Pass instruments to the surgeon as required.
- Swab as required.
- Remove soiled instruments or swabs from the surgical area.
- Retract tissue and cut sutures when required.
- Count swabs, needles and sutures as they are used and at the end of surgery.

Procedure: Handling and passing instruments

1. **Action:** Identify the procedure being performed.
   Rationale: The surgeon's instrument requirements can then be anticipated.
2. **Action:** Pass ringed instruments into the palm of the surgeon's hand with the points outwards and curves upwards.
   Rationale: The instrument is then ready for use, and sharp points or blades will not damage the surgical gloves.
3. **Action:** After use, clean with a swab and replace in the same position on the trolley.
   Rationale: If they are returned to the correct position on the trolley, instruments can quickly be found next time they are required.

Procedure: Swabbing

1. **Action:** Count all swabs before and during surgery.
   Rationale: It is essential to keep a record of all swabs used.
2. **Action:** Use a blotting action when swabbing tissue.
   Rationale: Do not use a wiping motion, as this will remove clots which have formed to control haemorrhage, and bleeding may restart.
3. **Action:** Dispose of used swabs.
   Rationale: Do not leave them on the trolley or at the surgical site because they may allow strike-through.
4. **Action:** Count all swabs before the incision is closed.
   Rationale: This ensures that none are accidentally left in the wound.

CARE AND MAINTENANCE OF SURGICAL INSTRUMENTS

Surgical instruments are commonly made of either chromium-plated carbon steel or stainless steel. Tungsten carbide inserts are often added to the tips of stainless steel instruments to increase strength and resistance to wear. Instruments with tungsten carbide inserts can be identified by their gold-coloured handles.

Good-quality instruments are expensive but will last for many years if they are handled and maintained correctly.

Procedure: Cleaning and maintaining instruments

1. **Action:** In accordance with COSHH regulations, protective clothing must be worn.
   Rationale: The risk of contamination by blood or tissue from a patient is minimized.
2. **Action:** Remove and dispose of any sharp items such as needles and scalpel blades.
   Rationale: To ensure safety of staff.
3. **Action:** Separate any delicate equipment.
   Rationale: These items should be cleaned separately to avoid damage.
4. **Action:** Rinse the instruments in cold water as soon as possible to remove blood and tissue.
   Rationale: Blood allowed to dry onto the instruments will lead to pitting of the instrument surface. Hot water should not be used because it causes coagulation of blood proteins.
5. **Action:** Soak the instruments in water containing a specified instrument-cleaning agent.
   Rationale: This cleans and decontaminates the instruments.
6. **Action:** Using a small brush, scrub each instrument, paying particular attention to serrations, joints and ratchets.
   Rationale: Debris may become trapped in these areas.
7. **Action:** The instruments may be put into an ultrasonic cleaner after manual cleaning, then thoroughly rinsed.
   Rationale: Ultrasonic cleaners are very efficient at removing debris that is inaccessible to manual cleaning.
8. **Action:** Dry the instruments thoroughly.
   Rationale: Water left in joints and ratchets may lead to corrosion.
9. **Action:** Inspect each instrument for damage, non-alignment of the tips or jaws, stiff hinges, bent ratchets, pitting, corrosion and loose screws. If any faults are identified, the instrument must be removed from the kit and either repaired or replaced.
   Rationale: Damaged instruments will be ineffective when used.

10. **Action:** Lubricate the instruments with a suitable preparation.

    Rationale: The life of the instruments will be prolonged, especially those with joints and ratchets.

SURGICAL KITS

It is common practice to have a number of surgical kits made up ready for use. Each kit should be clearly identified as to its contents. Colour-coded autoclavable plastic tape is often used to identify all the instruments belonging to the same kit. Fig. 7.10 illustrates some instruments commonly found in surgical kits.

CARE OF SPECIALIST EQUIPMENT

Diathermy

Diathermy is used either to cut or coagulate tissues. Unlike electrocautery, which uses an electric current to create a red-hot probe that is applied to the tissue, diathermy relies on alternating high-frequency currents to produce local heat at the site of application.

Monopolar or bipolar electrodes can be used to apply diathermy. Monopolar diathermy is used for cutting and coagulation and requires the patient to be 'earthed'. Bipolar diathermy allows more control over the depth and location of coagulation. It does not require the patient to be earthed, and it cannot be used for cutting.

Procedure: Diathermy

1. **Action:** Prepare the diathermy machine by placing a contact plate in a suitable position on the operating table. The plate should be connected to the diathermy machine.

   Rationale: This is done to 'earth' the patient. Contact gel can be applied to the plate before the patient is placed on to it. Alternatively, a rectal probe can be used. The current is transferred via the plate or probe to the ground. Electrical burns to the patient will then be avoided.

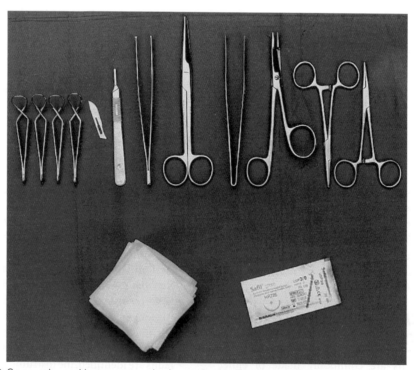

Fig. 7.10 Commonly used instruments: a basic suturing kit. Top (left to right): towel clips, scalpel blade and handle, rat-tooth forceps, Mayo scissors, dressing forceps, Gillies needle holders, Spencer Wells forceps. Bottom (left to right): swabs, suture materials. (Reproduced, with permission, from Bowden and Masters (2001), Butterworth-Heinemann.)

2. **Action:** Select the required electrodes. The cutting electrode can be a flat blade, scalpel blade or wire. A flat blade, ball electrode or dissecting forceps can be used to achieve coagulation diathermy. Dissecting forceps grasp the tissue, and the current is applied by touching the forceps with the electrode.
   Rationale: Selection of the correct electrode is required to ensure the required procedure can be performed.
3. **Action:** Do not prepare the surgical site with alcohol-based surgical solution.
   Rationale: Using an inflammable material such as alcohol in conjunction with diathermy is a fire hazard.
4. **Action:** Follow the manufacturer's instructions regarding sterilization, maintenance and operation of the unit.
   Rationale: Different components of the diathermy have specific maintenance requirements.

Cryosurgery

Cryosurgery is used to kill cells within a specific area with minimal damage to surrounding healthy tissue. This is achieved by the application of controlled extreme cold, as temperatures below $-20°C$ rapidly freeze the tissues, which eventually destroy the cells.

The patient may be required to have cryosurgery a number of times before the targeted cells are killed.

Procedure: Cryosurgery

1. **Action:** Wear protective clothing: apron, goggles and thick gloves. Avoid splashes.
   Rationale: Liquid nitrogen can cause severe cold burns.
2. **Action:** Prepare the surgical site aseptically. Surface lesions do not require asepsis; however, normal aseptic procedures should be carried out for deeper lesions.
   Rationale: This prevents infection of the site.
3. **Action:** Apply petroleum jelly to the tissues surrounding the site.
   Rationale: This protects surrounding healthy tissue from the effects of the freezing.
4. **Action:** After use, wash the probe in mild detergent.
   Rationale: A build-up of debris, particularly on the tip of the probe, can lead to corrosive deposits building up, which causes damage.
5. **Action:** Do not use corrosive or abrasive solutions when cleaning.

Rationale: These cause thinning of the metal components.
6. **Action:** Follow the manufacturer's instructions. Some probes may be sterilized.
   Rationale: Not all cryosurgery units can be sterilized.

Endoscopy

Endoscopy is the minimally invasive visual examination of an interior of a body cavity. A light source is used in combination with a series of optical lenses and mirrors.

Two types of endoscope are used in veterinary practice – rigid and flexible. They both contain fibre optic bundles and must be handled with care. It is important to note that individual manufacturer guidelines must be followed when cleaning endoscopes after use.

Procedure: General guidelines for cleaning an endoscope

1. **Action:** Wipe the endoscope immediately after use to remove gross contamination.
   Rationale: If not removed immediately after use, the endoscope parts may become damaged.
2. **Action:** A leak test should be performed prior to soaking.
   Rationale: Permanent damage may occur to the endoscope if cleaning liquid gets into the fibre optic bundle.
3. **Action:** Never immerse an endoscope in liquid unless the manufacturer's instructions specifically state that you can. Do not autoclave or place in a hot-air oven.
   Rationale: Considerable damage will occur to the delicate control section or light connector if liquid enters them.
4. **Action:** With the light source still attached, connect the water bottle and suction pump.
   Rationale: This will ensure effective cleaning of all parts.
5. **Action:** Prepare the recommended disinfectant.
   Rationale: This will ensure effective disinfection.
6. **Action:** With the tip of the endoscope in the solution, aspirate by depressing the suction button.
   Rationale: This ensures that patency is maintained.
7. **Action:** Clean the biopsy valve with a cotton bud and the biopsy channel with a specific cleaning brush, then clear rinse using suction.
   Rationale: This maintains patency of the biopsy channel.

8. **Action:** Disconnect the water bottle, block the water inlet and expel the water out of the channel by depressing the water/air button.

   Rationale: *Water must not be left inside the instrument, as it leads to deterioration of the working parts.*

9. **Action:** Wipe the insertion tube with lint-free swabs dampened with disinfectant. Rinse with clear water.

   Rationale: *Swabs must be lint-free to avoid leaving tiny threads.*

10. **Action:** Wipe the light guide tube with dampened swabs.

    Rationale: *Remove any residual disinfectant.*

11. **Action:** Apply an alcohol solution to the ocular lens and clean carefully.

    Rationale: *The alcohol will evaporate quickly without leaving smears.*

12. **Action:** Allow the endoscope to dry thoroughly by hanging it up on a secure hook.

    Rationale: *Any residual liquid will run downwards away from the controls.*

13. **Action:** Store in a carrying case or cabinet.

    Rationale: *This will protect the endoscope from damage.*

REFERENCES AND FURTHER READING

Ackerman, N., 2016. Aspinall's Complete Textbook of Veterinary Nursing, third ed. Elsevier, Oxford.

Aspinall, V., Aspinall, R., 2012. Clinical Procedures in Small Animal Veterinary Practice. Saunders, Oxford.

Cooper, B., Mullineaux, E., Turner, L., 2011. Textbook of Veterinary Nursing, fifth ed. BSAVA, Gloucester.

Martin, C., Masters, J., 2007. The Textbook of Veterinary Surgical Nursing. Butterworth-Heinemann, Edinburgh.

Tear, M., 2017. Small Animal Surgical Nursing, third ed. Elsevier Mosby, Missouri.

8

Surgical nursing procedures

Joanne Lee

CHAPTER CONTENTS

INTRODUCTION

It is outside the veterinary nurse's remit to diagnose a patient's condition but once a diagnosis has been made by a veterinary surgeon, it is often the responsibility of the veterinary nurse to manage the patient's condition by application of a dressing and bandage. If ever unsure of what is needed, refer to a more experienced colleague, be that a registered veterinary nurse or veterinary surgeon. Depending on the site and type of wound, the aim of bandaging is to cover and protect the area from contamination and the risk of infection, and to prevent the patient from interfering with the wound, both of which will delay the rate of healing. Bandaging is also used to immobilize fractured or dislocated bones to reduce discomfort and accelerate healing.

Many wounds will not require bandaging, and in some cases a bandage may draw the patient's attention to the area, leading to self-mutilation. This must be considered when deciding whether or not to apply a bandage. All wounds should be cleaned and dressed but every wound is different and should be assessed and treated as such. This chapter describes the steps involved in wound care and in applying the various types of bandages. It also covers the correct method of scaling and polishing an animal's teeth – a procedure that is often performed by the veterinary nurse.

WOUNDS AND WOUND MANAGEMENT

Wounds may heal by one of two ways:

First intention – the edges of the wound are close together, and there is little haemorrhage and no tissue loss. Epithelial cells and collagen slide across to form a strong join within a few days. Surgical, clean cuts and sutured wounds heal by this method.

Second intention – there is a gap between the cut edges, and there may be loss of tissue. Blood clots, inflammatory cells and collagen fill the gap and form a scab. Healing takes weeks or even months as the scab organizes and the wound contracts to pull the edges closer, enabling the epidermis to slide across from one side to another.

The rate of wound healing will be affected by:

- Movement
- Infection
- Tension
- Presence of foreign material
- Interference.

The purpose of a dressing is to provide an optimal environment for wound healing. There are many products on the market to promote moist wound healing. If desiccation (drying) of the wound surface occurs, this delays healing and may promote infection.

A bandage has multiple functions. These are to:

- Prevent nosocomial infections, i.e. those picked up during hospitalization
- Immobilize any fracture or dislocation to reduce pain and discomfort
- Prevent self-trauma
- Accelerate healing.

When a dressing and bandage have been applied, the patient should be kept under observation. Often, an Elizabethan collar is also required to prevent patient interference. If discharged into the care of the owner, dressing care instructions should be provided so that the owner knows how to care for the dressing and the potential problems that may occur.

Procedure: Wound management

1. **Action:** Ensure the patient is placed comfortably on soft bedding, either on a table or on the floor for larger patients.
   Rationale: Patient comfort and emotional wellbeing are the veterinary nurse's responsibility. If the patient is comfortable, it is less likely to resist.

2. **Action:** Ask a trained assistant to safely and humanely restrain the animal so that it is relaxed but secure, and so that the wound is accessible for treatment.
   Rationale: To prevent the patient harming itself or the veterinary nurse and prevent movement or

escape. The animal may resent the wound being touched.

3. **Action:** Wash your hands with a surgical scrub using the technique recommended by the World Health Organization (see Chapter 7, Fig. 7.2), and wear gloves and an apron. Consider changing gloves after lavage or if changing a heavily soiled dressing.
   Rationale: To prevent the introduction of infection into the wound.

4. **Action:** Control any haemorrhage (see Control of haemorrhage procedure in Chapter 9).
   Rationale: Haemorrhage should be controlled as a large loss of blood may cause hypovolaemic shock.

5. **Action:** Check for signs of shock and provide treatment (see Chapter 9).
   Rationale: Untreated, the patient's condition will deteriorate and could become life threatening.

6. **Action:** Assess the type of wound and treat accordingly (Table 8.1). Recognize signs of distress and act accordingly to minimize this.
   Rationale: Different types of wounds need different treatments, dressings and aftercare. A general anaesthetic/sedative may be necessary, and wound management can be painful, so appropriate pain management before, during and after the procedure needs to be considered.

7. **Action:** For open wounds, apply sterile aqueous jelly and clip hair away from around the wound.
   Rationale: The jelly prevents hair contamination. The hair is clipped to allow the area to be adequately cleaned.

8. **Action:** Clean the area surrounding the wound with a surgical scrub and warm water. Lavage the wound with copious amounts of warm, sterile isotonic solution by attaching a giving set to a bag of sterile fluid, connecting a three-way tap and a 20 ml syringe with an 18G needle. Apply a suggested pressure of 8 psi (Fig. 8.1). Continue until all debris has been flushed away.
   Rationale: The sterile fluid provides aseptic irrigation, whilst the pressure applied will remove foreign matter and contamination without forcing debris or bacteria into the wound. Isotonic solutions such as Hartmann's solution are a similar osmotic pressure to that of living cells, are non-toxic and do not cause cell rupture or electrolyte imbalance.

9. **Action:** Assess for devitalized, infected or contaminated tissue from the wound edge. If necessary, debridement can be carried out using a scalpel blade to remove necrotic tissue and expose healthy tissue.

TABLE 8.1	**Wound classification**	
Type	**Comments**	**Treatment**
Open wounds: There is a break in the covering of the body surface		
Incision	Clearly incised skin edges. Little trauma to surrounding tissue. Primary closure/first-intention healing is treatment of choice. Caused by sharp, cutting materials, e.g. scalpel or glass	Ensure that deeper structures are not damaged before wound closure. Wound edges held with little tension by sutures
Laceration	Torn skin edges, often caused by barbed wire or road traffic injury. Contamination and infection risk is high. The wound may heal by open healing/second-intention or delayed primary closure/third-intention healing	Determine appropriate dressing required which is dependent on wound. Wet-to-dry dressing may be needed to debride the wound in early stages. Closure may take place 2–3 days after presentation
Puncture	Often a bite/sting, stick injury or gunshot. Rapid healing on the surface may trap infection leading to abscess formation in the deeper tissues	If present, remove the cause of the injury. Keep the wound open to allow regular lavaging and dressing changes
Abrasion	Exposure of the underlying dermis tissue due to friction rubbing of the epidermis. Often caused by dragging in road traffic collisions. There is a risk of contamination of underlying tissues	Clean and dress the wound according to the degree of damage. Wet-to-dry dressings, which mechanically debride the wound and form a healthy tissue bed, may be indicated
Abscess	An accumulation of pus contained within an area of inflamed tissue. Often caused by puncture wound	The pus must be released from the tissue. The abscess should be lanced if not already burst. 'Pointing' is the thinning of the skin over the abscess site, and this is where lancing should occur. Express the pus. Lavage the wound with sterile saline until clear. Maintain the drainage by lavaging daily. The wound will heal by open healing/second-intention. Treatment with antibiotics may be indicated
Avulsion	Flap of skin partially separated by force from surrounding tissue. Often seen in road traffic accidents and dog fights	Assess the patient for any other injuries and assess the health of tissue for the possibility of delayed primary closure. Infection risk is high, so regular lavaging and dressing changes should be considered
Degloving	Tissue traumatically peeled off surrounding structure, similar to an avulsed wound. There may be damage to underlying tissue or bones	Assess the patient for any other injuries and assess the health of tissue for the possibility of closure or partial closure. Wet-to-dry dressings may be indicated to mechanically debride the wound and form a healthy tissue bed. Closure with surgical drain may need to be considered if there is a large area of dead space
Closed wounds: The injury does not penetrate the thickness of the skin		
Contusion	A bruise. Occurs when blood vessels are ruptured due to a blow to the skin surface. May also be seen in an open wound	Arrest the internal haemorrhage by applying a cold compress
Haematoma	A collection of blood under the skin causing swelling. The wound is soft and often painless. If left untreated, the blood will clot, contract and become 'knobbly'	Arrest the internal haemorrhage by applying a cold compress, and, if possible, apply a firm dressing. Surgical intervention may be necessary to drain the haematoma

Continued

TABLE 8.1	Wound classification—cont'd	
Type	**Comments**	**Treatment**
Other types		
Skin graft	A portion of skin is taken from one area of the body to fill a deficit in another part. There are two types: 1. A *pedicle graft* involves moving the entire skin thickness to another area. This heals by first-intention 2. A *free skin* graft involves transplanting the epidermis and part or all of the dermis. This heals by second-intention	Dress according to type
Ulcer	A local excavation of the surface of an organ or tissue. An ulcer contains inflammatory exudate within a crater. This heals by second-intention	Remove the cause of the injury and dress with a moist dressing, if anatomically possible. Treat bacterial infections
Tumour	Any abnormal swelling in or on part of the body that has no physiological use. May be benign or malignant	Before treatment, the type of tumour must be identified. Surgical intervention is often necessary
Fistula	A tract that passes from one skin surface to another and is lined with epithelial cells. Common sites are anal sacs as a result of infection, retrovaginal as a congenital abnormality and oronasally as a result of extraction of the upper canines	Treatment depends on the site. Surgical intervention may be required
Sinus	A blind-ending tract that runs from the skin surface to deep within a tissue. Often results from infection. Commonly caused by penetrating foreign bodies, e.g. grass seeds and anal furunculosis. Treatment depends on the cause	Remove foreign bodies surgically. Anal furunculosis may be treated by surgery, cryosurgery or by the use of immunosuppressant drugs
Hernia	A hole within a muscular wall that allows the passage of organs through it. May result in strangulation of the blood flow to the organs, which can become ischaemic and/or necrotic. Common sites are umbilical, inguinal and perineal	Surgical treatment to replace the organs, close the opening in the muscle and remove damaged tissue
Rupture	A tear within a muscular wall. Commonly seen within the diaphragm following a road traffic accident	Treat for shock and relieve pressure on the chest cavity by lifting the chest higher than the abdomen. Close the diaphragmatic tear surgically when the patient is stable

Rationale: Healthy tissue is needed to promote healing and minimize infection.

10. **Action:** Closure of the wound can take place if appropriate (Table 8.1). Suturing techniques are covered later in this chapter.

    Rationale: Primary closure/first-intention wound healing occurs with immediate closure of skin edges (usually with sutures). Open healing/second-intention healing occurs when closure is not possible. Healing is by granulation.

11. **Action:** Wounds treated with primary closure/first-intention healing should be dressed with a dry dressing. This should be covered with a primary layer of absorbent padding and then a secondary conforming bandage. Lastly, a tertiary layer of cohesive dressing should be applied for protection (Tables 8.2 and 8.3).

    Rationale: Application of this dressing will reduce swelling and seroma formation. The dry dressing will absorb any blood or exudate and will help protect the wound from infection and patient interference. It will also offer support, increasing patient comfort.

12. **Action:** Open healing/second-intention treatment of open wounds takes time and careful nursing.

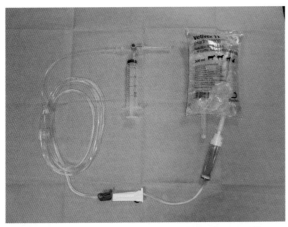

Fig. 8.1 Set-up of giving set and isotonic solution for wound lavage.

Accurate records should be kept for consistent management, and photographs should be taken, when possible, to record progression of wound healing. Daily dressing changes may be required with repeat lavaging, especially in the early stages, using wet-to-dry dressings (Table 8.2) for tissue debridement and to promote the development of granulation tissue.

> **Rationale:** *The wet-to-dry dressing will provide the ideal environment to promote a healthy bed for granulation and epithelialization, as well as debriding necrotic cells and contamination.*

13. **Action:** Once granulation has occurred, change the dressings to non-stick dressings (foam dressing), with a primary layer of absorbent padding, secondary layer of conforming bandage and tertiary layer

TABLE 8.2 Wound dressings

Type	Comments
Primary layer of most bandages is usually a wound dressing, which gives the wound the optimum conditions for healing. Materials may be as follows:	
Wet-to-dry dressings using lint or gauze	Soak the dressing in Hartmann's solution and apply to contaminated wounds. May be sutured into place. Allow to dry on the wound and then tear off under sedation or general anaesthesia to remove damaged and/or necrotic tissue, thereby debriding the wound and promoting granulation
Gamgee	A cotton-wool sheet covered on each side by gauze. Dry and non-sterile
Petroleum gauze	A moist dressing. Gauze impregnated with petroleum jelly. Inhibits epithelial growth
Perforated film dressing, e.g. Melolin	Absorbs exudate from lightly exuding wounds. Commonly used for surgical wounds (first-intention healing) over sutures
Foam dressing, e.g. Allevyn	A dry, sterile dressing that promotes a moist environment. Absorbs exudate; different dressings can absorb varying volumes of exudate, from low to high. Can combine with hydrogens or honey. Antimicrobial dressings are available that attack wound exudates and are useful in the treatment of MRSA
Hydrogels, e.g. Intrasite, Biodres	A moist gel, high in water content, applied into and onto the wound. Donates and transfers water
Hydrocolloids, e.g. Granuflex, Tagesorb	A moist, sterile dressing that rehydrates the wound and promotes debridement and granulation. Contraindicated in active infection
Calcium alginates, e.g. Kaltostat	A moist, haemostatic dressing derived from seaweed. A gel is formed over the wound that promotes wound healing by stimulating macrophages and fibroblasts
Semipermeable film dressing, e.g. Opsite, Bioclusive, Tegaderm	A sterile film dressing that retains moisture within the wound. No absorbency, but can be left in place for longer periods
Sodium chloride dressing (20% hypertonic saline)	Use on heavily infected, highly exudative wounds
Manuka honey	Available in impregnated dressing or alone in a tube. Bacteriostatic with a low pH
Silver-impregnated dressings	Broad-spectrum antimicrobial and effective against MRSA
Poultice	A dry dressing that is soaked in hot water and applied to a wound to draw out infection from the wound

MRSA, methicillin-resistant Staphylococcus aureus.

TABLE 8.3 Bandaging techniques

Type	Indications	Comments
Robert Jones	Support and immobilization of fore- and hindlimbs, commonly used in fractures. Reduction of pain, oedema and haemorrhage (Fig. 8.2)	A light but firm cylindrical bandage
Velpeau sling	Support and immobilization of the shoulder joint following luxation or surgery (Fig. 8.3)	
Ehmer sling	Support and immobilization of the hip following reduction of a luxation (Fig. 8.4)	
Ear	Support and protection of the ear following trauma, or post-operatively following resection or haematoma (Fig. 8.5)	One or both ears can be included. Ensure that the ear position is marked with a pen on the outer surface of the bandage
Chest	Support and protection of wounds and dressings. Useful for holding chest drains in place (Fig. 8.6)	
Limb	Support and protection of wounds, reduction of pain, swelling and movement (Fig. 8.7)	Ensure toes and dewclaws are padded. Work from distal to proximal. Include the whole foot and joint above the injury
Tail	Protection of wounds from environmental trauma and/or self-mutilation (Fig. 8.8)	Elastoplast may be applied directly to the hair to prevent this bandage from slipping
Ring	Indicated where there is a foreign body protruding from a wound. A ring bandage protects the wound while preventing further penetration by the object. Usually used in a first aid situation	Ready-made rings can be obtained. To make a ring, wind conforming bandage around your hand five times (size of ring depends on area of wound to be covered). Remove carefully, maintaining the ring shape, and wind the same bandage around the ring, creating a bound circle like a doughnut. Continue until you have the desired size and shape
Splint	Immobilization of an injury below the elbow or stifle	Limited to lower limbs. Immobilization cannot be achieved above the elbow and stifle due to the large mass of muscle that surrounds the bones. Application is often painful for the patient and is therefore limited to a first aid procedure. Common splints used in practice: Gutter splints – made of hard plastic, lined with foam and snapped off to the correct length Zimmer splints – made of pliable aluminium backed in a foam composite
Cast Permanent cast or bivalve cast	Immobilization of a limb	Common cast material: Plaster of Paris – bandage covered in gypsum (calcium sulphate) that sets hard when water is added Polyurethane-based and thermoplastic materials – lightweight, waterproof, short drying time and more radiolucent than plaster of Paris

of cohesive dressing (see Individual Bandaging Techniques, later).

Rationale: The primary layer absorbs any exudate; the secondary layer provides support; the tertiary layer acts as a protective outer layer, holding the others in place. Non-stick dressings are used to prevent disruption of the granulating tissue, absorb exudate and maintain a moist environment.

14. **Action:** Ensure that the dressing is comfortable and that the patient cannot interfere with it. An Elizabethan collar, topical sprays or supervised muzzling may be used. Observe for patient interference, odour, sores, discharge and slipping.

Rationale: Reasons for interference include the bandage being too tight (resulting in poor circulation and pain), sutures being too tight and boredom. Change the dressing when advised or if any concern arises.

15. **Action:** For dogs, protect from wet and dirt by covering with a bag when going outside for toileting purposes.

Rationale: Wet dressing material swells and can cause tissue compression and compromise tissue health.

16. **Action:** Explain the aftercare of the wound and dressing to the owner. Provide a dressing care leaflet to be referred to once the patient has returned home.

Rationale: If not monitored correctly, dressings themselves can cause tissue damage, so provide as much information to owners as possible so any problems can be spotted early.

Procedure: Bandaging techniques – general points

1. **Action:** Prepare all necessary equipment for the type of bandage being applied.

Rationale: Efficiency will allow you to complete the bandage without having to leave the animal.

2. **Action:** Ensure the patient is placed comfortably on soft bedding, either on a table or on the floor for larger patients.

Rationale: Patient comfort and emotional wellbeing are the veterinary nurse's responsibility. If the patient is comfortable, it is less likely to resist and try to escape.

3. **Action:** Ask a trained assistant to safely and humanely restrain the animal so that it is relaxed but secure, making sure the area for bandaging is accessible.

Rationale: The assistant will prevent the patient harming itself or the veterinary nurse and prevent movement or escape. The animal may resent the wound being touched.

4. **Action:** Apply a primary dressing to any wound that is present (Table 8.2).

Rationale: This layer is applied directly to the skin surface. It provides the optimal environment to encourage healing and protect the wound. Dressings can be moist or dry.

5. **Action:** Apply the bandage using a minimum of the three layers, as described previously. Check the tension of each layer.

Rationale: This will create a dressing with even tension. Excessive tension will be painful and delay healing.

6. **Action:** Ensure that the bandage is comfortable. Monitor the patient for interference, and monitor the affected area for odour, sores, discharge or slipping. An Elizabethan collar, topical sprays or supervised muzzling may be used.

Rationale: Interference can indicate the bandage is too tight, resulting in poor circulation. It also may indicate pain, sutures being too tight or boredom.

7. **Action:** Explain the aftercare of the wound and dressing to the owner. Provide a dressing care leaflet for them to refer to at home. Protect from wet and dirt by covering with a bag when outside. Change the dressing when advised, or if there are concerns over it.

Rationale: Dressing sores can cause prolonged healing for the patient and extra cost for the client. If the dressing gets wet, it may swell and constrict the tissues. It is important that owners know what to look out for.

INDIVIDUAL BANDAGING TECHNIQUES (TABLE 8.3)

Procedure: Robert Jones bandage

1. **Action:** Apply two strips of 2.5 cm-wide zinc oxide tape (or micropore tape if there are any concerns with skin integrity or allergies to zinc oxide tape) to the cranial and caudal aspect of the lower third of the limb. Allow another 10 cm of tape to overhang the toes, and gently stick to either side of a tongue depressor.

Rationale: These strips will later be included in the bandage and form the 'stirrups' (Fig. 8.2A). A tongue depressor facilitates easy separation later.

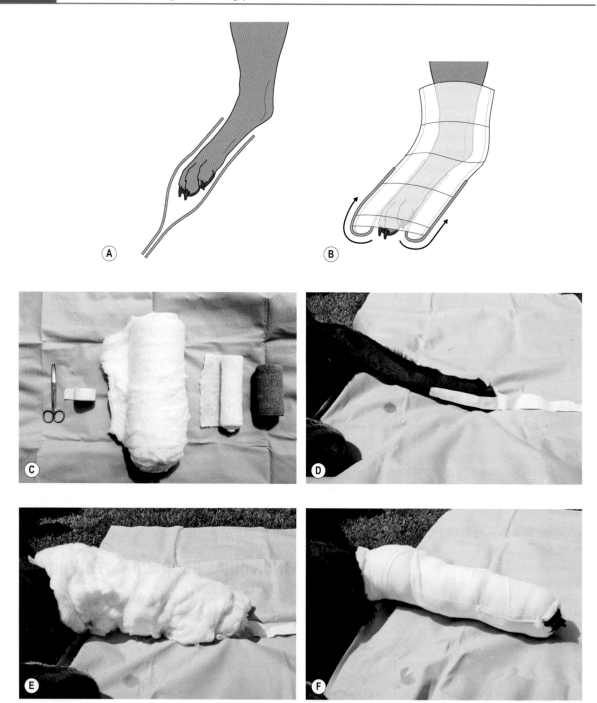

Fig. 8.2 The Robert Jones bandage. A, Stick the stirrups gently together. B, Stick the stirrups to the conforming bandage. C, Materials required for Robert Jones bandage. D, Zinc oxide tapes are applied to the limb to act as stirrups. E, Cotton wool is wrapped around the entire length of the limb. F, Conforming bandage is wrapped over the cotton wool, and the stirrups are twisted and stuck to the outside.

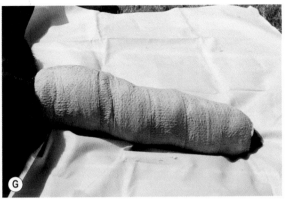
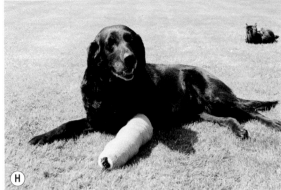

Fig. 8.2, Cont'd G, Cohesive bandage is applied as a protective layer. H, Patient with a correctly applied Robert Jones bandage.

2. **Action:** Apply cotton wool around the entire length of the limb. Pay particular attention to any bony prominences. Use at least three layers, depending on the size of the animal. Ensure that the cotton wool is of an even thickness throughout.
   Rationale: This layer provides the support. The greater the amount of cotton wool, the more immobilized the limb becomes. Larger animals will require more layers.
3. **Action:** Compress the cotton wool by bandaging firmly and evenly with a conforming bandage. Leave two toenails showing at the bottom.
   Rationale: Provides maximum support. The two toenails are used to assess circulation by checking the colour of the quick. It also may encourage the animal to use the limb to some degree.
4. **Action:** Continue applying conforming bandage until sufficient tension has been created.
   Rationale: The bandage should be approximately three times the width of the animal's leg. When it is 'flicked' with your finger, it should sound like a ripe melon.
5. **Action:** Separate the 'stirrup' tapes from each other. Twist the tape 180° and stick it to the conforming layer (Fig. 8.2B).
   Rationale: This will prevent the bandage from slipping down the limb.
6. **Action:** Apply a layer of cohesive bandage over the conforming bandage (Fig. 8.2C–H).
   Rationale: This will protect the other layers.

Procedure: Velpeau sling

1. **Action:** Apply cotton-wool padding to the carpal and metacarpal area of the affected limb.

   Rationale: This area will be held in flexion and needs to be padded for the comfort of the animal.
2. **Action:** Apply conforming bandage, appropriate to the animal's size, above the carpus for several turns (Fig. 8.3A).
   Rationale: This secures the bandage.
3. **Action:** Flex the elbow and shoulder and, at the same time, take the bandage over the shoulder, under the chest, medial to the other front leg and back to the carpus.
   Rationale: This will hold the shoulder and elbow in flexion against the body.
4. **Action:** Flex the carpus and include this in the bandage (Fig. 8.3B). Continue up over the shoulder and under the chest as before.
   Rationale: The carpus, elbow and shoulder should now be held in flexion against the chest.
5. **Action:** Continue in this manner until the whole limb is held securely.
   Rationale: The animal should not be able to move the limb, but make sure that the sling does not impede respiration.
6. **Action:** Apply a layer of cohesive bandage over the conforming bandage (Fig. 8.3C).
   Rationale: This will protect the other layers.

Procedure: Ehmer sling

1. **Action:** Apply cotton-wool padding to the metatarsal area of the affected limb.
   Rationale: This is the starting point of the sling and should be padded to provide comfort for the animal.

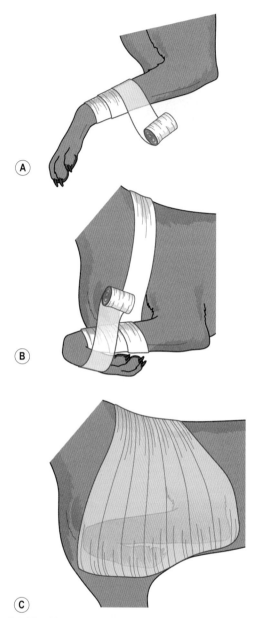

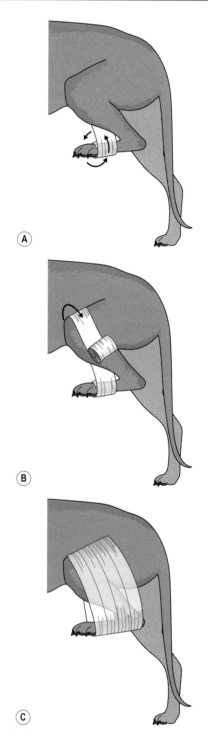

Fig. 8.3 The Velpeau sling. A, Wind the conforming bandage around the carpus. B, Flex the carpus. C, Apply a layer of cohesive bandage over the top.

2. **Action:** Apply conforming bandage, appropriate to the animal's size, around the padding for several turns (Fig. 8.4A). Ensure that the last bandage turn finishes on the lateral side of the metatarsals. *Rationale: This secures the bandage.*

Fig. 8.4 The Ehmer sling. A, Wind the bandage around the metatarsals. B, Bring the bandage over the lateral thigh. C, Apply a layer of conforming bandage.

3. **Action:** At this point, take the bandage up the medial aspect of the stifle, pad the top of the femur, and bring the bandage over to the lateral aspect of the thigh (Fig. 8.4B). The limb should be held in flexion.

   Rationale: This is halfway to the complete figure-of-eight that is the aim of the bandage.

4. **Action:** Take the bandage down to the medial aspect of the metatarsals and around to the lateral aspect. You are back at the starting point.

   Rationale: This figure-of-eight bandage ensures that the foot is rotated inwards and the hock outwards, which in turn pushes the femoral head into the acetabulum.

5. **Action:** Continue in this manner until the whole limb is securely held.

   Rationale: The animal should not be able to move the limb.

6. **Action:** Apply a layer of cohesive bandage over the conforming bandage (Fig. 8.4C).

   Rationale: This will protect the other layers.

Procedure: Ear bandage

1. **Action:** Apply cotton-wool padding to the top of the head, above the ear flap. Fold the affected ear(s) up on to the padding.

   Rationale: This will provide comfort and absorb any discharge. One or both ears can be folded on top of the head.

2. **Action:** Cover the ear(s) with cotton-wool padding. Ensure that the padding is the same size as the ear flap.

   Rationale: This helps to keep the bandage neat, with no pieces hanging over the face of the animal, whilst still large enough to be effective.

3. **Action:** Apply a layer of synthetic padding. Start at the top of the skull, run cranially around the ear that is down (if any), under the jaw and back up to the start point.

   Rationale: The idea is to keep the healthy ear exposed. This is achieved by using a figure-of-eight design, winding the bandage cranially then caudally around the healthy ear (Fig. 8.5A).

4. **Action:** Continue as above but apply the padding caudally around the healthy ear. Ensure that the bandage is not too tight around the larynx and trachea. Continue until the ear(s) and padding are covered.

   Rationale: Check that the bandage does not impede the animal's respiration.

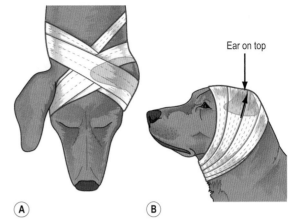

Ear on top

Fig. 8.5 The figure-of-eight design for an ear bandage. A, Wind the bandage around the head in a figure-of-eight. B, Mark the position of the ear with an arrow.

5. **Action:** Apply a cohesive bandage appropriate to the animal's size in the same manner. Continue until the padding layer is covered.

   Rationale: This will secure and protect the other layers.

6. **Action:** Clearly mark the bandaged ear and its direction with an arrow on the dressing (Fig. 8.5B).

   Rationale: This will help when the bandage is removed. The operator will know where the earflap is and will avoid injuring it.

Procedure: Chest bandage

1. **Action:** Start the bandage between the shoulder blades. Apply a layer of synthetic padding material cranially over the right lateral scapula. Bring the bandage through the front legs, caudal to the left scapula. Bring the bandage up to the start point.

   Rationale: This is halfway to achieving the desired figure-of-eight bandage.

2. **Action:** From the start point, take the bandage caudal to the right scapula, through the front legs, cranial to the left scapula. Bring the bandage over the left lateral scapula back to the start point.

   Rationale: The figure-of-eight is complete.

3. **Action:** Continue in this manner several times, moving the end point caudally by half the width of the bandage.

   Rationale: This ensures that the bandage does not slip backwards.

4. **Action:** Wind the bandage around the chest, working caudally, until the desired size is achieved (Fig. 8.6), monitoring tension as the dressing is applied.

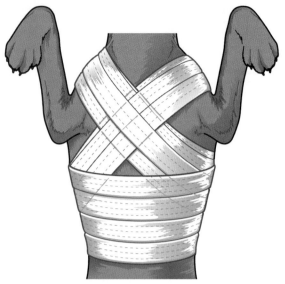

Fig. 8.6 Chest bandage.

Rationale: By checking tension, one can monitor that the bandage does not impede the animal's breathing.

5. **Action:** Apply a cohesive layer appropriate to the animal's size in the same manner. Continue until the padding layer is covered.
   Rationale: This will secure and protect the other layers.

Procedure: Limb bandage

1. **Action:** Apply cotton-wool padding between the digits and pads of the affected limb (Fig. 8.7A).
   Rationale: This will absorb sweat and prevent the digits from rubbing together.
2. **Action:** Apply a primary layer of synthetic padding. Start on the cranial aspect of the limb, over the toes to the caudal aspect, and return to the start (Fig. 8.7B). Turn the bandage by 90° (Fig. 8.7C) and cover the toes in a figure-of-eight. Work from distal to proximal. Overlap the bandage by half its width.
   Rationale: This layer is used for padding and support.
3. **Action:** Work proximally up the limb until over the joint that is above the injury (Fig. 8.7D). Do not return down the limb but cut any excess bandage off.
   Rationale: This will provide more support for the limb and, in turn, hold the bandage in place.
4. **Action:** Apply a secondary layer of conforming bandage, again working from distal to proximal.
   Rationale: This layer is used to support and hold the primary layer in place. Working distal to proximal

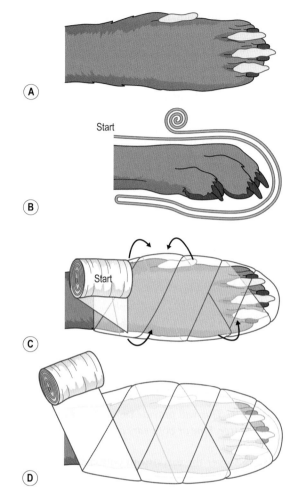

Fig. 8.7 Limb bandage. A, Pad the digits and pads with cotton wool. B, Bandage over the toes. C, Twist the bandage through 90°. D. Continue winding the bandage up the limb.

should prevent any tourniquet effect, which could trap fluid in the distal aspect of the limb.

5. **Action**: Apply a tertiary layer of cohesive bandage, again working from distal to proximal.
   Rationale: This layer is used to protect the other two layers from damp and daily wear and tear.

Procedure: Tail bandage

1. **Action:** Dress any wound on the tail and then cover by placing an empty syringe case over the end of the tail. Ensure the end of the case is pierced with a hole for ventilation (Fig.8.8).
   Rationale: This will prevent further trauma to the wound should the animal want to wag its tail!

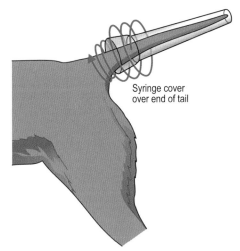

Syringe cover
over end of tail

Fig. 8.8 Tail bandage.

2. **Action:** Apply a layer of cohesive bandage from caudal to cranial over the syringe case.
   Rationale: Cohesive bandage has more grip on the hair than conforming bandage, making it less likely to come off. However, in shorthaired dogs, zinc oxide may have to be used to hold the bandage in place.
3. **Action:** Continue applying the bandage, working the animal's hair into each wind.
   Rationale: This will help the bandage to stay in place.

DRAINAGE SYSTEMS (TABLE 8.4)

Procedure: Use of the Penrose drain

1. **Action:** Clean and debride the wound (see Wound Management, earlier).

Rationale: This will reduce the risk of infection and increase the blood supply to the wound, increasing the rate of wound healing.
2. **Action:** Using a sterile scalpel blade, make an incision at the base of the wound (Fig. 8.9A), at the lowest point of the dead space. Work from the inside to the outside of the wound. The incision should be no wider than the width of the drain. Leave the tip of the blade protruding.
   Rationale: Excess fluid will drain to the lowest point of the wound, and this should be the site of the exit point.
3. **Action:** Using a pair of sterile artery forceps, grasp the tip of the blade. Retract the scalpel blade until the tips of the artery forceps are showing on the inside of the wound (Fig. 8.9B).
   Rationale: This technique maintains the incision.
4. **Action:** Release the blade and dispose of it safely in a sharps bin.
   Rationale: This leaves the artery forceps through the incision.
5. **Action:** Attach the end of the Penrose drain to the artery forceps and pull through (Fig. 8.9C). Release when 4–5 cm are showing.
   Rationale: This technique inserts the drain without the need to release and return to the incision, thus reducing soft-tissue damage and time taken.
6. **Action:** Take the other end of the drain and suture to the inside of the wound at the uppermost point of the dead space. Use a single suture to hold it in place.
   Rationale: This will enable the drain to be easily removed when it is no longer required.

TABLE 8.4	**Drainage systems**
Type	**Comments**
Closed drains	No exposure to the environment. Can be active (suction effect) or passive (reliant on gravity)
Thoracic – water trap	Fluid or air is drawn out from the thorax by gravity. It is prevented from returning by a water trap placed at least 80 cm away from the animal. Use in non-ambulatory patients only
Thoracic – Heimlich valve	Inlet is attached securely into the animal, whilst the outlet is attached to a giving set and bag
Urinary catheter	Drainage of the bladder. Can be indwelling and attached to a giving set and bag
Needle and syringe	Used in many situations as a low-pressure active drain
Open drains	Exposure to the environment. All types are passive
Penrose	Broad, hollow latex tubing. Fluid passes over the surface by capillary action
Seton	Usually a sterile gauze bandage packed into an area. A 'tail' is left protruding
Sump	Similar to a Penrose drain. Air passes inside to the wound, whilst fluid passes over the outside. Used in deep abscesses

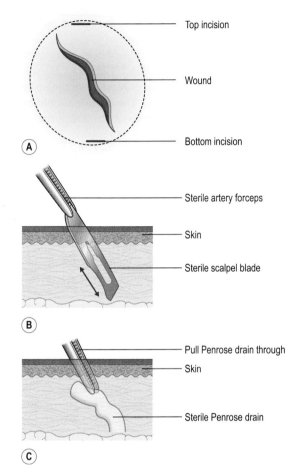

Fig. 8.9 The Penrose drain. A, Make an incision at the top of the wound. B, Incise from inside to outside. C, Pull the drain through.

7. **Action:** Suture the wound (see Suturing Techniques, later).
   Rationale: *The wound is separate from the drain.*
8. **Action:** Suture the Penrose drain to the skin at the lowest exit, at the point of the incisions made earlier. Use two single interrupted sutures, preferably in a nylon of a different colour to the wound sutures.
   Rationale: *The sutures hold the drain in place. The different colours allow easy identification of the sutures when it comes to removing them.*
9. **Action:** Cut the ends of the drain so that 2–3 cm protrude.
   Rationale: *A longer length than this increases the risk of contamination.*
10. **Action:** The wound can be dressed to absorb any exudate draining from the tubing. Ensure that the site is bathed and the dressing changed daily.

Rationale: *This reduces the risk of contamination and keeps the drain open.*
11. **Action:** Cover the drain with an absorbent dressing, which must be changed regularly.
    Rationale: *This holds the exudate, keeps the drain open and reduces the risk of contamination.*
12. **Action:** Advise the owner of the signs that may indicate infection and fluid build-up.
    Rationale: *Examine for signs of oedema, redness, pain, irritation and systemic illness.*
13. **Action:** Prevent the animal from removing the drain.
    Rationale: *Use an Elizabethan collar appropriate to the animal's size.*
14. **Action:** When removing the drain, prepare the area aseptically.
    Rationale: *There is a risk of contamination.*
15. **Action:** Remove the sutures on the lowest site and pull the drain out. The wound will heal by granulation.
    Rationale: *The suture in the top of the wound should give way, and the drain will be released.*

FRACTURE MANAGEMENT

Procedure: First aid procedure in a case of a suspected fracture

1. **Action:** Check the animal's airway, breathing and circulation (see Treatment of airway obstruction procedure in Chapter 9).
   Rationale: *This must be done before checking for other injuries. The animal will die within a few minutes without oxygen.*
2. **Action:** Restrain the animal in a comfortable position. Gently examine for injuries.
   Rationale: *An injured animal is more likely to try to escape and/or bite.*
3. **Action:** Control haemorrhage (see Control of haemorrhage procedure in Chapter 9).
   Rationale: *Loss of blood will cause the animal to go into shock (see Treatment of shock procedure in Chapter 9).*
4. **Action:** Examine the patient for fractures. This must be done gently to prevent further injury or cause pain.
5. **Action:** If possible, clean any wounds and apply a sterile dressing.
   Rationale: *This may not be possible if first aid treatment is not being performed in the practice.*

6. **Action:** Gently apply a splint or Robert Jones bandage to the affected limb (see Individual Bandaging Techniques, earlier).

   Rationale: *This will immobilize the limb, reducing pain and further damage.*

7. **Action:** If necessary, transport the animal to the surgery, constantly monitoring the patient's condition. Ensure that the animal is restrained adequately, safely and humanely.

   Rationale: *It is often easier to move the animal with two people. A stretcher may be necessary for large animals. If a spinal injury is suspected, then always use a rigid stretcher (see Chapter 1).*

8. **Action:** Treat the animal for shock.

   Rationale: *See Treatment of shock procedure in Chapter 9.*

9. **Action:** Administer analgesia as directed by the veterinary surgeon.

   Rationale: *The animal will be in pain.*

10. **Action:** When stable, the patient may be X-rayed to diagnose the extent of the injuries.

    Rationale: *An animal suffering from shock is not a good candidate for sedation/anaesthesia. Treatment for shock is of primary importance to stabilize the patient before administering an anaesthetic.*

11. **Action:** Any fractures may then be reduced, and fixation performed (Table 8.5).

TABLE 8.5 **Methods of fracture fixation**	
Type	**Comments**
External techniques	
Splints	See Individual bandaging techniques and Table 8.3
Casts	See Individual bandaging techniques and Table 8.3
Robert Jones bandage	See Individual bandaging techniques and Table 8.3
Internal fixation	
Intramedullary pins include:	Inserted into the medullary cavity
Steinmann pin	Straight pins with trocar tips designed to cut into the bone. Choose the correct size, as the pin must be a snug fit. Can have a tendency to migrate
Arthrodesis pin/wire	Small intramedullary pin. Small trocar tip on either end. Can have a tendency to migrate
Kirschner wire	Small intramedullary pin. One tip has buoyant point, the other a tracer tip. Can have a tendency to migrate
Rush pin	Curved pins, used in pairs
Cerclage wire	Made from stainless steel. Can be used as single sutures, in conjunction with pins or plates or as a tension band for avulsed fractures
Bone plates and screws include:	
Venables plate	Self-tapping screws are inserted into holes in the bone
Sherman plate	Similar to the Venables plate, but not as strong
Dynamic compression bone plate and ASIF/AO and cortical and cancellous screws	A tap is used to cut a thread in the bone for the screws. This gives a stronger hold. The holes in the plate are angled so that the screws can be placed in a 'neutral' or 'loaded' position. With appropriate placement of screws, the fracture site can be compressed
Lag screws	Half- or fully-threaded screws that draw fragments back into position
Locking plates	The screws are self-tapping. They are threaded so that they lock into threaded screw holes in the plates. Creating a strong fixation of plate to bone
External/internal fixation	
External fixator, e.g. Kirschner-Ehmer device and Ilizarov fixator	A series of pins screwed into the bone through the skin, held in place by scaffolding on the outside. Often used when wounds or infection are involved
Cage rest	Limited movement of the animal. Common treatment for a fractured pelvis

ASIF/AO, Association for the Study of Internal Fixation/Arbeitsgemeinschaft fur Osteosynthesefragen.

Rationale: There are several methods of treatment. Choice is dependent on location of fracture.

Procedure: Splinting a limb

1. **Action:** Apply cotton-wool padding between the digits and pads of the affected limb.
   Rationale: This will absorb sweat and prevent the digits from rubbing together.
2. **Action:** Apply a layer of synthetic padding to the affected limb. Pay particular attention to bony prominences.
   Rationale: To stabilize the injury, the joints above and below the injury must be included. The padding provides comfort; however, the splint must be in close contact to provide immobility.
3. **Action:** Apply the splint to the caudal aspect of the limb. Ensure that it is long enough to immobilize the joints above and below the injury.
   Rationale: There are many different types of splints available, e.g. foam or gutter splints.
4. **Action:** Apply a secondary layer of conforming bandage, working from distal to proximal.
   Rationale: This layer is used to support and hold the primary layer in place.
5. **Action:** Apply a tertiary layer of cohesive bandage over the top, working from distal to proximal.
   Rationale: This protects from daily wear and tear.

Procedure: Casting using plaster of Paris

The use of plaster of Paris as a means of fixing a fractured bone is relatively old-fashioned as there are now more efficient ways of repair; however, it is important to know how to use a plaster-impregnated bandage, should you be asked to apply it.

1. **Action:** Before applying the cast, ensure that the fracture has been reduced.
   Rationale: Reduction is necessary for optimum healing of the site.
2. **Action:** Cover the limb with tubular gauze appropriate to the animal's size. Ensure that the joints above and below the injury are covered. Allow 2 cm of extra gauze at either end.
   Rationale: This will be folded back later to create a smooth end.
3. **Action:** Apply a layer of synthetic padding, again leaving 2 cm at either end.
   Rationale: This is for the animal's comfort. Apply more padding to joints and bony prominences.

4. **Action:** Wearing gloves, unroll the plaster of Paris bandage by 10 cm and immerse in hand-hot water for a few seconds.
   Rationale: Gloves protect from the cast resin. The drying time is shortened if warm water is used.
5. **Action:** Squeeze out excess water from the bandage. Apply to the limb, working from distal to proximal. Overlap the bandage by half its width at each turn. Leave the middle two toes protruding from the end of the cast.
   Rationale: The colour of the nail quick and the skin of the toes can be used as guide to the health of the circulation.
6. **Action:** Ensure even coverage over the joints.
   Rationale: The cast can become weak over these points.
7. **Action:** Turn over the tubular gauze and padding at the ends. Smooth into the plaster of Paris.
   Rationale: This creates a neat and tidy cast.
8. **Action:** Smooth and mould the cast into the correct shape.
   Rationale: Any changes must be made before the bandage dries.
9. **Action:** The bandage must be completely dry before allowing the animal to bear weight on the limb.
   Rationale: Drying times vary; refer to manufacturer's instructions.
10. **Action:** Check the circulation regularly, using the protruding toes as a guide.
    Rationale: The toes should be warm to touch. Cold toes may indicate that the cast is too tight.

Procedure: Applying a bivalve cast in cats

The use of a bivalve cast (so-called because of its resemblance to the long-shelled mollusc) is particularly useful in cats or small dogs as it can be frequently and easily removed to check any underlying wounds.

1. **Action:** Before applying the cast, ensure the fracture has been reduced. General anaesthesia maybe required.
   Rationale: Reduction is necessary for optimum healing of the site. General anaesthesia allows for muscle relaxation, manipulation for appropriate fracture reduction and patient homeostasis.
2. **Action:** Place the patient in lateral recumbency, with the affected limb uppermost.

Rationale: This allows for optimal access of the limb and manipulation of the fracture site.

3. **Action:** Clip medium to long fur.
   Rationale: Clipping the fur ensures a secure fit.

4. **Action:** Cover the limb with orthopaedic stockinette or cling film. Ensure the joints above and below the injury are covered.
   Rationale: The stockinette or cling film prevents the casting material from sticking to the patient's fur.

5. **Action:** Wearing gloves, unroll the plaster of Paris bandage by 10 cm and immerse in hand-hot water for a few seconds.
   Rationale: Gloves will protect your hands from the cast resin. The drying time is shortened if warm water is used.

6. **Action:** Squeeze out excess water from the bandage. Apply to the limb, working from distal to proximal. Overlap the bandage by half its width on each turn. Leave the middle two toes protruding from the end of the cast.
   Rationale: The colour of the nail quick and the skin of the toes can be used as guide to the health of the circulation later on.

7. **Action:** Smooth and mould the cast into the correct shape.
   Rationale: Any changes must be made before the bandage dries.

8. **Action:** The bandage must be completely dry before an oscillating cast saw is used to cut it into two halves along the medial and lateral aspects of the cast. Once the cast has been cut, remove and discard the cling film.
   Rationale: It must be dry to prevent layers from coming away from one another. Note: Drying times vary; refer to manufacturer's instructions.

9. **Action:** Dress the limb as described in Splinting a limb. Using the two halves of the bivalve splint within the dressing.
   Rationale: The cast is perfectly contoured to the patient's limb and provides 360° support to the limb, while allowing frequent removal and replacement for possible wound inspection and management.

10. **Action:** Check the circulation regularly, using the protruding toes as a guide.
    Rationale: The toes should be warm to touch. Cold toes may indicate that the cast is too tight.

SUTURING TECHNIQUES (FIG. 8.10)

Procedure: Simple interrupted skin suture

1. **Action:** Ensure that the wound to be closed is clean and has a good blood supply (see Wound Management, earlier).
   Rationale: This reduces the risk of infection and increases the rate of wound healing.

2. **Action:** Select an appropriate suture material for the wound (Table 8.6).
   Rationale: This will depend on the type of tissue being sutured.

3. **Action:** Select an appropriate type of needle holder and grasp it using the thumb and ring finger.
   Rationale: This grip aids precision in placing and using the needle.

4. **Action:** Position the threaded needle at a right angle in the needle holder. Grasp the needle along two-thirds of its length.
   Rationale: This will prevent the needle from bending.

5. **Action:** Pick up a pair of rat-toothed forceps with the other hand. These should be held like a pencil.
   Rationale: The forceps are used to hold the skin stable.

6. **Action:** Stabilize the skin on the far side of the wound with the forceps. Push the tip of the needle through the skin towards you.
   Rationale: The 'bite', i.e. the distance from the skin edge to the point at which the tip of the needle enters the skin, should be equal to the skin thickness.

7. **Action:** Release the needle and skin. Regrasp the tip of the needle and pull through.
   Rationale: The needle is through the far side of the wound.

8. **Action:** Stabilize the near side of the wound with the forceps. Push the needle through the underside of the skin.
   Rationale: This 'bite' should be the same size as the first.

9. **Action:** Release the needle and skin. Regrasp the tip of the needle and pull through.
   Rationale: The needle has now passed through both sides of the wound.

10. **Action:** Tie the knot. Use a surgeon's knot on the first throw by looping the ends around each other twice. Follow with two single knots. These should be reef knots, not a granny knot.

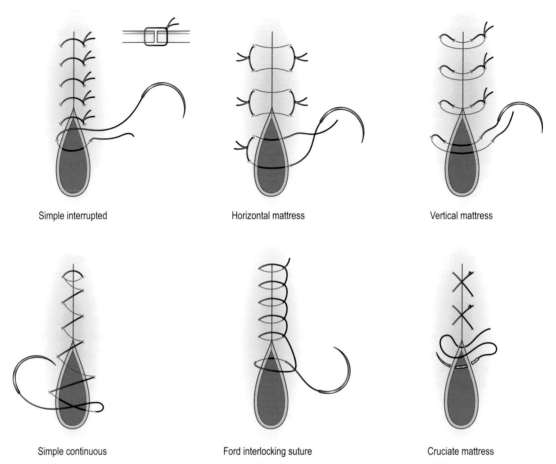

Simple interrupted   Horizontal mattress   Vertical mattress

Simple continuous   Ford interlocking suture   Cruciate mattress

Fig. 8.10 Common suture patterns used in the skin. (Redrawn from Lane and Cooper (2003), Butterworth-Heinemann.)

TABLE 8.6	**Suture materials**	
Type	**Characteristics**	**Indications**
Absorbable		
Chromic catgut	Derived from the intestines of cattle and sheep. A synthetic catgut is available. A monofilament that knots well. Occasional tissue reaction. Strength lasts for 14 days	Subcutaneous, subcuticular and muscle sutures
Polyglactin 910 (Vicryl)	A braided synthetic multifilament suture. High tensile strength lasting for 21 days. Totally absorbed in 70–90 days	Subcuticular, subcutaneous, muscle and mucous membrane
Polyglactin 910 (Vicryl Rapide)	Coated synthetic multifilament. Absorption rate 42 days, falls off after 7–10 days.	Subcuticular, subcutaneous and mucous membrane
Polyglycolic acid (Dexon)	As polyglactin, but absorption is longer. Knots can slip and become undone	Subcuticular, subcutaneous, muscle and mucous membrane

TABLE 8.6 Suture materials—cont'd

Type	Characteristics	Indications
Polydioxanone (PDS*11)	A synthetic monofilament. High tensile strength lasting for 42 days. Causes little tissue reaction	Subcutaneous, subcuticular and muscle sutures
Polyglecaprone 25 (Monocryl)	A synthetic, braided monofilament. The fastest absorbable suture. Minimal tissue reaction. Absorption rate 90–120 days	Subcuticular, subcutaneous, small intestine anastomoses and urological anastomoses
Non-absorbable		
Monofilament nylon (Ethilon)	Minimal tissue reaction, high tensile strength. Knots must have at least three throws for stability	Skin
Braided silk (Mersilk)	A natural suture material, made from cocoons of the silk worm *Bombyx mori*. Adequate tensile strength. Can attract infection. Occasional tissue reaction	Skin
Braided nylon (Nurolon)	Produced to mimic silk. Less tissue reaction, high tensile strength	Skin

Rationale: The knot can be tied by hand or by instrument. The latter is less time-consuming with practice. The skin edges should be brought together so that they are just touching. The first throw should never be pulled tight, as that is done with the later throws.

11. **Action:** Cut the ends of the suture as short as possible without risk of the knot undoing.
    Rationale: This will help prevent the animal biting the sutures, leading to removal.

12. **Action:** Repeat the suture along the length of the wound.
    Rationale: In a simple wound, work the stitches from left to right or right to left. If the wound is irregular, then place a few sutures along the wound and fill in the spaces. This will create an even closure.

For other types of suture pattern, see Fig 8.10. The method of holding the instruments is the same as is described above.

DENTISTRY

Procedure: Scaling and polishing the teeth

1. **Action:** Make sure that the patient is stable under a general anaesthetic and at the correct depth.
   Rationale: See Chapter 6, Anaesthetic procedures.

2. **Action:** Introduce an endotracheal tube of the correct size into the trachea. Tie the tube firmly behind the patient's head using a length of bandage.
   Rationale: It is essential that the animal is intubated to ensure that no fluid from the procedure enters the lungs. The tube must be secure.

3. **Action:** Apply an eye lubricant to both eyes.
   Rationale: Tear production is reduced when under an anaesthetic. This will help lubrication and decrease the risk of infection from the dental procedure.

4. **Action:** Position the patient in lateral recumbency, with the head slightly lower than the body. This can be achieved by tilting the table or raising the shoulders.
   Rationale: This will encourage fluid from the procedure to run out of the mouth.

5. **Action:** Make sure that any fluid is able to drain away from the animal. A tub table is ideal. Additional warming can be introduced, e.g. blankets, bubble wrap, warming devices.
   Rationale: This prevents the animal becoming wet and possibly hypothermic. Body temperature can reduce dramatically in anaesthetized and wet patients.

6. **Action:** Put on a face mask, gloves and goggles.
   Rationale: This prevents bacteria in the mouth, which could be disturbed by the procedure, from infecting the operator.

7. **Action:** Select a mouth gag appropriate to the animal's size (Fig. 8.11). Insert the top and bottom of the gag into the upper and lower canines respectively.
   Rationale: To keep the mouth open, enabling the operator to work.

8. **Action:** Pack the pharynx with a sterile throat pack appropriate to the animal's size.

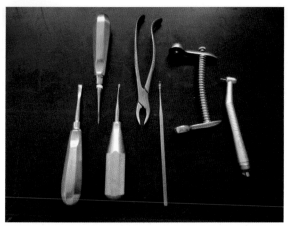

Fig. 8.11 Dental instruments. From left to right: periodontal probe, dental probe, hand scaler and curette, a pair of luxators, extraction forceps, mouth gag, ultrasonic scaler.

Rationale: To prevent fluid entering the lungs.

9. **Action:** Examine the teeth for signs of periodontal disease (Table 8.7).

   Rationale: Any problems must be referred to the veterinary surgeon.

10. **Action:** Using an ultrasonic scaler, scale the visible teeth on that side (Fig. 8.12). Refer to manufacturer's instructions. Spend no longer than 10 seconds on one tooth.

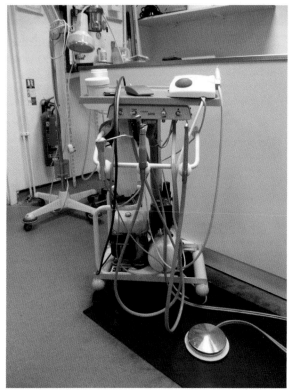

Fig. 8.12 Ultrasonic scaler showing the water/air source, the polisher and the drill.

TABLE 8.7	**Periodontal disease**	
Condition	**Description**	**Treatment**
Plaque	A soft layer composed of bacteria in an organic matrix that forms on the surface of a tooth	Brushing pet's teeth at home. Change diet if necessary
Calculus	A calcified deposit that forms on the surface of the teeth as a result of bacterial action on plaque	Scaling and polishing
Gingivitis	Inflammation of the gums, which become swollen and bleed easily. Caused by plaque at the base of the teeth	Removal of plaque and calculus by scaling and polishing. Short-term antibiotics to eradicate the infection
Periodontitis	Resulting from untreated gingivitis, the gum line recedes away from the base of the tooth	Extraction of the tooth. Treatment for gingivitis
Caries	Decay and crumbling of the tooth due to acid produced by bacteria	Extraction or filling
Fracture of the crown	Caused by trauma to the tooth	Extraction or filling
Retained deciduous teeth	Teeth are not shed before permanent ones erupt. May cause displacement of new teeth	Extraction

Rationale: The vibrating action of the ultrasonic scaler may damage the tooth if used for longer than 10 seconds. You may return to the tooth later if it is still not clean.

11. **Action:** With the aid of appropriate dental instruments (Table 8.8 and Fig. 8.11), check that all calculus (tartar) is removed.

    Rationale: Calculus is the hard, brown deposit on the teeth that forms from plaque as a result of bacterial action.

12. **Action:** Mop up any debris and excess fluid with damp cotton-wool swabs.

    Rationale: It is important to clean as you work; this prevents the fluid soaking the animal.

13. **Action:** Turn the animal over. Ensure that the anaesthetic circuit does not twist, and that the endotracheal tube is not pulled out.

Rationale: Dislodging or twisting the anaesthetic tubing is a common problem when moving the animal. It may be necessary to disconnect the circuit briefly.

14. **Action:** Repeat the scaling process on the other side.

    Rationale: It is possible to reach the inside of the far teeth.

15. **Action:** Polish the teeth with a polishing hand piece (refer to manufacturer's instructions), using prophylactic paste.

    Rationale: Polishing the teeth will leave them smooth, which in turn reduces the ability of bacteria to stick to the surface in the future.

16. **Action:** When both sides have been completed, clean up any excess paste, check that all teeth have been cleaned and remove the throat pack.

TABLE 8.8 Dental instruments (Fig. 8.11)

Name	Description	Use
Periodontal probe	A long thin instrument with a 90° bend in the head. It has graduations on the probe. It is blunt and smoothly rounded to reduce risk of soft tissue trauma	Used to examine and measure the subgingival margin, tooth mobility, inflammation and lesions
Dental probe	A long thin instrument with a rounded head. It has a sharp pointed end	Used to examine early caries, fractures and lesions and to detect subgingival calculus
Dental mirror	A long handle with a small, round mirror at the end	Used to visualize an area without repositioning the patient. Can be used as oral retractor of cheeks and tongue
Scaler	A long handle with a thin, bent head. It has a sharp, pointed tip that is more robust than a curette	Used to remove supragingival (above gum line) calculus ONLY. If used subgingivally, it will damage the tissue with its sharp tip
Curette	A modified hand scaler. Double-ended with mirror image for left and right (complimentary) curvature. Long handle with a thin, bent head. It has a rounded tip	Used to remove supragingival and subgingival calculus. Periodontal pockets deeper than 2 mm should be cleaned with curette rather than power scaler
Luxator/elevator	A thick handle with a rounded and/or curved tip. Various sizes available depending on the requirements of the patient	Used to break down the periodontal ligament, which holds the tooth in place
Periosteal elevator	A long, double-ended, thin handle with rounded or straight and/or curved tips. Various sizes are available depending on the requirements of the patient	Used when raising a periosteal flap to facilitate the removal of a tooth. A gingival retractor and guard
Extraction forceps	Various sizes available depending on the shape and size of the tooth	Used to lift a tooth out after being loosened by elevation. Do not use to remove 'set-in' teeth, as the tooth can snap off, leaving the root still embedded

Rationale: It is very important to always check that no teeth have been overlooked.

17. **Action:** Ensure the animal is clean and dry before finishing.

    Rationale: A dental scale and polish is a very wet procedure. If necessary, use a hair dryer to dry the animal's fur.

REFERENCES AND FURTHER READING

Anderson, D., 2003. Wound dressings unravelled. Companion Animal Practice. 25 (2): BVA, pp. 70–83.

Anderson, D., 1996. Wound management in small animal practice. Companion Animal Practice. 18 (3), 115–128.

Ackerman, N., 2016. Aspinall's Complete Textbook of Veterinary Nursing, third ed. Elsevier, Oxford.

Aspinall, V., 2011. The Complete Textbook of Veterinary Nursing, second ed. Elsevier, Oxford.

Chivers, E., 2010. Wound healing and management of open wounds. The Veterinary Nurse. 1 (2), 106–114.

Conner, J., McKerrel, J., 1995. A Guide to Animal Bandaging. Millpledge, Retford.

Cooper, B., Mullineaux, E., Turner, L., 2011. Textbook of Veterinary Nursing, fifth ed. BSAVA, Gloucester.

Grierson, J., 2009. External coaptation in small animal practice. Practice. 31, 218–225.

Hotson-Moore, A. (Ed.), 1999. Manual of Advanced Veterinary Nursing. BSAVA, Gloucester.

Hotston Moore, A., Rudd, S. (Eds.), 2008. Manual of Canine and Feline Advanced Veterinary Nursing. BSAVA, Gloucester.

Kirk, M., 2014. Initial stabilisation and treatment of traumatic wounds. The Veterinary Nurse. 5 (8), 442–447.

Lane, D.R., Cooper, B. (Eds.), 2003. Veterinary Nursing, third ed. Butterworth-Heinemann, Oxford.

O'Dwyer, L., 2007. Wound Management in Small Animals. Butterworth-Heinemann, Oxford.

O'Dwyer, L., 2015. Hard to heal wounds: dealing with the problematic wound. The Veterinary Nurse. 6 (6), 316–329.

Pead, M.J., Langley-Hobbs, S.J., 2007. Acute management of orthopaedic and external soft tissue injuries. BSAVA manual of canine and feline emergency and critical care, pp. 251–259.

Tracy, D.L. (Ed.), 1994. Small Animal Surgical Nursing, second ed. Mosby, London.

Young, A., 2008. Wound care and management. Veterinary Nurses Times CPD. 2 (5), 5–8.

9

First aid procedures

Trish Scorer

CHAPTER CONTENTS

INTRODUCTION

Under the Veterinary Surgeons Act of 1966, anyone may perform first aid on an animal to save life, prevent suffering or prevent the condition from deteriorating but only until such time as a veterinary surgeon is able to attend to the animal. Although, by law, lay people and veterinary nurses are able to perform the same procedures, the veterinary nurse will have greater knowledge, training and clinical experience to be able to assess the situation, deal with the frightened animal and apply the relevant techniques.

Procedure: Triage of the emergency patient

1. **Action:** Call a veterinary surgeon as soon as possible.
   Rationale: This must be done at the first available opportunity. While you are waiting, you can assess for airway, breathing and circulation (ABC).

2. **Action:** Ensure that the environment is safe to treat the animal.
   Rationale: Do not attempt to treat the animal if there is any risk to you, e.g. fire, risk of electrocution, traffic, radiation or falling masonry.

3. **Action:** Stand back from the animal and evaluate the situation. What are you presented with?
   Rationale: You must remain calm and in control. The owners are likely to be panicking. Avoid rushing in to help before you have assessed the situation.

4. **Action:** Make sure that the patient is handled and restrained appropriately. If the animal is breathing normally but is potentially aggressive, it may be necessary to apply a muzzle (see Chapter 1).
   Rationale: This is made easier if you have an assistant. The animal is likely to be frightened and in pain, and its immediate reaction may be to escape and/or bite.

5. **Action:** Check that the animal has a patent airway (see Cardiopulmonary Resuscitation Techniques (CPR), later).
   Rationale: *The animal may be trying to breathe but if the airway is blocked, respiration will be difficult.*

6. **Action:** Check the animal is breathing. If not, check that the heart is beating and begin cardiopulmonary resuscitation (see CPR, later).
   Rationale: *Lack of oxygen to the body will kill the animal within a few minutes.*

7. **Action:** Check that the animal has a heartbeat. If not, begin cardiopulmonary resuscitation (CPR).
   Rationale: *If the heart is not beating, blood will not circulate around the body to supply the vital organs.*

8. **Action:** Once the patient is stable, check for haemorrhage and control it (see Control of haemorrhage, later).
   Rationale: *Loss of blood may cause the animal to go into shock.*

9. **Action:** Examine the patient for fractures and immobilize (see Chapter 8).
   Rationale: *This must be done before attempting to move the patient to reduce pain and prevent the injury deteriorating.*

10. **Action:** Check the patient's capillary refill time, mucous membrane colour, pulse and temperature. Record all the information (see Chapter 2).
    Rationale: *These all indicate the condition of the animal.*

11. **Action:** Examine the patient for other wounds.
    Rationale: *These can be cleaned and dressed as appropriate once the patient is stable.*

12. **Action:** Treat for shock.
    Rationale: *See Treatment of shock, later.*

Examples of conditions requiring emergency treatment are shown in Table 9.1.

Procedure: Control of haemorrhage

1. **Action:** Place the animal in a comfortable position on a table or at a comfortable height for you.
   Rationale: *If the animal feels uncomfortable, it will try to escape.*

2. **Action:** Ask an assistant to restrain the animal so that it is relaxed and secure and the wound is accessible for treatment (see Chapter 1).

Rationale: *The assistant will be able to react quickly if the animal tries to escape. The animal may resent the wound being touched.*

3. **Action:** Clean your hands with a surgical scrub (see World Health Organization (WHO) hand-washing technique in Chapter 7) and put on sterile gloves.
   Rationale: *It is important not to introduce infection into the wound.*

4. **Action:** Assess what type of haemorrhage you are presented with (Table 9.2).
   Rationale: *The extent of the haemorrhage depends on the type of blood vessels that have been damaged, e.g. an arterial bleed is much more serious than a capillary bleed.*

5. **Action:** Control the haemorrhage using one of the methods described in Table 9.3.
   Rationale: *The method used will depend on your location and the materials to hand, e.g. you may be in the surgery or at the roadside.*

6. **Action:** Once haemorrhage has been controlled, check for signs of shock and treat if necessary (see Treatment of shock, later).
   Rationale: *Blood loss will reduce the circulating blood volume. This is hypovolaemic shock, which must be treated or the animal may die.*

7. **Action:** Monitor the animal closely. If blood soaks through the dressing you have applied, place further dressing material on top.
   Rationale: *Removing the previous dressing may pull off any clot formed and restart the haemorrhage.*

Procedure: Treating burns and scalds

1. **Action:** Ensure the environment is safe to treat the animal.
   Rationale: *Do not attempt to treat the animal if there is any risk to you, e.g. fire, risk of electrocution, radiation or falling masonry.*

2. **Action:** Prevent further damage to the patient by removing the source of the burn.
   Rationale: *This may mean moving the patient away or moving the source from the patient.*

3. **Action:** Place the animal in a comfortable position.
   Rationale: *The animal may be in extreme pain and may try to escape and/or bite.*

4. **Action:** Ask an assistant to restrain the animal so that it is relaxed and secure and the burned area is accessible for treatment.

TABLE 9.1 Conditions requiring emergency first aid

Condition	Definition	Symptoms
Death	Absence of a heart beat for more than 3 minutes. Until death is confirmed, emergency treatment must continue (see CPR)	No heart beat No respiration (Cheyne–Stoke respiration may be present) Pupil is fixed and dilated No corneal reflex Cornea is dry and glazed. Mucous membranes are cyanotic and dry Body temperature cools. Rigor mortis sets in after a few hours
Unconsciousness	Occurs when the animal's brain is unable to respond to sound and touch. Usually the patient is flaccid and still, but occasionally the brain becomes overactive, e.g. epilepsy, and the patient's muscles convulse. There are two types of unconsciousness: 1. Stupor – animal is aware of surroundings 2. Coma – patient cannot be roused Treatment starts by evaluating the patient's airway, breathing and circulation (ABC) (see Triage of the emergency patient)	Heart beat present, but may be slow Respiration present Pupil may be reactive to light but slow (compare both pupils' reactions, as a difference may indicate brain damage) Nystagmus (side-to-side or up-and-down movement) or strabismus (squint) may be present Cornea is moist The eyeball position, as in anaesthesia, can indicate the depth of unconsciousness Muscles are flaccid
Epilepsy	A type of unconsciousness. Occurs when there is abnormal electrical activity in the brain. Various causes include brain damage, poisoning, infection and metabolic disease, e.g. liver or kidney failure Treatment of epilepsy is covered in Chapter 3	There are three phases: 1. Pre-ictal phase – patient may be anxious or excitable 2. Ictal phase – patient collapses and has convulsions. Body is tense with limbs extended and often paddles its limbs. Head and neck are extended. The jaws champ and saliva becomes foamy. Eyes are fixed and stare ahead. Respiratory rate is increased. The patient may urinate and defecate 3. Post-ictal phase – patient calms down but is dazed and exhausted
Collapse	A collapsed patient is unable and/or unwilling to stand up. Ensure constant monitoring, as this can progress into unconsciousness Evaluate the patient's airway, breathing and circulation (see Triage of the emergency patient)	Vital signs may be normal. Animal will respond to sound, light and touch
Asphyxia/respiratory failure	Occurs when the lungs are unable to oxygenate the blood. Causes may include trauma, airway obstruction, neoplasia, anaesthetic overdose and poisoning Evaluate the patient's airway, breathing and circulation (see Triage of the emergency patient and Treatment of airway obstruction)	Cyanosis Dyspnoea Tachypnoea Orthopnoea Tachycardia Collapse leading to unconsciousness

TABLE 9.2   Types of haemorrhage

Type	Identification	Treatment
Arterial	Bright red and pumps out in spurts. Bleeding point is easy to identify	Very serious. Haemorrhage must be arrested immediately. Use directed digital pressure on the ends of the vessels until a more long-term method can be instigated
Venous	Darker red and flows in a steady stream. Bleeding point is easy to identify	Slightly less serious than an arterial bleed. However, haemorrhage must be arrested quickly. Use direct digital pressure or a pressure bandage
Capillary	Multiple pinpoint haemorrhages. The wound will ooze with little force. Commonly seen in incisional wounds	Less serious than arterial and venous haemorrhage. However, capillary bleeding over a long period of time can be serious. Use of a pressure bandage is recommended
Mixed	Commonly seen. This is a combination of the above	Treatment depends on the extent of the haemorrhage
External	Haemorrhage on the outside of the body. Easy to identify	Treatment depends on the extent of the haemorrhage
Internal	Haemorrhage inside the body. Difficult to identify and therefore treat	Treatment depends on the area affected. Possible treatments are a pressure bandage, ice pack, immobilization of the area and/or treatment for hypovolaemic shock

TABLE 9.3   First aid treatment of haemorrhage

Type	Method	Comments
Direct digital pressure	With a clean finger and thumb, apply pressure to the wound on either side. Care must be taken not to push a foreign body or bone fragments deeper	Quick and easy; however, this is a temporary measure, and a pressure bandage must be applied as soon as possible
Pressure bandage	Apply direct pressure by using a sterile dressing and firmly applied bandage. Ensure breathing is not impeded	Deep wounds may need packing with sterile gauze before bandaging. If foreign bodies or bone fragments are suspected, use a ring pad to remove the pressure from the site
Pressure points	An artery is pushed against a bone in order to reduce the flow of blood in that vessel. Can be used in the brachial, femoral and coccygeal arteries	The artery is not always easy to find. Venous bleeding will still continue. This is a temporary measure, and a pressure bandage must be applied as soon as possible
Tourniquet	A ready-made or improvised strap is applied above the haemorrhage on a limb. Pressure should be such that it just stops the haemorrhage	This is used as a last resort. The tourniquet should be applied for no longer than 15 minutes, before resting for 1 minute and then reapplying closer to the wound

Rationale: The assistant will be able to react quickly should the animal try to escape. The animal may resent the wound being touched.

5. **Action:** Clean your hands with a surgical scrub using the WHO method (see Fig. 7.2) and put on sterile gloves.

   Rationale: It is important not to introduce infection into the wound.

6. **Action:** Cool the area with cold water or sterile saline if available. A shower hose can be used for large areas as long as it is not too pressurized. A bag of saline and giving set can be used for smaller areas. Continue for at least 10 minutes.

   Rationale: This will cool the area, limiting the number of cells destroyed. The use of an ice pack is not recommended as it puts pressure on the burnt area.

7. **Action:** Keep the patient warm by wrapping it in dry blankets. Avoid the use of direct heat, i.e. lamps and pads. Care must be taken, as the animal will be in severe pain.

   Rationale: Although the burned area must be cooled, the patient must be warmed to reduce shock. Direct heat causes vasodilation in one specific area, drawing blood away from other areas. It is better to warm the whole room.

8. **Action:** Clean the area gently with sterile saline.

   Rationale: The area is extremely painful, and proper cleaning and clipping may only be achieved under a general anaesthetic. General anaesthesia is only recommended if the patient is stable.

9. **Action:** Dress the wound. This may be with wound gel, paraffin tulle and/or saline-soaked swabs.

   Rationale: The wound must be kept moist at all times.

10. **Action:** Apply a light, non-adhesive dressing on top.

    Rationale: Heat must be able to escape and moisture loss must be avoided, so the dressing must be minimal. Excessive fluid loss may result in hypovolaemic shock.

11. **Action:** Apply a polythene bag or cling film over the dressing.

    Rationale: This will prevent moisture evaporating from the area.

12. **Action:** Gently place a cold wet towel on top. Replace regularly.

    Rationale: This will keep the area cool.

13. **Action:** Observe and treat for shock.

    Rationale: Fluid therapy is essential to replace the fluid lost from the wound.

14. **Action:** Consult the veterinary surgeon on the administration of antibiotics and analgesia.

    Rationale: A burn is extremely painful and susceptible to infection, so analgesia and antibiotic cover are recommended.

Procedure: Treating frostbite

1. **Action:** Ensure the environment is safe to treat the animal.

   Rationale: Do not attempt to treat the animal if there is any risk to you.

2. **Action:** Place the animal in a comfortable position.

   Rationale: The animal will be in pain and may try to escape and/or bite.

3. **Action:** Ask an assistant to restrain the animal so that it is relaxed and secure and the frost burns are accessible for treatment.

   Rationale: Common places for frostbite are anywhere that the blood supply is reduced, e.g. on the ear tip, nose, paws, pads and scrotum.

4. **Action:** Clean your hands with a surgical scrub using the WHO method (see Fig. 7.2) and put on sterile gloves.

   Rationale: It is important not to introduce infection into the wound.

5. **Action:** Apply warm, body temperature water (38–40°C) to the areas. Continue until all areas are warmed to body temperature.

   Rationale: This will gradually warm the area, reducing the number of cells destroyed.

6. **Action:** Do not rub the area.

   Rationale: This will shatter frozen cells.

7. **Action:** Observe and treat for shock.

   Rationale: See Treatment of shock, later.

8. **Action:** Consult the veterinary surgeon on the administration of antibiotics and analgesia.

   Rationale: Frostbite wounds are susceptible to infection, so antibiotic cover is recommended.

Procedure: Treatment of airway obstruction

Patients with an obstructed airway may display:

- Laboured breathing with an expiratory push of the diaphragm
- Cyanosis
- Anxiety.

Auscultation of the chest reveals high-pitched wheezes throughout the lung field. In severe life-threatening situations the animal is:

- Cyanotic
- Breathing open-mouthed
- Collapsed
- Asphyxiating.

1. **Action:** Calm the patient. This may be by gentle handling and reassurance but sedation may also be necessary to facilitate treatment.

   Rationale: The patient will be highly stressed if it is still conscious.

2. **Action:** Remove any visual foreign bodies from the mouth and pharynx by manual removal, suction and/or the Heimlich manoeuvre (Fig. 9.1).

   Rationale: The animal may be unconscious but trying to breathe. Examples of common obstructions

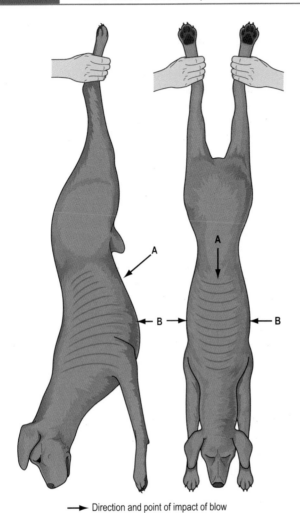

→ Direction and point of impact of blow

Fig. 9.1 The Heimlich manoeuvre A, Standard version; B, modified version. (Redrawn from Lane and Cooper (2003), Butterworth-Heinemann.)

include vomit, balls, toys, blood, water and leaves (if the animal has fallen into water).

3. **Action:** If the animal has water or a foreign body blocking the trachea, then the Heimlich manoeuvre can be used.
   Rationale: This technique is designed to force foreign matter from the trachea.

4. **Action:** Hold the animal up by its hind legs, or hang larger animals upside down over a table or door frame (Fig. 9.1).
   Rationale: The obstructing material may move downwards towards the mouth by the force of gravity.

5. **Action:** Administer a sharp punch to the abdominal wall, above the xiphisternum and angled down towards the diaphragm (Fig. 9.1).
   Rationale: This will force air down the respiratory tract from the lungs to the trachea, to dislodge the blockage.

6. **Action:** Repeat up to four times.
   Rationale: Repeating the procedure too many times can inflict damage.

7. **Action:** If the blockage is removed, then place patient in lateral recumbency with head tilted upwards to facilitate airway patency. If appropriate, remove the foreign material from the mouth. Administer 100% oxygen by the 'flow by' method. This is done by placing the oxygen outlet next to the patient's nose/mouth.
   Rationale: Be aware that the animal may recover quickly and try to escape. It is a good idea to have an assistant close by and ready to restrain the animal if this happens.

8. **Action:** If attempts to remove the blockage are unsuccessful, provide an emergency airway by pushing a wide-gauge needle through the ventral midline of the neck into the trachea.
   Rationale: Please note, placement needs to be below the blockage so that inspired air can reach the lungs. This will act as an air inlet/outlet until a proper tracheostomy can be performed.

9. **Action:** Prepare the animal for a tracheostomy by clipping and scrubbing the ventral throat area (see Tracheostomy procedure, later). Prepare all equipment necessary for the procedure.
   Rationale: This is a surgical procedure that must be carried out by the veterinary surgeon. (N.B.: The term tracheostomy seems to be interchangeable with the term tracheotomy, although some texts describe a tracheotomy as a temporary opening and a tracheostomy as a permanent opening in the trachea.)

Procedure: Tracheostomy

This procedure creates a temporary opening in the trachea that allows the animal to breathe when there is upper-airway obstruction. It is usually done as an emergency procedure under local anaesthetic or sedation. The patient may present with increased inspiratory effort, dyspnoea, cyanosis, open-mouthed breathing and orthopnoea (extension of the neck in sternal recumbency and abduction of the elbows). If the patient has an acute upper-airway obstruction and there is no time to prepare for a tracheostomy, i.e. patient is close to death and requires urgent first aid, then a wide-gauge hypodermic needle can be pushed through the ventral midline of the trachea as a temporary measure.

1. **Action:** Prepare the necessary equipment to perform the tracheostomy. This will include surgical scrub and clippers, tracheostomy tube, laryngoscope, endotracheal tube, surgical kit, suture material, drapes and Gelpi retractors.

   Rationale: Preparation will save time in this emergency procedure. Please note that the components of the tracheostomy tube may vary from different manufacturers. Familiarization with its components will save time when placing it.

2. **Action:** Place the patient in dorsal recumbency on the table with neck extended over a sandbag.

   Rationale: This is the optimal position for the procedure because the trachea can be palpated, and the skin overlying it is taut.

3. **Action:** Clip and clean the area with surgical scrub and warm water until aseptic.

   Rationale: This is a surgical site and should be aseptic. There may not be time for scrubbing up if the patient's life is at risk.

4. **Action:** A small incision is made in the skin between the fifth and sixth tracheal rings in the ventral midline of the neck. This is usually done with a size 15 scalpel blade.

   Rationale: This is the optimal site for the tube. It is away from the larynx, and the tube will not be disturbed as the patient moves its neck.

5. **Action:** Separate the pair of longitudinal neck muscles, which overlie the trachea.

   Rationale: This exposes the cartilaginous tracheal rings.

6. **Action:** Incise between the tracheal rings and insert the tracheostomy tube.

   Rationale: The incision should be one-third of the circumference of the tracheal rings.

7. **Action:** Secure the tube in place with sutures placed cranially and caudally.

   Rationale: Sutures in this position will ensure equal tension on the tube and prevent it pulling out.

8. **Action:** The tube and surrounding area must now be cared for correctly (Box 9.1).

   Rationale: The wound is liable to infection, which may compromise the patient's recovery.

BOX 9.1 Care of the tracheostomy tube

1. Patients with a tracheostomy tube require critical care – monitor the patient immediately after placement and for 24 hours a day
2. Use a pulse oximeter or a capnograph to make sure the animal is maintaining adequate ventilation once oxygen supplementation is withdrawn
3. Ideally the patient should have humidified air to inhale
4. Avoid patient interference with the tube
5. Avoid fluffy bedding and cat litter as this can be sucked up into the tube
6. Do not feed sloppy, dry or flaky food
7. Never put a lead or collar on the patient
8. Ensure that the patient does not occlude the tube when sleeping
9. Before beginning any procedure with the tube, administer 100% oxygen to the patient for 5 minutes
10. Clean the tube regularly, ideally every 2–3 hours; this could potentially need doing every half hour to prevent occlusion by blood, mucous and/or exudate
11. Wear sterile gloves when cleaning the tube
12. Clean around the tube entry site with surgical scrub and then dry
13. Unlock and remove the inner tube. Clean thoroughly and rinse through with hot water and shake it dry
14. Replace the inner tube
15. Administer 100% oxygen to the patient for 5 minutes
16. The tracheostomy tube can be suctioned to remove excess secretions, but it does carry risks. The introduction of negative pressure to the trachea may remove air from the lungs, leading to hypoxia and collapse of alveoli. To minimize the risk, pre- and post-oxygenation should be carried out, and suctioning should be kept to a maximum of 15 seconds
17. The use of regular coupage of the chest may help with dislodgement of secretions but carries the risk of dislodging the tube. Check the tube carefully before and after any coupage

CARDIOPULMONARY RESUSCITATION (CPR) TECHNIQUES

Following an assessment of current literature, the Reassessment Campaign on Veterinary Resuscitation (RECOVER) has developed guidelines for CPR in small animals. These are available to view at http://www.acvecc-recover.org/.

The RECOVER initiative identified five areas to be investigated (Boxes 9.2–9.4):
- Preparedness and prevention
- Basic life support
- Advanced life support
- Monitoring
- Post-arrest care.

Procedure: Diagnosis of cardiopulmonary arrest (CPA)

Presentation of an unresponsive, apnoeic patient should prompt an emergency reaction as follows.

1. **Action:** Assess the patient's airway, breathing and circulation (ABC). The absence of effective ventilation, audible heart sounds and/or a pulse support the diagnosis of CPA. This must be done quickly but effectively.
   Rationale: Lack of blood to the cells, pumped around by the heart, very quickly results in cell death and, eventually, death of the patient. Do not spend too long checking for a pulse as research has shown that rescuers often believe a pulse is present when one is not. CPR should be started immediately where a pulse cannot be readily identified.
2. **Action:** Monitoring equipment such as Doppler blood pressure system, electrocardiogram (ECG)

BOX 9.3   Preparation for cardiopulmonary resuscitation

1. An organized and efficient response is crucial. This should include a 'whole team' approach where every member of staff knows what to do
2. Identify 'at risk' patients and establish a monitoring plan. This should occur for any patient admitted for treatment
3. Consider the layout of the area. If in a practice, is there a designated area for CPR, or will you take equipment to the patient? A source of oxygen is necessary
4. It is essential that there is enough room for all members of the resuscitation team to work
5. Good lighting is essential for the procedures and monitoring to be carried out
6. Consider the size and height of staff members. The table height for chest compressions may need to be altered, or a footstool may be required. It may be easier to do CPR on the floor
7. There must be access to an organized and audited crash box that is regularly restocked
8. Monitoring equipment will help monitor the effectiveness of the treatment
9. CPR algorithm charts and emergency drug dosing charts improve adherence to the guidelines (available to download from RECOVER website)

BOX 9.4   Cardiopulmonary resuscitation training

1. Formal training of the resuscitation team is essential (3–5 people to cover all tasks)
2. Training must include cognitive and psychomotor skills
3. Refresher training every 6 months is recommended
4. The use of mock-ups on mannequins every 3–6 months to keep up awareness of CPR guidelines is recommended
5. It is recommended that there is a trained team leader. She/he will distribute tasks, enforce rules and procedure and give clear and focused communication
6. After any case in which cardiopulmonary resuscitation has been used, a debriefing session to evaluate and reflect on the team performance should be held

---

BOX 9.2   Definitions for cardiopulmonary resuscitation terminology

1. Cardiopulmonary resuscitation (CPR) – an emergency procedure consisting of external cardiac massage and artificial respiration
2. Cardiopulmonary arrest (CPA) – cessation of effective cardiac output and respiration
3. Return of spontaneous circulation (ROSC) – re-establishment of sustained cardiac output
4. Basic life support (BLS) – chest compressions and ventilation
5. Advanced life support (ALS) – drug therapy and post-resuscitation care

and capnograph to measure end tidal carbon dioxide ($EtCO_2$) can be used to support diagnosis.

Rationale: These are useful if available but do not rely on them alone.

Procedure: Basic life support (BLS) – chest compressions

BLS should be instigated as soon as possible following diagnosis of cardiopulmonary arrest.

1. **Action:** Use CAB concept (circulation, airway and breathing) as a starting point in BLS.

   Rationale: Evidence suggests that the outcome worsens with the delay of initiation of chest compressions. This is because ventilation will be ineffective if there is no cardiac output, causing no oxygen to be delivered to the tissues, resulting in cell death.

2. **Action:** Place the patient in lateral recumbency (left or right). If the patient is a barrel-chested dog, e.g. an English Bulldog, then place in dorsal recumbency.

   Rationale: This is the optimum position for CPR. There are two main theories to explain why external chest compressions lead to blood flow during CPR:

   - The **cardiac pump theory** suggests that the cardiac ventricles are directly compressed, opening the pulmonic and aortic valves and providing blood flow.
   - The **thoracic pump theory** suggests that chest compressions increase overall intrathoracic pressure, secondarily compressing the aorta and collapsing the vena cava, leading to blood flow out of the thorax. Elastic recoil of the chest creates negative pressure, improving filling of the ventricles in between compressions.

3. **Action:** Start chest compressions according to the species and breed of patient you are presented with.

   Rationale: It is vital that the correct position is adopted to facilitate the optimal CPR for the type of patient:

   A. **For round-chested, medium, large and giant dogs** use the thoracic pump theory as it is difficult to compress the heart directly. Put the dog in lateral recumbency and place your hands on the widest portion of the chest (Fig. 9.2) to give maximum compression.

   B. **For narrow-chested dogs,** e.g. greyhounds, use cardiac pump theory. Put the dog into lateral

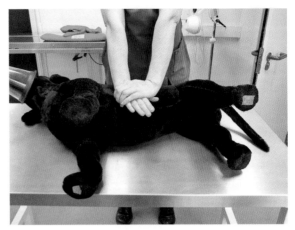

Fig. 9.2 Thoracic pump method in a large dog.

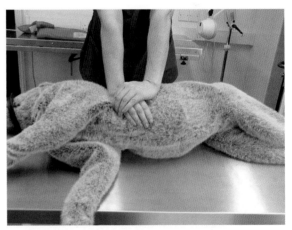

Fig. 9.3 Cardiac pump method in a narrow-chested dog.

recumbency and place both your hands directly over the heart (Fig. 9.3).

   C. **For barrel-chested dogs,** e.g. English Bulldogs, use cardiac pump theory. Put the dog into sternal recumbency and place both your hands directly over the heart (Fig. 9.4).

   D. **For cats and small dogs** use cardiac pump theory. This may be carried out using either:

   i. One-handed circumferential compressions by wrapping your fingers around the sternum at the level of the heart (Fig. 9.5), or

   ii. Two-handed cardiac pump method (Fig. 9.6).

4. **Action:** The compressor should lock his or her elbows with one hand over the other. The shoulders should be directly over the hands. Avoid leaning on the chest in between compressions.

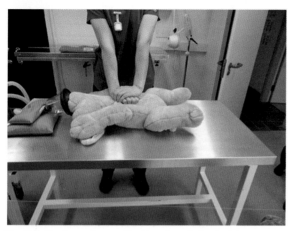

Fig. 9.4 Cardiac pump method in a barrel-chested dog.

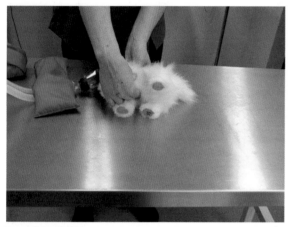

Fig. 9.5 One-handed circumferential compressions in a kitten.

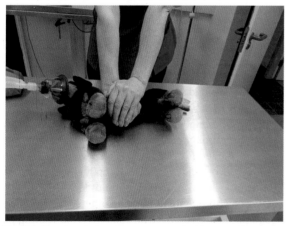

Fig. 9.6 Two-handed cardiac pump method in a small dog.

Rationale: This position should allow the strength to come from the core rather than the arms and facilitate more consistent compressions. Relaxing in between compressions allows full elastic recoil of the chest.

5. **Action:** Compressions should be at a depth of one-third to one-half the width of the chest at a rate of 100–120 compressions per minute.

   Rationale: This is a set rate regardless of the patient's size or species. The use of a metronome or song with a regular beat, e.g. 'Staying Alive', is recommended to maintain the correct timing.

6. **Action:** Chest compressions should be carried out in 2-minute cycles. The person should then be replaced and compressions continued.

   Rationale: This should prevent the compressor becoming too tired, leading to the risk of the compressions become less effective.

Procedure: Basic life support (BLS) – ventilation

Both hypoxia and hypercapnia reduce the likelihood of the return of spontaneous circulation (ROSC), so securing a patent airway and providing ventilation are essential during CPR. Evidence suggests that early intubation and ventilation are likely to be of benefit, especially in patients that are in arrest due to non-cardiac problems such as anaesthetic problems.

1. **Action:** Intubate the patient as soon as possible once chest compressions have been started. This is easier with two or more people.

   Rationale: Lateral intubation can be practised on 'regular' patients to increase the rate of success in an emergency situation.

2. **Action:** Begin ventilation with oxygen at a rate of 10 breaths/min, with a tidal volume of 10 ml/kg and a short inspiratory time of 1 second.

   Rationale: These are the recommended respiratory rates regardless of species or size of patient.

3. **Action:** For non-intubated patients, use the mouth-to-nose technique. With the patient still in lateral recumbency, extend the head and neck and pull the tongue forwards.

   Rationale: This is the optimum position for maximum air intake.

4. **Action:** Grasp the nose firmly in the left hand so that the thumb and fingers curl around the nose and mouth and hold the mouth closed (Fig. 9.7).

   Rationale: This creates an air-tight seal.

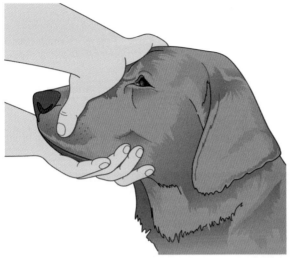

Fig. 9.7 Mouth-to-nose resuscitation: holding the nose. (Redrawn from Lane and Cooper (2003), Butterworth-Heinemann.)

5. **Action:** Place the right hand under the lower jaw.
   Rationale: The weight of the head is now supported.
6. **Action:** Blow down the nose. This should be at a rate of two breaths for every 30 chest compressions. Turn your head away after each blow to avoid inhaling the expired air and saliva.

Rationale: This should be done in 2-minute cycles, and then the operator should be changed to avoid exhaustion.

Procedure: Treatment of poisoning

1. **Action:** Take a comprehensive history from the owner of the animal (Table 9.4).
   Rationale: The history may be taken over the telephone or when the animal is brought into the surgery. It will provide information to help identify the poison and the time at which it was taken.
2. **Action:** Inform the veterinary surgeon.
   Rationale: This must be done at the first available opportunity so that treatment can start as soon as possible.
3. **Action:** If the animal is still in contact with the poison, then remove it from the source. This is likely to be done by the owners – explain clearly what you expect them to do as they may be panicking.
   Rationale: For example, if the animal has the poison on its coat or is close to the source, e.g. gas. If the coat is contaminated, wipe the poison away with paper towelling until professional advice can be sought. The use of an Elizabethan collar or towel wrapped around the patient will prevent further ingestion. Licking of the paws may be prevented by bandaging or putting socks on the animal.

TABLE 9.4 Questions to ask the owner in a case of poisoning	
Question	**Rationale**
Do you know the cause of the poisoning?	Time is saved if the owner can give you the details of the poison or bring the packet or container to the surgery
Do you know at what time the patient ate, or came into contact with, the poison?	This will determine whether inducing emesis will be effective
Did the patient eat anything unusual prior to the onset of symptoms?	If a sample is available, then advise the owner to bring it to the surgery
Was the patient missing prior to the onset of symptoms? If so, then where?	If the owner knows that the patient has been in a certain place, e.g. shut in a garden shed or garage, then this should be searched for a possible source
Is there any substance on the patient's coat, or around or in its mouth?	Advice can be given to obtain a sample and prevent further absorption
Is there any medication, human or animal, which is damaged or missing?	This may help identify the poison. If a sample is available, then advise the owner to bring it to the surgery
Did the owner use any product in the house or garden prior to the onset of symptoms?	This may help identify the poison. If a sample is available, then advise the owner to bring it to the surgery

If the poison is known, the Veterinary Poisons Information Service can be contacted with the consent of the veterinary surgeon. The telephone number is 02073 055055. A charge will be made for the use of this service; however, many veterinary practices subscribe yearly. Owners should call the Animal Poison Line on 01202 509000 – standard charges apply.

4. **Action:** Identify the poison (Table 9.5). Ask the owner to bring in the packet or label if applicable.
   Rationale: *The type of poison will determine your actions. The information may be obtained by questioning the owner.*
5. **Action:** Prevent further absorption of the poison. An emetic (Table 9.6) and/or a demulcent (Table 9.7) may be used. *Never* induce vomiting if the poison is corrosive or the patient is unconscious or fitting.

Rationale: *If the identity of the poison is known and it is non-corrosive, then advise the owners to induce emesis at home. Emesis is ineffective if the substance was ingested over 4 hours previously.*
6. **Action:** Collect a clearly labelled sample of any poison, vomit and/or urine/faeces. This may be used for analysis at a later date.
   Rationale: *Analysis may aid identification of the substance.*

TABLE 9.5 **Toxic agents**			
Type	**Causes**	**Effects**	**Treatment**
Medicines			
Acepromazine (ACP) misuse	Accidental overdosing with tablets in the house Idiosyncratic reaction to the drug	Depression or collapse (cats may become hyperaesthetic) Vasodilatation leads to decreased blood pressure and increased susceptibility to heatstroke on warm days Brachiocephalic dogs are especially likely to suffer Increased likelihood of fits in epileptic animals	Induce vomiting if many tablets have been eaten (unlikely, since few surgeries prescribe more than a few tablets for specific occasions) Treat symptoms of collapse/ shock, heatstroke and epilepsy
Abnormal response (potential of anaphylactic reaction)	Allergic-type response to medication, e.g. vaccination, antibiotics	Depression, occasionally vomiting and diarrhoea, swelling of injection sites Severe reactions result in collapse, with signs of shock	Swellings may have cold compresses applied Treat for shock if collapsed and maintain treatment if unconscious Prepare corticosteroid injection
Non-steroidal anti-inflammatory drugs (NSAIDs)	Owners using human preparations on their animals (dosing their pets with so-called painkillers). Dogs 'stealing' owners' medications *Aspirin* – particularly toxic in cats *Ibuprofen, flurbiprofen* and *naproxen* – may be rapidly fatal in some dogs *Phenylbutazone* – more toxic to cats than dogs	*Aspirin* – depression Gastric irritation, leading to vomiting and anorexia. Cats may show some incoordination *Ibuprofen* and *flurbiprofen* – gastric ulceration and perforation in dogs lead to vomiting and haematemesis, followed by diarrhoea with melaena. Kidney damage may cause acute and fatal renal failure. Dehydration due to fluid losses. *Naproxen* – gastric inflammation and ulceration leading to vomiting and melaena. Anaemia due to low-grade blood loss Dehydration	Stop medication with the drugs *Before symptoms show*, induce vomiting as soon as possible *If showing symptoms*, give absorptive preparations and/ or demulcents. Dosing with activated charcoal is vital in cases of aspirin poisoning, and it should be given immediately after vomiting ceases. Prepare intravenous fluids Prepare *cimetidine* for intravenous injection in cases of naproxen poisoning

TABLE 9.5	**Toxic agents—cont'd**		
Type	Causes	Effects	Treatment
Paracetamol	Owner-administered dose or tablet packet chewed	Dogs tolerate paracetamol well, but cats are easily poisoned by as little as half a 500 mg tablet. Poisoning with paracetamol results in haemoglobin being changed to methaemoglobin, which is incapable of transporting oxygen *Signs* Cyanosis Depression or excitement Incoordination due to hypoxia Facial swelling	Induce vomiting if no symptoms shown Give absorptive material by mouth but *not* before consulting veterinary surgeon – if *N-acetyl cysteine* is to be used, the absorptive material may also prevent the absorption of this antidote Provide oxygen if any sign of cyanosis; ensure that the animal rests as much as possible. Prepare *methionine* or *N-*acetyl cysteine (human preparation Parvolex) for oral administration
Salbutamol	Human preparations that are used to treat asthma and for premature labour	Stimulation of the sympathetic nervous system, causing peripheral vasodilatation and rapid heart rate (tachycardia) Panting respiration Muscle weakness	General first aid treatment, but beta blockers may be needed if the heart rate becomes excessively high
Calcipotriol	Vitamin D derivative contained in psoriasis creams and ointments, chewed by pups	Similar to vitamin D overdose. Poisoning leads to hypercalcaemia and hyperphosphataemia, causing acute nephritis and damage to gastrointestinal tract *Signs* Haemorrhagic diarrhoea, polyuria and polydipsia Collapse with or without convulsions. Death may occur within 24 hours	Induce vomiting if ingested within the past 2–4 hours Prepare activated charcoal solution. Prepare Hartmann's solution for intravenous administration – it is important to flush the calcium and phosphates through the kidneys to minimize renal damage Prepare furosemide diuretic injection
Herbicides Chlorates	Ingestion of weedkillers or drinking from contaminated puddles – this substance does not degrade readily after use	Vomiting and diarrhoea with abdominal pain. Cyanosis of mucosae, turning to a muddy brown colour (blood becomes chocolate in colour because poison causes the formation of methaemoglobin – see Paracetamol)	General first aid treatment Prepare *methylene blue* injection

Continued

TABLE 9.5 Toxic agents—cont'd

Type	Causes	Effects	Treatment
Dinitro compounds	Ingestion of 2,4-dinitrophenol (2,4-D) or dinitro-orthocresol (2,4,5-T)	Depression, listlessness, muscle weakness. Rapid respiration and dyspnoea Hyperthermia with sweating Urine is almost fluorescent yellow/green	General first aid treatment Monitor rectal temperature to detect hyperthermia
Paraquat	Ingesting weedkiller (although this product is rapidly absorbed on to the soil after application, which renders it harmless). Paraquat has been used in malicious poisonings, but most cases are due to accidents	Inflammation of the mouth and tongue Vomiting and diarrhoea, with abdominal pain Depression and progressive respiratory distress and cyanosis over a period of days, resulting in death	*Induce vomiting* as soon as ingestion of this chemical is suspected. Even though this is an irritant poison, the effects of the absorbed poison are so severe that treatment is usually hopeless, and the only hope is to remove the poison from the alimentary tract as soon as possible. Administering Fuller's earth is also helpful because the poison will bind to the Fuller's earth and be rendered inactive
Insecticides			
Borax	Ant killers (e.g. Nippon), which are based on honey and therefore very attractive to dogs	Vomiting and diarrhoea Collapse, convulsions and possible paralysis Poisoning may be fatal	General first aid treatment
Organophosphates	Overdosing with insecticidal sprays, chewing insecticidal collars, etc.	Vomiting and diarrhoea Salivation Constricted pupils. Muscular twitching, excitement, followed by weakness, incoordination. Depression or convulsions	General first aid treatment Prepare *atropine sulphate* for injection
Organochlorines	Woodworm treatments and other insecticides (aldrin, dieldrin, gamma benzene hexachloride, etc.). Many products are now withdrawn from sale, but old stocks still exist	Involuntary twitching of muscles, especially facial, fore- and hindlimbs, and convulsions Behavioural changes, e.g. aggression, pacing, apprehension, frenzy	Wash off contamination Administer absorptive material and/or liquid paraffin to decrease absorption *Fatty foods and drinks* (including milk) *must not be given* as they may increase absorption of the poison Prepare *barbiturate* injection to control convulsions

TABLE 9.5   Toxic agents—cont'd

Type	Causes	Effects	Treatment
Molluscicides			
Carbamate Metaldehyde	See Organophosphates Ingestion of slug bait, which some dogs and cats seem to find very palatable	Incoordination leading to hyperaesthesia and convulsions Rapid pulse and respiration, and possibly cyanosis	General first aid treatment Dosing with liquid paraffin may delay absorption of poison, as long as it is given before the patient shows any symptoms (do not dose the unconscious patient) Prepare *barbiturate* injection to control convulsions
Rodenticides			
Alphachloralose	Rat baits and preparations to control pigeon and seabird populations	Poison acts by lowering the body temperature Progressive depression, incoordination and coma with hypothermia	General first aid treatment, but warmth is essential
Calciferol	Ingestion of rat bait	See Calcipotriol (medicines)	
Anticoagulant preparations	Rat baits. Several different compounds come under this heading: warfarin, coumatetralyl, chlorophacinone, difenacoum, brodifacoum, bromadiolone	Interference with clotting mechanism results in haemorrhages in the mucosae, bruising and haematomas, swollen joints, etc.	General first aid treatment Prepare injections of vitamin K. Large and repeated dosing may be necessary
Household items			
Alcohol	Ingestion of alcoholic drink or fermenting grain (especially likely with pups)	Hyperaesthesia, incoordination, collapse and even death	Induce vomiting and provide general first aid treatment
Chocolate	Ingestion of theobromine (a stimulant) found in chocolate. Severity will depend on the amount of theobromine in the chocolate compared to the weight of the patient. Dark chocolate is more toxic than milk chocolate	Vomiting Diarrhoea Nervous excitement progressing to fits and coma Tachycardia Seizures Panting	Induce vomiting (may not be effective if chocolate ingested because of its sticky consistency). Gastric lavage may be required. Prepare activated charcoal solution
Disinfectants. Household disinfectants, when diluted to correct strength, do not cause a problem, but are often used undiluted or are	Phenols – *cats are particularly susceptible to poisoning by phenols.* Licking paws after walking on wet surfaces recently cleaned with undiluted or incorrectly diluted solutions	*These are corrosive poisons with a strong, distinctive odour*, e.g. pine disinfectants Convulsions, coma and death in acute poisoning cases	*Do not induce vomiting* General first aid treatment, including thorough washing of contaminated fur As for phenols

Continued

TABLE 9.5   Toxic agents—cont'd

Type	Causes	Effects	Treatment
incorrectly diluted by overzealous owners	of disinfectant Grooming coat after accidental spraying or splashing with strong disinfectant solutions	Less acute cases may have inflamed mouths (stomatitis) and occasionally ulcers in the mouth. Animals may also vomit and have diarrhoea and abdominal pain	
	Quaternary ammonium compounds – as for phenols	These are also corrosive poisons, but are odourless Depression and anorexia. Occasionally vomiting Salivation, stomatitis and mouth ulcers, especially on the tongue tip Skin ulcerations if compound not washed off quickly	
Ethylene glycol (antifreeze)	Ingestion of water drained from car radiators (dogs seem particularly prone to drink this)	Incoordination, depression and rapid breathing. Toxic effect on the kidney leads to progressive acute renal failure	General first aid treatment Ethanol is the specific antidote, and intravenous injections may be prepared if available at the surgery
Lily plants (in cats)	All parts of the lily are poisonous to cats, including the water they are in. Even a small amount can be toxic. Cats can ingest the pollen from their coat/feet if they come into contact	Toxic effect on the kidneys causing: Vomiting Depression Dehydration Diarrhoea	Early treatment can be effective. Induce vomiting. Intravenous fluid therapy and blood testing. Symptomatic treatment
Petroleum products	Usually a problem in cats which have fallen into containers of sump oil drained from cars Accidental spillages of petrol, paraffin, etc. Caking of tar in the paws	These are very corrosive poisons with a distinctive odour Depression, vomiting, collapse and death if enough ingested If submersed in the liquid, may also suffer an aspiration pneumonia, which is very severe because of the extremely irritant nature of the inhaled liquid Inflammation of the in-contact skin and mouth, especially the tongue if the animal has been allowed to groom	Do not induce vomiting General first aid treatment, including giving olive oil by mouth to decrease the absorption of the toxins

Adapted and reproduced with permission from Cooper and Lane (1999), Butterworth–Heinemann.

TABLE 9.6 Emetic agents

Agent	Method
Washing soda crystals	Two crystals on the back of the tongue
Apomorphine	Only given under the direction of the veterinary surgeon; 0.1 mg/kg subcutaneously
Xylazine	Only given under the direction of the veterinary surgeon; 3.0 mg/kg intramuscularly
Mustard	Not as effective as above; two teaspoonfuls in a cup of warm water

TABLE 9.7 Demulcent agents – used to bind poison in gut

Agent	Method
BCK granules	1–3 heaped teaspoons orally. May need to mix with food or water and syringe in
Charcoal	1 g/kg orally. May need to mix with food or water and syringe in
Kaolin	1–2 ml/kg orally

7. **Action:** Treat the symptoms shown by the patient. Administer drugs as directed by the veterinary surgeon.
   Rationale: *If the patient is collapsed or unconscious, administer oxygen. If advised, administer demulcents (Table 9.7) to bind the poison.*
8. **Action:** Administer an antidote if it is available.
   Rationale: *Very few poisons have an antidote. If there is one, it must be given under the direction of a veterinary surgeon.*
9. **Action:** Administer fluids orally if the animal is conscious or set up an intravenous drip.
   Rationale: *Oral fluids will dilute any poison that has been absorbed. In some cases, the administration of fluids will reduce damage to the tissues by flushing out the poison via the urine.*
10. **Action:** Make the patient warm and comfortable. Monitor the patient's rectal temperature. Ensure that the body temperature is maintained.
    Rationale: *Some poisons will depress or raise the body temperature.*

11. **Action:** Monitor the patient continually.
    Rationale: *Any changes in the patient's condition must be acted upon quickly.*
12. **Action:** If the owner implies that the poisoning was malicious, maintain a diplomatic silence and do not express opinions that could be used in a subsequent legal case.
    Rationale: *The case history and the laboratory results may be used as evidence in a legal case, should the poisoning be malicious. Make sure that all records are accurate and kept safely.*

Procedure: Treatment of bites and stings

1. **Action:** Place the animal in a comfortable position on a table.
   Rationale: *If the animal feels uncomfortable, it will try to escape.*
2. **Action:** Ask an assistant to restrain the animal so that it is relaxed and secure and the area is accessible for treatment.
   Rationale: *The assistant will be able to react quickly should the animal try to escape. The animal may resent the area being touched.*
3. **Action:** Clean your hands with a surgical scrub (see Fig. 7.2).
   Rationale: *It is important not to introduce infection into the wound.*
4. **Action:** Assess the type of wound (Table 9.8).
   Rationale: *Treatment depends on the cause of the injury. There may be multiple bites or stings.*
5. **Action:** Treat the area with the appropriate action.
   Rationale: *Refer to Table 9.8.*
6. **Action:** Monitor the patient continually.
   Rationale: *Any changes in the patient's condition can be acted upon quickly.*

Procedure: Treatment of electrocution

1. **Action:** Assess the environment that you are in – is there any risk to you or to others?
   Rationale: *Never touch an electrocuted animal until the power supply is disconnected as you may get an electric shock via the animal.*
2. **Action:** If the power cannot be disconnected, then push the animal from the source with a *dry, wooden pole*.
   Rationale: *Such a pole will not conduct the electricity.*
3. **Action:** Check the patient's airway, breathing and circulation. Resuscitate as appropriate.

TABLE 9.8 Treatment of bites and stings

Type	Symptoms	Complications	Treatment
Wasp sting	Commonly seen in dogs. Stings are usually around the mouth and nose, and also the feet. The result is a painful swelling and, if in the mouth area, excessive salivation. Stings to the pharynx can inhibit respiration. The stinger is *not* left in the animal	Some animals may be allergic to the sting and may show an excessive reaction, anaphylaxis. Collapse, dyspnoea and symptoms of shock may be seen	Wash the area with warm water and apply a dilute solution of water and acetic acid (vinegar). If the patient is collapsed, then treat as for shock. If the patient is dyspnoeic, then treat for asphyxia (see Treatment of airway obstruction)
Bee sting	Commonly seen in puppies, who are prone to curiosity, and adult dogs. Stings are usually around the mouth and nose, and also the feet. The result is a painful swelling and, if in the mouth area, excessive salivation. Stings to the pharynx can inhibit respiration. The stinger is left in the animal as the bee dies	Some animals may be allergic to the sting and may show an excessive reaction (anaphylaxis). Collapse, dyspnoea and symptoms of shock may be seen	The stinger has a pumping sac attached. This must be removed carefully to avoid further liquid entering the site. Hold the sting at the point of entry with a pair of tweezers and remove. Wash the area with warm water and apply a solution of water and bicarbonate of soda (1 teaspoon in 0.5 litre water)
Snake bite – the adder (*Vipera beris*) is the only venomous snake is Britain	Commonly seen in dogs. Bites are usually around the head and neck. The area is painful and oedematous. Two fang marks may be visible. The patient may be dull and depressed, and may collapse	The severity of the reaction depends on the type of snake, the amount of venom injected and the patient's reaction to the venom	Call a vet. Keep the patient as still as possible. Thoroughly wash with warm water, but do *not* rub. This will push the venom deeper into the tissue. Apply a cold compress to reduce tissue perforation. Administer antivenom and medication under the directions of the veterinary surgeon
Toad skin venom	Commonly seen in dogs that have picked up the toad in their mouths. Excessive salivation may be seen	Occasionally the animal may swallow the toad	Constant observation of the patient. Occasionally, nervous symptoms may develop. Administer medication as directed by the veterinary surgeon

Rationale: The animal may be found collapsed or even dead. Electric shocks may induce cardiac arrest.

4. **Action:** When stable, examine the patient for burns and other injuries. Treat as appropriate.
   Rationale: Burns may appear on the entry and exit points of the electric current. Pieces of skin that touch other skin, e.g. toes or scrotum, may also be affected.

Procedure: Treatment of shock

1. **Action:** Assess the animal for clinical signs of shock (Tables 9.9 and 9.10).
   Rationale: From this examination you can assess the severity of the problem.
2. **Action:** Restore the circulating blood volume to its original level by using intravenous fluid therapy.

TABLE 9.9 Clinical signs of shock

Symptom	Reason
Rapid, weak pulse	The heart is working harder because of low blood volume/pressure
Quiet heart sounds	Poor cardiac filling
Pale mucous membranes	Vasoconstriction due to the blood going to the vital organs, e.g. heart, brain and lungs
Increased capillary refill time	Vasoconstriction due to the blood going to the vital organs, e.g. heart, brain and lungs
Cold extremities	Due to vasoconstriction and low metabolic rate
Depressed level of consciousness	Reduced blood flow to the brain
Reduced urine output	Reduced blood flow to the kidneys

TABLE 9.10 Types of shock

Type	Cause
Cardiogenic	Cardiac output is reduced, e.g. reduced cardiac filling, pericarditis or reduced cardiac emptying, cardiomyopathy
Hypovolaemic	Low circulating blood volume, e.g. haemorrhage, excessive vomiting or diarrhoea
Vasculogenic	The capacity of the blood vessels increases due to vasodilation

a. Neurogenic – trauma to the central nervous system
b. Anaphylactic – an abnormal reaction to an antigen. Causes widespread histamine release, which in turn causes vasodilation
c. Endotoxic – endotoxins from bacteria release chemicals that cause vasodilation

Rationale: This will increase blood pressure and therefore improve the circulation to the body tissues.

3. **Action:** The fluid used should resemble that which is lost. In cases of severe shock, the use of a plasma expander is recommended (see Chapter 4).

   Rationale: Replace blood with blood or a plasma expander, and replace electrolytes with a crystalloid solution such as Hartmann's solution. Plasma expanders increase the osmotic pressure of blood, which draws fluid into the blood vessels, increasing circulating blood volume.

4. **Action:** Provide oxygen to the patient via a closed anaesthetic circuit.

   Rationale: This will correct hypoxia caused by low haemoglobin levels due to blood loss.

5. **Action:** Provide warmth. This should be by indirect heat, i.e. a warm environment and/or conserving body heat with bubble wrap and blankets.

   Rationale: Direct heat will increase surface dilation of the capillaries and take blood away from the vital organs to the skin surface.

6. **Action:** Monitor the patient closely.

   Rationale: Any changes in the patient's condition can be noted and treated.

7. **Action:** Administer medication under the direction of a veterinary surgeon.

   Rationale: Drugs used may include sodium bicarbonate to correct metabolic acidosis, corticosteroids, anticoagulants, adrenaline (epinephrine) and antibiotics.

For treatment of injuries to the different body systems, refer to Table 9.11.

DYSTOCIA – DIFFICULT BIRTH

Procedure: Diagnosis of dystocia

1. **Action:** Ensure that you are familiar with the gestation period and the timings of the stages of parturition for the species with which you are dealing (Table 9.12).

   Rationale: This will enable you to make an accurate assessment of any problems concerning parturition when contacted by the owner.

2. **Action:** Take an accurate history from the owner of the dam – this may be face-to-face or over the telephone. Make particular note of the breed and age of the bitch or queen, the date of mating, the current behaviour of the dam and the timing of each incident.

TABLE 9.11   Injuries to the body systems potentially requiring first aid

Area	Possible causes	Symptoms	Treatment
Respiratory system			
Nose	Trauma	Head shaking, epistaxis, mouth-breathing, crepitus, deformity and/or dyspnoea	Cold compress to control swelling/haemorrhage Oxygenation if dyspnoeic. Rest to lower blood pressure. Constant monitoring in case of concussion
	Foreign body, e.g. grass/grass seed	Sneezing, head shaking, epistaxis, discharge and/or mouth-breathing	Remove if visible. Prepare for general anaesthetic/sedation
	Tumour	Head shaking, epistaxis, mouth-breathing, crepitus, deformity and/or dyspnoea	Cold compress to control haemorrhage. Oxygenation if dyspnoeic. Rest to lower blood pressure
Pharynx and oesophagus	Foreign body, e.g. grass, fish hook, string, balls and sticks	Gagging, retching, salivation, dysphagia, dyspnoea and/or asphyxia	Remove if visible Prepare for GA/sedation. Fish hooks must be cut out (not pulled). Treat asphyxia (see Treatment of airway obstruction). The Heimlich manoeuvre may be required
Larynx and trachea	Foreign body, e.g. grass, balls and sticks	Gagging, retching, salivation, dyspnoea and/or asphyxia	Remove if visible Treat asphyxia (see Treatment of airway obstruction). The Heimlich manoeuvre may be required
	Trauma, e.g. dog bites, strangulation from a caught collar	Open and closed wounds, pain, swelling, emphysema (air in tissues) dyspnoea, air hissing and/or asphyxia	Clean and dress wounds. Ensure that no fluid enters the trachea. Cover holes in the trachea with clean cling film before dressing. Treat dyspnoea with oxygen. Treat asphyxia (see Treatment of airway obstruction). Treat for shock
Lungs and chest wall	Trauma, e.g. bites, gunshot wounds	Open and closed wounds, pain, swelling, emphysema (air in tissues) dyspnoea, air hissing and/or asphyxia	Clean and dress wounds. Ensure that no fluid enters the trachea. Cover holes in the trachea with clean cling film before dressing. Treat dyspnoea with oxygen. Treat asphyxia (see Treatment of airway obstruction). Treat for shock
	Fluid in the alveolar spaces	Dyspnoea and asphyxia	Treat dyspnoea with oxygen. Treat asphyxia (see Treatment of airway obstruction). Treat for shock

TABLE 9.11	Injuries to the body systems potentially requiring first aid—cont'd		
Area	**Possible causes**	**Symptoms**	**Treatment**
	Paraquat poisoning	Dyspnoea and cyanosis	See Treatment of poisoning
	Trauma resulting in a pneumothorax and/or haemothorax	Open and closed wounds, pain, swelling, emphysema (air in tissues) dyspnoea, air hissing and/or asphyxia	Clean and dress wounds. Ensure that no fluid enters the thorax. Do *not* remove any penetrating foreign bodies. The use of a ring pad will prevent displacement of the foreign body and/or fractures. Cover holes with clean cling film before dressing. Treat dyspnoea with oxygen. Treat asphyxia (see Treatment of airway obstruction). Treat for shock
Diaphragm	Trauma, e.g. road traffic accident	Commonly seen in cats. Dyspnoea, abdominal respiration and lung collapse	Treat dyspnoea with oxygen. Encourage abdominal organs back into place by lifting the patient up under the shoulders. Rest with the head and shoulders higher than the body
Digestive system			
Mouth	Stings	Swelling and salivation	See Treatment of bites and stings
	Foreign body, e.g. bones, sticks, string and fish hooks	Gagging, retching, salivation, dysphagia, dyspnoea and/or asphyxia	Remove if visible. Prepare for GA/sedation. Fish hooks must be cut out (not pulled). Treat asphyxia (see Treatment of airway obstruction). The Heimlich manoeuvre may be required
	Trauma	Fractures, crepitus and/or wounds	Compress wounds if possible. Fractures will need immobilizing under GA
Stomach and intestines	Infection	Vomiting and/or diarrhoea. Pain and dehydration	Supportive therapy such as intravenous fluids. Nil by mouth Treat shock
	Gastric dilatation and volvulus. The stomach distends with gas and then twists (volvulus) at the cardia and pylorus	Restlessness, vomiting and belching. Swelling of the abdomen, laboured breathing, progressing to collapse and death	Call a vet as soon as possible. Relieve pressure in the stomach by passing a stomach tube. Use a roll of bandage as a mouth guard to prevent chewing. If that is unsuccessful, then insert a wide bore needle into the upper left abdominal wall at the point of maximum distension
	Intussusception or foreign body, e.g. toys, bones and balls	Vomiting, pain and dehydration	Supportive therapy such as intravenous fluids. Nil by mouth. Treat shock. Prepare for X-rays and surgery

Continued

TABLE 9.11	Injuries to the body systems potentially requiring first aid—cont'd		
Area	**Possible causes**	**Symptoms**	**Treatment**
Rectum	Prolapse caused by tenesmus or diarrhoea	Protrusion of the rectum through the anal sphincter. Common in hamsters. Can be partial or total. Swelling can occur if left for too long	Moisten the area with warm saline and lubricate with liquid paraffin. Attempt to replace by turning the prolapse back on itself. Ensure that hands are scrubbed. Prevent further straining with an analgesic suppository or local anaesthetic. Prevent self-trauma with the use of an Elizabethan collar
Anus	Impacted faeces or foreign body, e.g. bones	Tenesmus, discomfort, haemorrhage and licking the area	Lubricate the area with liquid paraffin. Remove with fingers or forceps. Wear gloves
Perineum	Fly strike	Smelly, inflamed and burnt area. Eggs and maggots visible	Remove *all* maggots Clip and clean the area. An application of an insecticide can be used. Treat for shock if extensive
Urogenital system			
Prolapsed uterus and polyps	Sometimes seen at time of oestrus	Red mass protruding from the vulva	Ensure hands are scrubbed. Lubricate with liquid paraffin and apply gentle pressure to replace. Prevent self-trauma with the use of an Elizabethan collar
Penis	Paraphimosis – penis is engorged with blood and too big to slide back into the prepuce	Swelling and redness	Apply a cold compress on to the area. This will reduce the blood supply and the size of the penis. Lubricate and replace
	Trauma, e.g. cuts or haemorrhage from an over-amorous dog	Open wounds and haemorrhage	Apply a cold compress on to the area. Pinching the skin in front of the scrotum will reduce the haemorrhage
	Foreign body, e.g. grass/grass seed	Swelling, pain and anuria	Remove if visible. GA/sedation may be required. Prepare theatre
Special senses			
Eye	Foreign body, e.g. grass seed	Blepharospasm (eye screwed up), photophobia (fear of light), tears, redness and rubbing	Remove by flushing with sterile saline and/or use a damp cotton bud GA/sedation or local anaesthetic may be necessary. Do *not* remove a penetrating foreign body

TABLE 9.11		Injuries to the body systems potentially requiring first aid—cont'd	
Area	**Possible causes**	**Symptoms**	**Treatment**
	Prolapse	The eyeball is outside the patient's head. It will become more inflamed the longer it is out	Replace the eyeball as soon as possible. With scrubbed hands, lubricate the eyeball and lids with 'false tears'. Pull back the eyelids and attempt to replace. Never put any pressure on the eyeball. Advise an owner to keep the eyeball damp with a cloth soaked in cooled boiled water before bringing to the surgery
	Chemical splashes	Blepharospasm (eye screwed up), photophobia (fear of light), tears, redness and rubbing	Flush with copious amounts of sterile saline. Dilute vinegar may be used to neutralize alkali splashes, and sodium bicarbonate will neutralize acid splashes. Follow with sterile saline
Ear	Trauma	Open wounds or haematoma	Control haemorrhage with a cold compress or pressure bandage. Clean and dress wounds. Apply an ear bandage. The haematoma may need draining under a GA
Metabolic disorders			
Hypocalcaemia	Low blood calcium. Commonly seen in bitches at the peak of lactation (usually 2–3 weeks). Calcium is depleted from the blood stream to go into the milk. This leaves little calcium for the rest of the body	Restlessness, panting and shivering, progressing into collapse, hyperaesthesia and eventually death	Extra calcium must be provided in the diet. If the patient is already hypocalcaemic, then an injection of intravenous calcium 10% must be given under the direction of the veterinary surgeon. Wean the offspring immediately
Hypoglycaemia	Occurs in diagnosed diabetics, where there is an imbalance between the insulin given and glucose available. This can be due to an overdose of insulin, anorexia, strenuous exercise and/or extreme temperatures	Slowed metabolic rate, lethargy, incoordination and dry mucous membranes, leading to collapse, hyperaesthesia, convulsions and eventually death	If the animal is conscious, administer oral glucose solution. Honey or sugar is the best alternative. If the animal is unconscious, then an intravenous injection of glucose must be given under the direction of a veterinary surgeon. Glucose can also be given via a stomach tube. This is metabolized at a slower rate
Uraemia	Usually occurs in old dogs and cats with chronic renal failure. The kidneys, which normally excrete toxins, are not working, so the toxins remain in the blood	Polydipsia and polyuria, loss of weight, vomiting, halitosis and mouth ulcers, progressing into epileptiform fits and death	Make the patient comfortable. The use of intravenous fluids can help to alleviate the symptoms

Continued

TABLE 9.11	**Injuries to the body systems potentially requiring first aid—cont'd**		
Area	**Possible causes**	**Symptoms**	**Treatment**
Hyperthermia	Often caused by heatstroke, e.g. dogs left in hot cars. The temperature regulating centre in the brain is unable to control the body temperature	Restlessness, panting, salivation and distress, progressing into collapse, coma and death. High rectal temperature	Cool the patient as soon as possible. Use a cold shower or hosepipe. Ice packs and wet towels are useful. Monitor rectal temperature every 15 minutes. Cool until normal temperature is reached. Continue to monitor every 30 minutes in case temperature rises again
Hypothermia	Often seen in young or small animals under anaesthetic. Heat loss is greater due to their large surface area compared to body mass	Lethargy, reluctance to move or feed, cold to touch, progressing to collapse and death	Warm the animal as soon as possible. Use a warm environment, blankets, heat pad and/or hot water bottle. Monitor rectal temperature every 15 minutes until normal temperature is reached. Continue to monitor every 30 minutes in case it falls again

GA, General anaesthetic.

TABLE 9.12	**Stages of parturition**
Stage	**Symptoms**
Preparation	Nesting, restlessness, may seek out the company of the owner. Prepartum hypothermia due to declining levels of plasma progesterone concentration may occur, and the body temperature may fall to below 37°C within 24–36 hours of birth. Relaxation and softening of the vulva
Stage 1: Start of contractions until the cervix is fully dilated. May last for 24 hours in the bitch, but is difficult to assess as start of contractions is very gradual	Onset of uterine contractions, which push against the dilating cervix. Allantoic fluid may drain from the vulva due to the rupture of the allantochorion (first water bag). The dam may appear uncomfortable and restless. Vomiting, shivering and/or loss of appetite may occur
Stage 2: Full dilation of the cervix until the delivery of the fetus. Normally, puppies may be born every 20–30 minutes, while kittens may be born every 30–60 minutes	Stronger uterine contractions push the fetus through the dilated cervix and into the vagina. The fetus may be in anterior or posterior presentation, and the amniotic sac surrounding the puppy or kitten may rupture. This is normal and allows the neonate to breathe when born. The dam may break the sac, but if not, the sac must be broken rapidly
Stage 3: Delivery of the placenta. Usually complete within 30–60 minutes	Placenta is expelled from the vulva and may be eaten by the dam. Stages 2 and 3 may be mixed up in multiparous (litter-bearing) species
Puerperium: period during which the uterus involutes (contracts) and returns to normal. It may last for several weeks	A dark discharge known as the lochia may drain from the dam for up to a week after parturition. As long as this is odourless, and the dam is well, there is no need to worry

Rationale: This information will help you to assess the stage of parturition (Table 9.12) and whether there is a cause for concern (Table 9.13 and Box 9.5). Certain breeds are more prone to dystocia than others.

3. **Action:** Ask the owners if they have done anything to assess or assist the dam, e.g. taking the body temperature at regular intervals, watching behaviour patterns such as restlessness or nesting, administering herbal remedies such as raspberry tea.

   Rationale: Some experienced breeders/owners may have methods by which they assist their animals through parturition, and it is important that you are aware of what has been done and at what stage. The information will also help to diagnose the type of dystocia (Table 9.13).

4. **Action:** Make sure that you write down all the details.

   Rationale: You must pass this information to the veterinary surgeon and writing it down will ensure you do not forget.

5. **Action:** If you are concerned, then the owner must be asked to bring the dam into the surgery for the veterinary surgeon to examine.

   Rationale: As a veterinary nurse you may monitor the progress of the dam, but it is the veterinary surgeon who ultimately diagnoses the problem and prescribes the treatment.

BOX 9.5 Causes for concern

1. A bitch has passed 70 days of gestation and shows no sign of starting parturition
2. A queen passed 65 days of gestation and shows no sign of starting parturition (N.B.: Persians and Siamese often go up to 70 days' gestation)
3. Dam is restless, strains forcefully but infrequently
4. Straining begins and then ceases
5. Black/green discharge with no sign of parturition beginning
6. Parturition has not started within 48 hours of a drop in body temperature
7. Straining for over an hour with no progress
8. Has produced several fetuses, the last more than 2 hours ago, and the dam is restless
9. Has produced a few fetuses, the last more than 2 hours ago, and a large litter is expected

---

6. **Action:** Once the dam has been admitted, she may be placed in a quiet kennel to await the veterinary surgeon.

   Rationale: Many parturient dams may cease to make progress when they are in unfamiliar or noisy environments. Try to put her in a quiet area away from other dogs or cats, ensuring that the area is in subdued light and warm.

TABLE 9.13 Types of dystocia

Type	Comment
Maternal – resulting from factors in the dam	1. Primary uterine inertia – contractions may fail to start or start weakly and then cease. May be due to very large litters, very small litters or may be seen in fat, unfit bitches. This is rare in cats 2. Secondary uterine inertia – contractions may start but then stop. May be due to exhaustion caused by obstruction or during delivery of a large litter. In both cases, oxytocin and calcium borogluconate may be given by the veterinary surgeon to strengthen contractions. Caesarean section may be required 3. Obstruction of the birth canal – due to abnormalities such as pelvic deformity, neoplasm or torsion of the uterus. If the obstruction cannot be rectified, then a caesarean section is required contractions. Caesarean section may be required

Fetal – resulting from factors caused by the fetus	1. Oversized fetuses may result from:
	  (a) Breed conformation, e.g. large head size, brachycephalic breeds
	  (b) Large fetuses as a result of a small litter
	  (c) Abnormalities such as fetal monsters
	2. Incorrect presentation – the fetus may be misaligned so that it is unable to progress through the birth canal

7. **Action:** The veterinary surgeon will assess the dam to check that she is pregnant. This may be done by ultrasonography or radiography.

   Rationale: An obese bitch or queen may appear to be pregnant, especially if her owner is convinced that she is!

8. **Action:** Wearing gloves and using a water-soluble lubricant, the veterinary surgeon will then gently examine the bitch via the vagina.

   Rationale: This is to check for the presence of a puppy in the birth canal. This is impossible in the queen, although a kitten in the birth canal may be palpable externally.

9. **Action:** Depending on the results of this examination, the appropriate treatment will be given (Table 9.13).

   Rationale: In most cases of dystocia, oxytocin will be administered and the dam left for about 30 minutes in a quiet cage to see if this will have an effect on contractions. If progress has still not been made, a caesarean section will be performed.

REFERENCES AND FURTHER READING

Ackerman, N., 2016. Aspinall's Complete textbook of Veterinary Nursing, third ed. Elsevier, Oxford.

Aspinall, V., 2011. The Complete Textbook of Veterinary Nursing, second ed. Elsevier, Oxford.

Cooper, B., Mullineaux, E., Turner, L., 2011. Textbook of Veterinary Nursing, fifth ed. BSAVA, Gloucester.

ECPD, 2014. Tracheostomy. [ONLINE] Available at: http://www.ecpd-vetnurse.com/wpcontent/uploads/2014/01/Tracheostomy-Notes.pdf. [Accessed 4 April 2017].

Fletcher, D., Boller, M., Brainiard, B., et al., 2012. RECOVER evidence and knowledge gap analysis on veterinary CPR. Part 7: Clinical guidelines. [ONLINE] Available at: http://onlinelibrary.wiley.com/doi/10.1111/j.1476-4431.2012.00757.x/abstract. [Accessed 4 April 2017].

Hotston-Moore, A., 1999. Manual of Advanced Veterinary Nursing. BSAVA, Gloucester.

Lane, D., Cooper, B., 1999. Veterinary Nursing. Butterworth-Heinemann, Oxford.

Lane, D., Cooper, B., 2003. Veterinary Nursing. Butterworth-Heinemann, Oxford.

Linklater, A., 2016. Primary Survey (Triage) and Resuscitation. [ONLINE] Available at: http://www.msdvetmanual.com/emergency-medicine-and-critical-care/evaluation-and-initialtreatment-of-the-emergency-patient/primary-survey-triage-and-resuscitation. [Accessed 4 April 2017].

O'Dwyer, L., 2013. Staying Alive – What's New in CPR? [ONLINE] Available at: http://ecpdvetnurse.com/2013/02/05/staying-alive-whats-new-in-cpr-online-vet-nurse-cpd/. [Accessed 4 April 2017].

10

Diagnostic imaging

Suzanne Easton

CHAPTER CONTENTS

INTRODUCTION

The term *radiography* covers all the procedures involved in the production and processing of a radiograph. The veterinary nurse is often given the responsibility for positioning the patient, setting up the X-ray machine ready for the exposure and processing the radiograph, either in an automatic or in a manual processor. It is important that the quality of the resulting radiograph is such that it aids the diagnosis of the veterinary surgeon – if it does not, there is little point in the technique. To achieve a high standard of radiography, the nurse must have a clear understanding of the steps involved in each procedure and how each step contributes to the final product. In addition, health and safety considerations are of particular importance when dealing with ionizing radiation, and the veterinary nurses must always be aware of the danger to themselves and to others in the vicinity of the machine. The Ionising Radiations Regulations 2017 must be strictly observed.

Nowadays, radiography is not the only diagnostic imaging technique available in a veterinary practice. Ultrasonography – the use of high-frequency sound waves to create an image – is becoming commonplace, and the veterinary nurse is likely to be responsible for the preparation of the patient and for setting up and maintaining the machine. The advantage of diagnostic ultrasound is that there is little danger to the patient or to the personnel involved in its use. Many referral practices have access to magnetic resonance imaging (MRI) and computerized tomography (CT) machines which increase the accuracy of the diagnostic process.

This chapter describes the procedures involved in the use of X-rays, ultrasound, MRI and CT scans.

RADIOGRAPHY

Procedure: Setting up the X-ray machine

1. **Action:** Place the X-ray machine in the designated room or controlled area.
   Rationale: To ensure that the local rules are followed, the X-ray machine must be used in a specifically designated area as outlined in the rules.
2. **Action:** Make sure that the radiation warning signs are displayed and visible.
   Rationale: Warning signs must be displayed when X-rays are being used. The position of these warning signs will be specified in the local rules.
3. **Action:** Plug the machine into the mains.
   Rationale: Most machines rely on mains electricity to work.
4. **Action:** Switch the X-ray machine on at the console or the main body of the machine.
   Rationale: The machine must be plugged in prior to switching on the machine.
5. **Action:** Check that the mains voltage compensation is accurate.
   Rationale: Mains voltage compensation ensures that the voltage received by the machine remains constant despite fluctuations within the mains voltage.
6. **Action:** Adjust the mains voltage compensation if needed.
   Rationale: Without adjustment of the mains voltage, radiographic exposure factors will not be accurate.
7. **Action:** Set the X-ray tube to the correct height above the film.
   Rationale: The X-ray tube should always be at a standard distance from the film – the film focal distance. This depends on the height of the table and the length of the stand supporting the tube.

8. **Action:** Set the exposure factors suitable for the examination, the patient type and the equipment being used.

   Rationale: *Exposure factors depend on the type of machine, the film/screen combination, the size of the patient and the region being examined.*

Procedure: Preparing the X-ray room for a radiographic examination

1. **Action:** Place the X-ray machine in the room and ensure that the correct exposure factors are set.

   Rationale: *Setting the exposure factors prior to positioning the patient ensures that, once the patient is positioned, an exposure can be made immediately.*

2. **Action:** Place the cassette on the table and centre it under the centre of the X-ray tube.

   Rationale: *The cassette should be placed securely on the table to prevent it falling on to the floor and breaking.*

3. **Action:** If a stationary grid is being used, place this in the correct position over the cassette.

   Rationale: *Incorrect use of the grid will result in poor-quality/non-diagnostic images.*

4. **Action:** Place sandbags, ties and foam pads so that they can be easily reached if needed to position the patient.

   Rationale: *Sandbags, ties and foam pads are used to hold the patient in the required position.*

5. **Action:** Remove unnecessary equipment from the room.

   Rationale: *This includes any objects that may cause an accident or be needed at a later part of the examination.*

6. **Action:** Remove any distractions from the room.

   Rationale: *Anything that may prevent the animal cooperating or cause unnecessary distress.*

Procedure: Preparing the patient for a radiographic examination

1. **Action:** Ensure that there is a valid clinical indication for the examination.

   Rationale: *Under the Ionising Radiations Regulations 2017, all examinations must be clinically justified, and all exposures must be kept to a minimum.*

2. **Action:** Use some form of chemical restraint – either sedation or general anaesthesia – as appropriate to the patient.

   Rationale: *Suitable chemical restraint should be used, unless the patient is considered to be an anaesthetic risk. Manual restraint should be used only in extreme circumstances, as it poses a risk to the health and safety of personnel.*

3. **Action:** Remove any artefacts from the patient, e.g. leads, collars, clips, matted or wet hair.

   Rationale: *Artefacts may distract the attention from and overlie the main point of interest.*

4. **Action:** If required for the procedure, ensure that any preparation of the patient, e.g. fasting, use of an enema or emptying the bladder, has taken place.

   Rationale: *In some examinations, the presence of faeces or urine, or food in the stomach, may restrict the view of the diagnostic points.*

5. **Action:** Position the animal correctly for the radiograph.

   Rationale: *If the animal is conscious and/or sedated, it may be necessary to calm the animal while it is positioned.*

POSITIONING THE PATIENT
(TABLES 10.1 AND 10.2, FIG. 10.1)

THORAX

Procedure: Lateral thorax (Fig. 10.2)

1. **Action:** Place the patient in right lateral recumbency.

   Rationale: *This is the conventional position for a thoracic radiograph.*

2. **Action:** Extend the forelegs and secure them using sandbags or ties.

   Rationale: *Extending the forelegs prevents the soft-tissue mass of the shoulder girdle impeding the view of the thoracic contents.*

3. **Action:** Place a pad under the sternum.

   Rationale: *This prevents rotation of the chest and ensures that it is in the same horizontal plane as the spine. This prevents distortion of structures in the thorax.*

4. **Action:** Place sandbags over the neck and hind legs to hold them in place.

   Rationale: *The hind legs should be secure but should not be extended as this rotates the chest.*

5. **Action:** Centre the beam (indicated by the cross on the light beam diaphragm) midway between the sternum and spine, level with the caudal border of the scapula.

TABLE 10.1 Positioning aids

Type	Use	Radiographic density
Troughs – range of sizes	To restrain animal on its back. Prevents rotation of the trunk	Radiolucent
Foam wedges – range of shapes and sizes Covered in plastic for ease of cleaning	For lateral views to provide support and prevent rotation of the trunk, and for accurate limb positioning. May be useful for supporting the spine and trunk to achieve a horizontal plane	Radiolucent
Sandbags – loose filling allows bending and twisting. Covered in plastic for ease of cleaning	Can be wrapped around to hold limbs in position or placed over the neck	Radiopaque – do not place in the primary beam
Tapes or ties – range of lengths	Looped around limbs to pull them into position and tie them to cleats on the table	Radiolucent
Wooden blocks	For raising the cassette up to the area of interest	Radiopaque – do not place in the primary beam

TABLE 10.2 General principles of positioning

Action	Rationale
Centre the primary beam over the main point of interest	To prevent distortion of the area by an oblique view
Place the area of interest as close as possible to the film	To prevent gross magnification of the part due to an excessive object–film distance. The image may also be blurred
Ensure that the centre of the primary beam is at right angles to the film	To avoid distortion of the image. This is important when examining joint or intervertebral disc spaces
Collimate the beam to as small an area as is realistically possible	To reduce the amount of scattered radiation
Take two views at right angles to each other	To assist in accurate location of a lesion and to visualize the area completely
Try to contain the whole area of interest on a single film	To reduce the number of exposures. If this means that important parts are viewed obliquely, e.g. whole spine, it is better to take views of several smaller areas
When imaging the spine, the body must be supported so that the vertebrae are in the same horizontal plane	To prevent distortion and magnification of individual vertebrae and of the intervertebral disc spaces

Rationale: This ensures that the centre of the primary beam coincides with the base of the heart.

6. **Action:** Collimate the beam to include the front of the shoulder and the edge of the sternum.
   Rationale: All regions of the lung field will be included.

7. **Action:** Expose on inspiration.
   Rationale: The lungs are fully inflated during inspiration, which provides better contrast between the air and the soft tissues.

Procedure: Dorsoventral thorax (Fig. 10.3)

1. **Action:** Place the patient in sternal recumbency.
   Rationale: This is particularly used for examination of the heart.

2. **Action:** Support the chin on a pad.
   Rationale: This keeps the head, neck and spine in a horizontal plane. The patient may also be more comfortable.

3. **Action:** Place a sandbag over the neck.
   Rationale: To prevent movement.

4. **Action:** Extend the forelegs and adduct them with the elbows out to the sides.
   Rationale: This prevents the muscle mass of the shoulder girdle overlying the thoracic cavity.

5. **Action:** Centre the beam (indicated by the cross of the light beam diaphragm) in the midline on the caudal border of the scapula.
   Rationale: This ensures that the heart base is in the centre of the image.

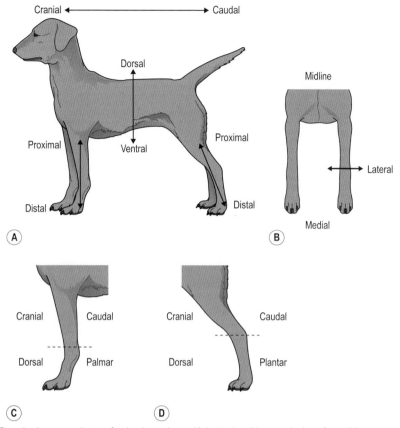

Cranial ← → Caudal

Dorsal

Ventral

Proximal

Distal

Proximal

Distal

(A)

Midline

Lateral

Medial

(B)

Cranial   Caudal

Dorsal   Palmar

(C)

Cranial   Caudal

Dorsal   Plantar

(D)

Fig. 10.1 Standard nomenclature for body regions. (Adapted, with permission, from Masters and Bowden (2001), Butterworth Heinemann.)

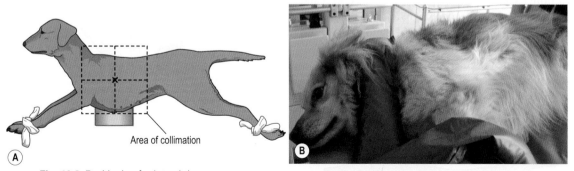

Area of collimation

(A)

(B)

Fig. 10.2 Positioning for lateral thorax.

6. **Action:** Collimate the beam to include the skin surfaces laterally, the thoracic inlet and the diaphragm.
   Rationale: *The image will include the cranial and caudal extent of the lung field.*
7. **Action:** Expose on inspiration.

Rationale: *The lungs are fully inflated during inspiration, which provides better contrast between the air and the soft tissues.*

N.B.: A ventrodorsal view of the thorax may be used to examine the lungs; however, if the animal is in

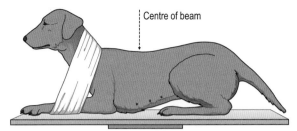

Fig. 10.3 Positioning for dorsoventral thorax.

respiratory distress, this position should be avoided as it may make respiration even more difficult.

ABDOMEN

Procedure: Lateral abdomen (Fig. 10.4)

1. **Action:** Place the patient in right lateral recumbency.
   Rationale: This is the conventional position for viewing the abdomen.
2. **Action:** Place a pad under the sternum.
   Rationale: A pad will support the sternum to keep the body in a horizontal plane.
3. **Action:** Extend the fore- and hindlimbs and secure them with sandbags or ties.
   Rationale: To prevent movement.
4. **Action:** Centre the beam (indicated by the cross of the light beam diaphragm) at the 11th/12th intercostal space, just cranial to the last rib.
   Rationale: This ensures that the entire abdomen is included.
5. **Action:** Collimate the beam to include the dorsal and lateral skin edges, the diaphragm and the pubic symphysis. If the patient is large, then move the beam towards the diaphragm or pubic symphysis, depending on the area of interest.
   Rationale: The top of the liver should be included in all radiographs of the complete abdomen.

6. **Action:** Expose on expiration.
   Rationale: During expiration, the diaphragm relaxes into its characteristic dome shape and the lungs contract, providing the maximum amount of space for the abdominal contents.

Procedure: Ventrodorsal abdomen (Fig. 10.5)

1. **Action:** Place the patient in dorsal recumbency.
   Rationale: Care must be taken if the animal is only lightly anaesthetized.
2. **Action:** Extend each foreleg cranially and secure with a tie or sandbag placed over the carpus.
   Rationale: This prevents rotation of the body. Do not place sandbags over the axillae as this can be uncomfortable.
3. **Action:** Make sure that the body does not rotate, to ensure that the sternum and spine are maintained in vertical alignment.

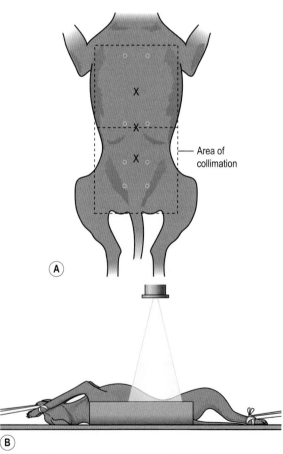

Fig. 10.5 Positioning for ventrodorsal abdomen.

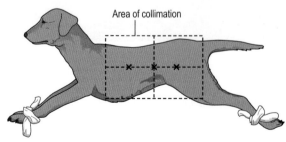

Fig. 10.4 Positioning for lateral abdomen.

Rationale: The use of a trough or sandbags placed on either side may help to support this position.

4. **Action:** Centre the beam (indicated by the cross of the light beam diaphragm) on the midline at the level of the umbilicus. This point may be adjusted towards the diaphragm or the pubic symphysis in larger breeds of dog.

   Rationale: This ensures that the whole abdominal area is included.

5. **Action:** Collimate the beam to include the lateral skin surfaces, the diaphragm and the pubic symphysis.

   Rationale: The cranial border of the liver must be shown in an abdominal radiograph.

6. **Action:** Expose on expiration.

Rationale: During expiration, the diaphragm relaxes into its characteristic dome shape and the lungs contract, providing the maximum amount of space for the abdominal contents.

PELVIS

Procedure: Lateral pelvis (Fig. 10.6)

1. **Action:** Place the patient in right lateral recumbency.

   Rationale: This is the only way of providing a true lateral projection of the pelvis.

2. **Action:** Place pads between the hind legs.

   Rationale: This ensures that the pelvis does not rotate.

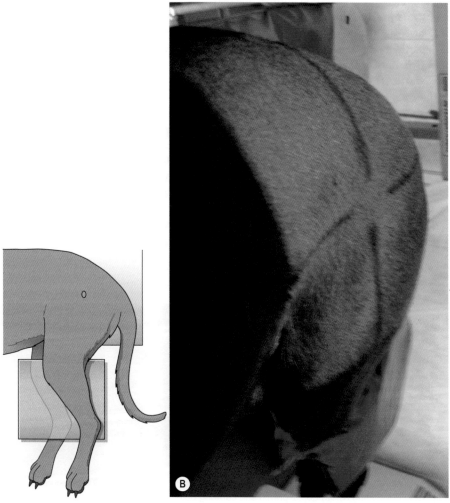

Fig. 10.6 Positioning for lateral pelvis.

3. **Action:** Centre the beam (indicated by the cross of the light beam diaphragm) over the greater trochanter of the left femur.

   Rationale: This ensures that the wings of the ilium and the acetabulum are visible.

4. **Action:** Collimate the beam to include the entire pelvic area.

Procedure: Ventrodorsal pelvis (extended hip position) (Fig. 10.7)

This is the position required by the British Veterinary Association/Kennel Club hip dysplasia scheme. It is important to make sure that the radiograph is correctly positioned as those that are not will be returned to the veterinary surgeon. The radiograph must also be labelled with the dog's Kennel Club registration number, the date of radiography and left and/or right markers.

1. **Action:** Place the patient in dorsal recumbency, ensuring that the body is straight.

   Rationale: This may be helped by the use of a trough or sandbags placed on either side of the upper abdomen. If the upper body is straight, the pelvis should also be straight. If the pelvis rotates, a foam pad may be placed under the lower hip.

2. **Action:** Extend the hind legs caudally so that the hips and stifles are fully extended. Secure with ties at the hocks.

   Rationale: This will further ensure that the pelvis is straight.

3. **Action:** Rotate the hind legs medially so that the femurs lie parallel to each other and the patellae are centred over the distal femurs.

   Rationale: Rotation of the femur places the femoral head into the acetabulum, which gives an indication of the degree of hip dysplasia.

4. **Action:** Hold the femurs together by placing a tie around the level of the mid-femurs. Sticky tape may be a convenient way of doing this.

   Rationale: The use of ties will ensure that the patient remains in this position.

5. **Action:** Added security may be achieved by placing another tie around the legs at the level of the mid-tibia. Again, sticky tape may be of use.

6. **Action:** Centre the beam (indicated by the cross on the light beam diaphragm) in the midline over the pubic symphysis.

   Rationale: This should provide equal detail on either side of the pelvic girdle.

7. **Action:** Collimate the beam to include the wings of the ilium and the proximal half of the femurs.

   Rationale: This should demonstrate the entire pelvic girdle and the hip joints. The obturator foramina should be of equal size. Any inequality may be due to tilting of the pelvis and poor positioning.

SKULL

Procedure: Ventrodorsal skull (Fig. 10.8)

1. **Action:** Place the patient in dorsal recumbency.

   Rationale: This ensures that the skull is as close as possible to the film.

2. **Action:** Extend the neck.

   Rationale: Extension makes sure that the head is horizontal.

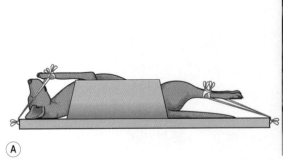
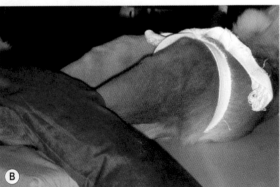

(A)   (B)

Fig. 10.7 Positioning (ventrodorsal pelvis) and centring point for assessment of hip dysplasia. Part A redrawn from Lane and Cooper (2003), Butterworth-Heinemann.

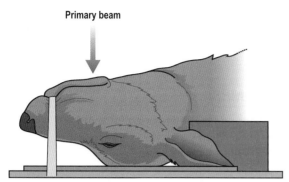

Primary beam

Fig. 10.8 Positioning for ventrodorsal skull to show the position of the hard palate.

3. **Action:** Place a foam pad under the neck.
   Rationale: This forces the head back, so that the hard palate is parallel to the table top.
4. **Action:** Centre the beam (indicated by the cross on the light beam diaphragm) in the midline at a point halfway along the interpupillary line.
   Rationale: This point may vary with the area to be examined.
5. **Action:** Collimate the beam to include the entire skull.
   Rationale: If necessary, collimate more tightly over the area of interest, e.g. tympanic bulla.

Procedure: Open-mouth rostrocaudal view of the tympanic bullae (Fig. 10.9)

1. **Action:** Place the animal in dorsal recumbency, with the hard palate perpendicular to the cassette. Tip the nose slightly past the vertical.

Rationale: This position ensures that the bullae are as close as possible to the cassette. By tilting the head, the skull bones do not obstruct the view of the tympanic bullae.
2. **Action:** Hold the mouth open to form a V-shape, using tapes around each jaw, or place an old needle case (with one end cut off to create a hole) between the teeth of the upper and lower jaws.
   Rationale: In this position, the mandible and the maxilla are removed from the area of interest.
3. **Action:** Orientate the primary beam parallel to the hard palate and centre it (indicated by the cross of the light beam diaphragm) on the base of the tongue.
   Rationale: The tympanic bullae are located directly behind the base of the tongue in this position.
4. **Action:** If the animal is intubated, remove the endotracheal tube before exposure.
   Rationale: The endotracheal tube will be superimposed on the tympanic bullae if it is not removed.

Procedure: Dorsoventral intraoral view of the nasal chambers (Fig. 10.10)

1. **Action:** The patient must be fully anaesthetized.
   Rationale: The cassette must be placed in the patient's mouth and without anaesthesia, the animal will chew on the film.
2. **Action:** Place the animal in sternal recumbency.
   Rationale: This position ensures that the maxilla does not overlie the nasal chambers and provides a comfortable supported position for the animal.
3. **Action:** Extend the neck.

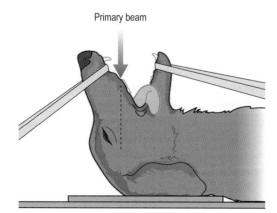

Primary beam

Fig. 10.9 Positioning for open-mouth rostrocaudal view.

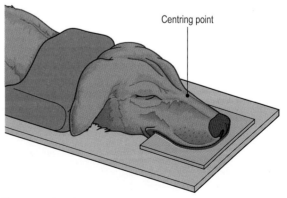

Centring point

Fig. 10.10 Positioning for dorsoventral intraoral view of the nasal chambers.

Rationale: The position of the head is straighter if the neck is extended.

4. **Action:** Place a sandbag over the neck.
   Rationale: This prevents the head from rotating.

5. **Action:** Place a non-screen film, corner first, as far into the mouth as possible.
   Rationale: Non-screen film is used as it provides excellent definition.

6. **Action:** Centre the beam (indicated by the cross on the light beam diaphragm) on a line midway between the external nares and the interpupillary line.
   Rationale: This allows visualization of the entire area of the nasal chambers.

7. **Action:** Place a left/right marker on the relevant side.
   Rationale: This ensures that any lesion can be related to the relevant nasal chamber. Most non-screen film cannot be labelled after processing, so this must be done prior to exposure.

Procedure: Nasopharynx (Fig. 10.11)

1. **Action:** Place the patient in lateral recumbency.
   Rationale: This will provide radiographic access to the nasopharynx.

2. **Action:** Place pads under the nose and under the neck.
   Rationale: These maintain the skull in a horizontal line and prevent rotation.

3. **Action:** Pull the forelegs caudally to lie against the wall of the thorax, using ties.
   Rationale: This pulls the shoulders and associated soft-tissue structures away from the area of interest.

4. **Action:** Centre the beam (indicated by the cross on the light beam diaphragm) on the mid-cervical area to include the pharynx and thoracic inlet.
   Rationale: The areas cranial and caudal to the pharynx must be included.

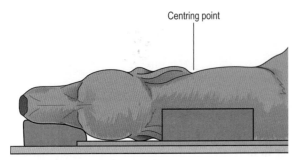

Centring point

Fig. 10.11 Positioning for nasopharynx.

5. **Action:** If the animal is intubated, remove the endotracheal tube before exposure.
   Rationale: The endotracheal tube may mask a stricture or a mass.

THE LIMBS

Procedure: Mediolateral view of a distal limb extremity (Figs 10.12A, 10.13B and 10.13C) – general rules

1. **Action:** Place the patient in lateral recumbency, with the limb to be X-rayed closest to the cassette, e.g. for the right forelimb, place the body in right lateral recumbency.
   Rationale: This ensures that the area is in close contact with the film, minimizing distortion of the image.

2. **Action:** Extend the uppermost limb caudally (forelimb) or cranially (hindlimb) and support it on the flank using a tie.
   Rationale: The limb and any associated tissue that is not required are pulled out of the area of interest.

3. **Action:** The limb to be X-rayed should lie parallel to the cassette. It may be necessary to prevent rotation of the limb by using a pad.
   Rationale: Rotation of the limb should be avoided as the image should show a true mediolateral view.

4. **Action:** Stifles and elbow joints should be flexed.
   Rationale: Flexion enables a full examination of the joint.

5. **Action:** Centre the beam (indicated by the cross on the light beam diaphragm) at the level of the joint or mid-shaft.
   Rationale: Accurate centring will avoid distortion.

6. **Action:** Collimate the beam to include the joint above and below the long bone, or a small area above and below the joint in question.
   Rationale: Viewing adjacent structures may aid diagnosis.

Procedure: Dorsopalmar or dorsoplantar view or craniocaudal view of a limb (Fig. 10.13) – general rules

1. **Action:** Place the patient in sternal (forelimb) or dorsal (hindlimb) recumbency so that the limb under investigation is parallel to the cassette.
   Rationale: Joints of the hindlimb are better imaged with the patient in dorsal recumbency. This allows the limb to be extended more easily, whilst still keeping the limb in good contact with the film.

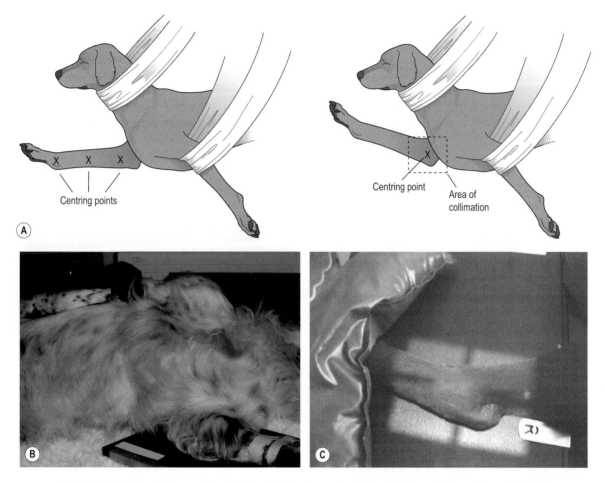

Fig. 10.12 A, Positioning for mediolateral view of a distal extremity. B, Position for mediolateral view of distal left elbow. C, Position for mediolateral view of right hock.

2. **Action:** Keep the limb under investigation straight.
   Rationale: On extension, the limb may rotate inwards. To prevent this, it may be necessary to lift and rotate the opposing limb.
3. **Action:** Centre the beam (indicated by the cross on the light beam diaphragm) at the level of the joint or the mid-shaft.
   Rationale: This must be accurate to avoid distortion.
4. **Action:** Collimate the beam to include the joint above and below the long bone, or a small area above and below the joint under investigation.
   Rationale: Viewing adjacent structures may aid diagnosis.

Procedure: Lateral shoulder (Fig. 10.14)

1. **Action:** Place the patient in lateral recumbency, making sure that the limb to be examined is closest to the cassette.
   Rationale: Lateral recumbency gives adequate access to the shoulder joint.
2. **Action:** Extend the head and neck and secure by placing a sandbag over the neck – be careful to avoid interfering with normal respiration.
   Rationale: This ensures that an endotracheal tube lying in the trachea and larynx is pulled away from the area of the shoulder.
3. **Action:** Pull the affected leg cranially and secure with a tie.

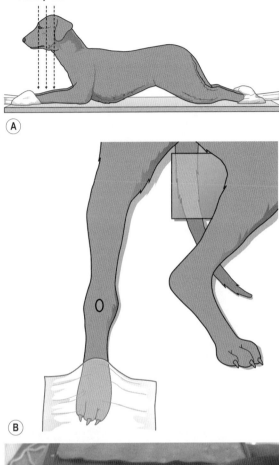

Primary beam

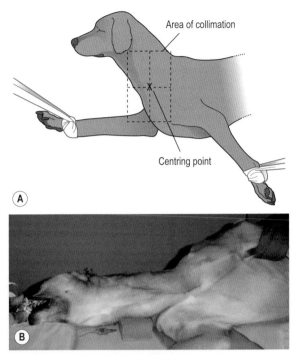

Area of collimation

Centring point

Fig. 10.14 Positioning for lateral shoulder.

Fig. 10.13 Positioning for A, craniocaudal view of distal forelimb, B, dorsoplantar view of distal hindlimb and C, dorsopalmar view of distal right forelimb.

Rationale: This ensures that the area of the shoulder joint is not overlain by the soft tissues of the other shoulder.

4. **Action:** Pull the opposing limb caudally and secure with a tie.
   Rationale: This draws the soft tissues of the opposing limb away from the shoulder joint to be examined.

5. **Action:** Centre the beam (indicated by the cross on the light beam diaphragm) through the joint space of the shoulder.
   Rationale: Palpating the greater tuberosity of the humerus on the lateral aspect of the bone will provide the correct location.

6. **Action:** Collimate the beam to include the proximal third of the humerus and the distal part of the scapula.
   Rationale: This will cover the complete shoulder joint.

Procedure: Craniocaudal shoulder (Fig. 10.15)

1. **Action:** Place the patient in dorsal recumbency and support in a cradle or with sandbags.
   Rationale: This allows extension of the limb while preventing obstruction by the chest wall.

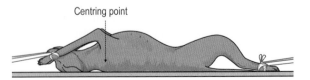

Centring point

Fig. 10.15 Positioning for craniocaudal shoulder.

2. **Action:** Fully extend the limb to be examined cranially and secure with a tie.
   Rationale: Full extension of the limb will demonstrate the joint, without the elbow overlying the area.
3. **Action:** Rotate the thorax until the limb is in the craniocaudal position.
   Rationale: Rotation of the thorax enables the limb to be placed in a true craniocaudal position.
4. **Action:** Centre the beam (indicated by the cross on the light beam diaphragm) over the acromion of the scapula.
   Rationale: The acromion can be palpated on the lateral aspect of the joint, at the distal end of the spine of the scapula. The joint will be in the centre of the radiograph and demonstrated without distortion.
5. **Action:** Collimate the beam to include the proximal third of the humerus and the distal part of the scapula.
   Rationale: This will cover the complete shoulder joint.

SPINE

Procedure: Lateral spine (Fig. 10.16)

1. **Action:** Place the patient in right lateral recumbency.
   Rationale: This will provide an image on which to base a diagnosis.
2. **Action:** Place supporting pads under the natural curves of the spine, i.e. the neck and the lumbar region. Place a pad under the nose.
   Rationale: These supports keep the spine horizontal and parallel with the tabletop. Placing a pad under the nose keeps the head in line.
3. **Action:** Place pads under the sternum and between the limbs.
   Rationale: These prevent rotation, which will pull the spine out of its horizontal position.
4. **Action:** If the cervical spine is to be examined, pull the forelimbs caudally.
   Rationale: This ensures that the soft tissues of the shoulder do not overlie the spine.

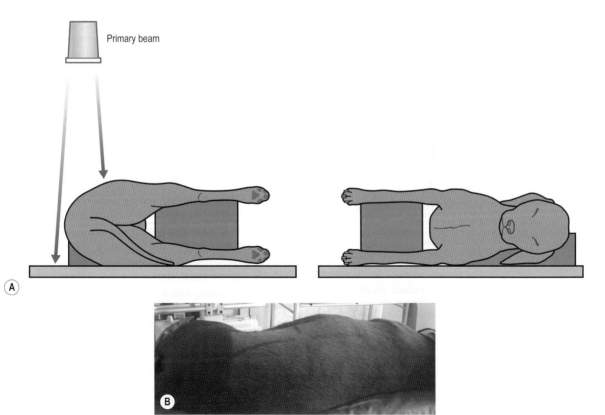

Primary beam

Fig. 10.16 Positioning for lateral spine.

5. **Action:** Centre the beam (indicated by the cross of the light beam diaphragm) over the area of interest.

   Rationale: Centring must be accurate, and care must be taken to avoid trying to cover too large an area at one time – divergence of the beam at the edges of the field will cause artificial narrowing of the joint spaces.

6. **Action:** Collimate the beam to cover about three vertebrae either side of the centre. Include muscle mass but not fat and skin. If the entire spine is to be examined, each image should overlap with the ones on either side.

   Rationale: By ensuring overlap, a complete study of each vertebra can be achieved with a minimum of distortion.

Procedure: Ventrodorsal spine (Fig. 10.17)

1. **Action:** Place the patient in dorsal recumbency supported in a trough or with sandbags.

   Rationale: Support must be provided to prevent rotation. This is even more important if a spinal injury is suspected.

2. **Action:** The spine must be positioned so that the sternum and the spine are in the same vertical plane.

   Rationale: Lack of alignment and rotation will affect the image and may provide an incorrect diagnosis.

3. **Action:** Extend the fore- and hindlimbs and secure with ties.

   Rationale: This provides additional support and prevents rotation of the spine.

4. **Action:** Centre the beam (indicated by the cross of the light beam diaphragm) over the area of interest.

   Rationale: Try to select the areas that correspond to those radiographed in the lateral view. In this way you have two planes per area of the spine.

5. **Action:** Collimate the beam to cover about three vertebrae either side of the centre. Include the transverse

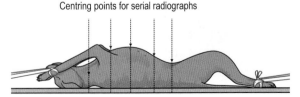

Centring points for serial radiographs

Fig. 10.17 Positioning for ventrodorsal spine.

processes and muscle mass, but not fat and skin. If the entire spine is to be examined, each image should overlap with the ones on either side.

Rationale: By ensuring overlap, a complete study of each vertebra can be achieved with a minimum of distortion.

USE OF CONTRAST MEDIA

Procedure: Use of barium in the evaluation of the gastrointestinal tract

1. **Action:** Prepare the barium sulphate. It may require mixing with a prescribed amount of water or may be ready-made. This must be done in the preparation room, away from the patient.

   Rationale: Barium should not be prepared near to the X-ray table as it may contaminate the table or the patient.

2. **Action:** Ensure that the patient is prepared as appropriate, e.g. fasted, given an enema. Do not sedate the animal.

   Rationale: Good patient preparation prevents the formation of artefacts on the radiograph, e.g. stomach contents mixed with barium. The use of sedatives will artificially slow gastrointestinal function and may affect the final diagnosis.

3. **Action:** Take plain radiographs before the introduction of contrast material.

   Rationale: These can be used for comparison with the contrast radiographs. Contrast media may mask some diagnostic features.

4. **Action:** If the patient is to be given a barium swallow, mix the barium with a small amount of normal food. Place a small amount of normal food on the top to entice the animal to eat.

   Rationale: The use of food allows the processes of eating and swallowing to be seen more clearly.

5. **Action:** If the patient is to be given a barium follow-through or meal, draw up approximately 5 ml/kg of liquid barium into a syringe. The patient may lap up the liquid or be force-fed with it.

   Rationale: A larger volume of barium is needed to prevent dilution as it passes down the gastrointestinal tract.

6. **Action:** If the patient is to be given a barium enema, the barium must be as liquid as possible. Introduce the barium into the rectum using a catheter (retrograde filling). Air may be introduced to provide a double contrast examination (Fig. 10.18).

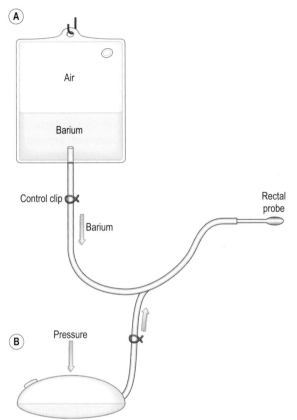

Fig. 10.18 Barium enema bag. In position A, the barium flows under gravity into the colon. In position B, barium empties from the colon into the bag, and then pressure on the bag will distend the colon with air for the double contrast effect. (Adapted, with permission, from Cooper and Lane (2000), Butterworth Heinemann.)

> *Rationale: Barium is used to outline the colon and must be as liquid as possible. Air can be used to enhance the image.*

7. **Action:** Always use the correct volume and consistency of contrast material.
   Rationale: If the wrong type and volume of contrast material are used, the radiographs may not be diagnostic.

8. **Action:** Select the correct patient position and collimate accurately.
   Rationale: Incorrect positioning may miss the area of interest and alter the appearance of the pathology present. Collimation will enhance the image.

Procedure: Barium swallow

1. **Action:** The patient remains conscious, but mild sedation may be needed.
   Rationale: The use of general anaesthesia is not recommended as the animal will be unable to swallow. Sedation should be avoided as this may slow the passage of ingesta down the gastrointestinal tract. If the animal seems likely to object to the taking of serial radiographs, sedation may be necessary.

2. **Action:** Place the patient in right lateral recumbency and take a plain radiograph.
   Rationale: Plain radiographs can be used to compare with the contrast radiographs.

3. **Action:** Offer the patient food mixed with barium or restrain the patient as described in Chapter 1 and place a syringe full of liquid barium into the corner of the mouth, avoiding spillage. Administer in one bolus.
   Rationale: The barium must be given as a bolus to aid visualization on the radiograph. Any spillage of barium may appear as an artefact on the radiograph.

4. **Action:** Place the patient in right lateral recumbency and take the X-ray of the oesophageal/thoracic area.
   Rationale: Food takes 15–30 seconds to pass down the oesophagus, so the radiograph must be taken quickly. Any barium remaining in the oesophagus will line the mucosa and outline any lesions.

Procedure: Barium meal or follow-through

1. **Action:** The patient should be fasted for 12 hours. Water should be withheld for 2 hours.
   Rationale: The presence of food and water will affect stomach function and the appearance and movement of the barium.

2. **Action:** Moderate sedation may be needed.
   Rationale: The patient may object to serial radiographs being taken. Acepromazine has the least effect on gut motility.

3. **Action:** Take plain radiographs – lateral and ventrodorsal views.
   Rationale: These provide a comparison with contrast radiographs. Taking two views allows accurate location of any lesions.

4. **Action:** Restrain the patient and place a syringe containing barium into the corner of the mouth, avoiding spillage. Administer slowly. It may be necessary to use a stomach tube.
   Rationale: The barium must be administered over a short period, so the procedure must be carried out quickly and cleanly. Any spillage of barium may appear as an artefact on the radiograph.

5. **Action:** If fluoroscopy is available, it may be used to observe the movements of the stomach.
   Rationale: Fluoroscopy produces 'live' X-rays and can be used for real-time investigations.
6. **Action:** Take a series of radiographs – right lateral, left lateral, ventrodorsal and dorsoventral centred over the mid-abdomen – immediately after administration of the barium.
   Rationale: These four views ensure that all parts of the stomach are examined.
7. **Action:** Repeat these views 10 minutes later and then at 30-minute intervals until the stomach is empty.
   Rationale: These time intervals allow the movement of barium to be monitored without missing too much detail.
8. **Action:** To demonstrate the small intestine, radiographs should be taken every hour until the stomach is empty.
   Rationale: This ensures that the complete intestinal tract is demonstrated.

Procedure: Barium enema (Fig. 10.18)

1. **Action:** The patient should be fed on a low-residue diet for 3 days.
   Rationale: This will ensure that a minimum amount of faeces is present in the colon.
2. **Action:** Prepare the patient by giving a non-irritant enema 2–3 hours before the examination.
   Rationale: This removes the faeces and ensures that barium does not adhere to anything other than the wall of the colon. The presence of faeces may obscure much of the abdominal detail.
3. **Action:** The patient should be given a general anaesthetic or heavy sedation.
   Rationale: This is essential to allow catheterization of the rectum and the introduction of barium, which can be uncomfortable.
4. **Action:** Place the patient in ventrodorsal and right lateral recumbency and take plain radiographs of the abdomen.
   Rationale: These will demonstrate any pathology present and may be used for comparison with the contrast radiographs.
5. **Action:** Hang an old drip bag containing a 50–50 mixture of barium and water from a drip stand.
   Rationale: This mixture allows the barium to flow into the colon.

6. **Action:** Insert a Foley catheter into the rectum. This is attached by means of a length of rubber tubing to the drip bag. Attach a clamp to control the flow from the bag.
   Rationale: Control of the barium flow is essential to prevent back flow and overfilling of the colon.
7. **Action:** Adjust the clamp to allow barium to flow slowly into the rectum and colon. Continue until the barium just begins to leak out around the catheter.
   Rationale: Hanging the bag from a drip stand allows the barium to flow into the rectum by gravity.
8. **Action:** Place the patient in right lateral, left lateral and ventrodorsal recumbency – take radiographs.
   Rationale: These views allow the entire colon to be demonstrated.
9. **Action:** kV should be increased above that used for the plain radiographs.
   Rationale: This ensures that the edges of the barium are clearly delineated, which aids interpretation of the radiograph.
10. **Action:** If a double contrast technique is used, lower the drip bag and allow barium to flow back into the bag by gravity.
    Rationale: If the radiograph is taken with both barium and air in the colon, it will not be diagnostic.
11. **Action:** Gently squeeze the bag, forcing air into the rectum and colon.
    Rationale: Air distends the colon, whilst the remains of the barium stick to the colonic mucosa.
12. **Action:** Repeat the radiographs as in step 8.
    Rationale: Reduce the kV as air is of a lower density than barium.

Procedure: Intravenous urography (Fig. 10.19)

1. **Action:** The patient should be starved for 12 hours. Water should be withheld for 2 hours prior to the procedure.
   Rationale: This procedure is performed under a general anaesthetic; starvation ensures that the patient does not vomit and choke.
2. **Action:** Administer an enema.
   Rationale: The presence of faeces in the colon may mask the view of the kidney and ureters.
3. **Action:** Administer a general anaesthetic to the patient.
   Rationale: Intravenous iodine may cause an unpleasant feeling of nausea and may be irritant

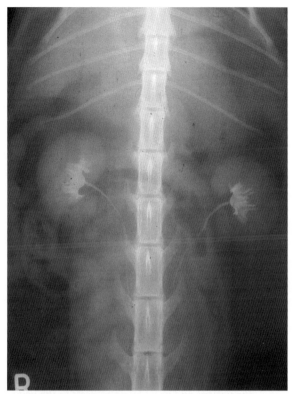

Fig. 10.19 Radiograph of a ventrodorsal abdomen showing the effects of intravenous urography.

if perivascular leakage occurs. A large number of radiographs may be needed. If the patient is anaesthetized, these are all made easier.

4. **Action:** Take plain radiographs in right lateral and ventrodorsal recumbency, centred on the umbilicus.
   Rationale: These views will demonstrate all the areas of the urinary tract and can be used for comparison with the later contrast radiographs.

5. **Action:** Introduce a urinary catheter into the bladder and empty it by gentle compression on the bladder or by drawing urine out by syringe. Introduce a small amount of air.
   Rationale: The presence of urine in the bladder will dilute the contrast medium. Air in the bladder enables the ureters passing over the bladder and the position of the neck of the bladder to be seen.

6. **Action:** Restrain the patient for an intravenous injection – see Chapter 1.
   Rationale: The cephalic vein is the easiest intravenous route to use in the dog and the cat.

7. **Action:** Inject either:
   - Bolus of warmed contrast medium (iodine 300–400 mg/ml) at a dose of 850 mg iodine/kg bodyweight (approx. 1 ml/kg)
   - Infusion of warmed contrast medium (iodine 150–200 mg/ml) at a dose of 1200 mg iodine/kg bodyweight. May be given using a giving set over a period of 10–15 minutes.
   Rationale: Bolus intravenous urography is recommended for kidney examination. Infusion intravenous urography is used for patients with urinary incontinence and ureteric problems. Warming the iodine solution reduces its viscosity and makes intravenous injection easier.

8. **Action:** As soon as the intravenous injection has been completed, take a ventrodorsal radiograph of the abdomen, centring on the area of the umbilicus.
   Rationale: Clear colourless iodine appears as a radiopaque material within the urinary system. The kidneys will fill with iodine, demonstrating the size and shape of the kidneys. A ventrodorsal view enables a comparison of both kidneys to be made.

9. **Action:** Take another radiograph after 5 minutes.
   Rationale: The pelvis of each kidney will be outlined by contrast material.

10. **Action:** Place the patient in right lateral recumbency and take another radiograph after 10 minutes.
    Rationale: The ureters will be filled, and their size and position can be evaluated.

11. **Action:** Place the patient in right lateral recumbency and take another radiograph after 15 minutes. Centre at the level of the neck of the bladder.
    Rationale: The bladder will be filling and the trigone area should be visible.

12. **Action:** Further radiographs can be taken if abnormalities are detected or if excretion rates are slowed.
    Rationale: Taking additional views can be decided on the basis of individual findings.

Procedure: Urethrogram (retrograde urethrography) – male

1. **Action:** Administer an enema to the patient (but this is not essential).
   Rationale: The presence of faeces may alter the position of the bladder or urethra.

2. **Action:** Administer a sedative to the patient. In some cases, a general anaesthetic may be given.

Rationale: This procedure can be performed with care in a conscious animal but it may cause the urethra to constrict – the interpretation of the radiograph should take this into account.

3. **Action:** Place the patient in right lateral recumbency and take a plain radiograph centred for the neck of the bladder and collimated to include the entire urethra.

   Rationale: This may indicate any lesions that may later be masked by the contrast material.

4. **Action:** Introduce a urinary catheter into the bladder and drain the urine. Remove the catheter.

   Rationale: The presence of urine in the bladder will dilute the contrast medium.

5. **Action:** Select a Foley catheter and flush with contrast material before it is inserted.

   Rationale: This flushes air out of the catheter. If air is present in the catheter when it is inserted into the urethra, the air may appear to be in the urethra and affect the diagnosis.

6. **Action:** Place the patient in right lateral recumbency.

   Rationale: This is the most comfortable position for the patient and provides easy access to the penis and urethra.

7. **Action:** Gently introduce the Foley catheter into the penile urethra and inflate the cuff.

   Rationale: Inflating the cuff prevents back flow of contrast material out of the urethra.

8. **Action:** Inject 5–15 ml of iodine (150 mg/ml) slowly up the catheter.

   Rationale: The addition of K-Y jelly to the contrast material will increase the degree of urethral distension and may produce a better image.

9. **Action:** Stand back from the patient and take a lateral radiograph. Pull the hind legs cranially to show the ischial arch and pull them caudally to show the penile urethra.

   Rationale: If it is necessary to prevent leakage of the contrast material by occluding the end of the penis manually, your hands and forearms must be protected from scattered radiation by a lead sheet or gloves during the exposure.

Procedure: Urethrogram (retrograde vaginourethrography) – female

1. **Action:** Administer an enema to the patient (but this is not essential).

   Rationale: The presence of faeces may alter the position of the bladder or urethra.

2. **Action:** Administer a general anaesthetic to the patient.

   Rationale: The use of Allis tissue forceps later in the procedure is painful, so a general anaesthetic is recommended.

3. **Action:** Place the patient in right lateral recumbency and take a plain radiograph centred on the neck of the bladder and collimated to include the entire urethra.

   Rationale: This will demonstrate any lesions and provide a comparison with later contrast radiographs.

4. **Action:** Introduce a urinary catheter into the bladder and drain the urine. Remove the catheter.

   Rationale: The presence of urine in the bladder will dilute the contrast medium.

5. **Action:** Select a Foley catheter and flush with contrast material.

   Rationale: This flushes air out of the catheter. If air is present when the catheter is inserted into the vestibule, the air may appear to be in the vestibule and affect the diagnosis.

6. **Action:** Place the animal in right lateral recumbency.

   Rationale: This is the most comfortable position for the patient and provides easy access to the vagina and vestibule.

7. **Action:** Insert the Foley catheter through the vulval lips and into the vestibule and inflate the cuff.

   Rationale: Inflating the cuff prevents back flow and leakage of contrast material out of the vagina and vestibule.

8. **Action:** Hold the catheter in place and attach a pair of Allis tissue forceps across the vulva.

   Rationale: This procedure prevents further loss of the contrast material but can be painful in a conscious bitch.

9. **Action:** Inject up to 1 ml/kg bodyweight of iodine (150 mg/ml) slowly up the catheter.

   Rationale: The contrast material enters the vagina under pressure and care must be taken not to overfill the vagina and urethra as rupture can occur.

10. **Action:** Stand back from the patient and take a lateral radiograph.

    Rationale: If it is necessary to prevent leakage of the contrast material by occluding the vulva manually, your hands and forearms must be protected from scattered radiation by a lead sheet or gloves during the exposure.

Procedure: Cystography – pneumocystogram, positive contrast cystogram, double contrast cystogram

1. **Action:** Administer an enema to the patient.
   Rationale: The presence of faeces may alter the position of the bladder.
2. **Action:** Administer a general anaesthetic – although the procedure can be performed under sedation.
   Rationale: This is not necessarily a painful procedure, but it may be easier to position the animal if it is sedated or anaesthetized. The urethra may constrict when a fully conscious animal is catheterized, and interpretation of the radiograph should take this into account.
3. **Action:** Place the patient in right lateral recumbency and take a plain radiograph centred on the neck of the bladder.
   Rationale: This can be used as a comparison with later contrast radiographs.
4. **Action:** Introduce a urinary catheter into the bladder and drain the urine.
   Rationale: The presence of urine in the bladder will dilute the contrast material.
5. **Action:** With the patient in right lateral recumbency, gently introduce room air into the bladder using a syringe and a three-way tap at a rate of approximately 10 ml/kg bodyweight.
   Rationale: The bladder should feel moderately distended when the abdomen is palpated. Care must be taken to avoid rupturing the bladder.
6. **Action:** Take a lateral radiograph.
   Rationale: This is known as a pneumocystogram – the bladder will appear as a dark mass in the caudal abdomen. This is used to detect the presence of calculi in the bladder.
7. **Action:** For a positive contrast cystogram, introduce diluted iodine contrast material at a rate of 10 ml/kg bodyweight after draining the urine from the bladder. Take a lateral radiograph. kV must be increased.
   Rationale: The bladder appears as a radiopaque mass in the caudal abdomen. kV must be increased as positive contrast is denser than the air in the pneumocystogram.
8. **Action:** For a double contrast cystogram, inject 2–15 ml of iodine (150 mg/ml) into the empty bladder via the catheter and gently roll the patient from side to side.
   Rationale: Rolling the patient ensures that the iodine covers the bladder mucosa.
9. **Action:** Inflate the bladder with air until it feels taut. Take a lateral radiograph.
   Rationale: The bladder mucosa appears covered with positive contrast, whilst the lumen appears dark with a shadow of residual contrast material in the centre. This technique is used to evaluate the thickness of the bladder wall, the presence of lesions such as tumours and the presence of calculi.
10. **Action:** In all cases, exposure should be carried out immediately after the contrast material has been injected.
    Rationale: This procedure does not require anyone to remain in the room, so in the interests of radiation safety, normal procedures should be followed.

Procedure: Myelography – cisternal and lumbar puncture (Fig. 10.20)

1. **Action:** Administer a general anaesthetic to the patient.
   Rationale: This procedure is potentially painful and requires accurate placing of a spinal needle in the subarachnoid space. Any sudden movements could have serious consequences.
2. **Action:** Place the patient in lateral recumbency and take plain radiographs of the area under investigation.
   Rationale: This will provide preliminary indications as to the diagnosis and enables exposure factors to be set.
3. **Action:** Clip the neck caudal to the skull (cisternal) or over the lumbar spine (lumbar) and prepare the site as for a surgical procedure.

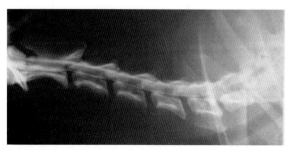

Fig. 10.20 Lateral radiograph of the spine showing the effects of myelography.

Rationale: Care must be taken to prevent the introduction of infection into the spinal cord.

4. **Action:** Select a non-ionic contrast material (200–300 mg/ml iodine) and gently warm it. Dose rate is 0.3–0.45 ml/kg bodyweight, depending on size.

   Rationale: Non-ionic iodine provides the least amount of irritation to the spinal cord. Warming reduces the viscosity of the liquid, making it easier to inject.

5. **Action:** For cisternal puncture: raise the table to about a 10° tilt, with the patient's head at the raised end.

   Rationale: This ensures that contrast material does not flow up into the ventricles of the brain, which could cause pain due to a rise in cerebral pressure and result in fitting.

6. **Action:** Flex the head to an angle of 90° so that the chin touches the sternum.

   Rationale: The needle is to be inserted into the cisterna magna, which is the cranial end of the subarachnoid space just behind the skull. Flexing the neck opens up access to this space.

7. **Action:** Insert a spinal needle of a suitable length, depending on the patient's size, between the skull and the atlas (Fig. 10.21). Advance it until cerebrospinal fluid (CSF) drips from the needle. Collect a sample of CSF.

   Rationale: The presence of CSF indicates that the needle is in the correct position. Analysis of the sample of CSF may be an added diagnostic aid.

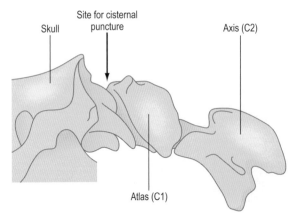

Fig. 10.21 Myelography: site for cisternal puncture. (Redrawn from Lane and Cooper (2003), Butterworth-Heinemann.)

8. **Action:** Inject the required amount of contrast material slowly. Remove the needle and extend the neck. Take radiographs.

   Rationale: Slow injection prevents a sudden increase in pressure.

9. **Action:** For lumbar puncture: flex the vertebral column by pulling the hind legs forward.

   Rationale: The site used is at the level of the L4–5 or L5–6 junction. This position should not be used if there is any indication of spinal instability.

10. **Action:** Insert a spinal needle of a suitable length into the appropriate junction and note the twitch of the legs and anus.

    Rationale: This twitch indicates that the needle has passed through the spinal cord.

11. **Action:** Little or no CSF should appear through the needle. If this is the case, inject a small amount of contrast material.

    Rationale: Lack of CSF does not indicate incorrect needle placement. A small amount of contrast material is injected to test for correct needle placement.

12. **Action:** A test radiograph may be taken in lateral recumbency centred over the needle.

    Rationale: This will show whether the small amount of contrast material has reached the correct site.

13. **Action:** Inject the remainder of the contrast material. Remove the needle and straighten the spine. Keep the head raised. Take the radiographs.

    Rationale: If the needle is left in position, it may damage the spinal cord. Keeping the head raised prevents the flow of contrast material towards the brain.

14. **Action:** In either technique, once the contrast material has been introduced, take lateral views of the spine starting at the site of injection and move caudally. In the area of the cervical spine, remove the endotracheal tube from the larynx.

    Rationale: The entire spine should be examined as additional lesions may be found. The endotracheal tube will lie over the spinal cord and make interpretation more difficult.

15. **Action:** When the contrast material has reached the main point of interest, take ventrodorsal and oblique views.

    Rationale: Lateral, ventrodorsal and oblique views allow accurate identification and location of the lesion.

16. **Action:** During recovery, the patient must be placed in its kennel with its head raised.
    Rationale: *This prevents flow of contrast material into the ventricles of the brain, which could cause a painful rise in pressure and increase the risk of fits.*

TECHNIQUES FOR PROCESSING RADIOGRAPHS

Procedure: Manual processing (Fig. 10.22)

1. **Action:** Put on a pair of rubber gloves and a plastic apron.
   Rationale: *Processing chemicals can be irritant, and you should protect your hands and your clothes. Goggles will also protect your eyes from splashes.*
2. **Action:** Check that the levels and the temperatures of the developer and fixer tanks are correct. If appropriate, check the temperature of the surrounding water bath.
   Rationale: *If the levels of chemicals in the tanks are low, the upper parts of the film will not be processed. The temperature of the developer should be 20°C and the fixer 20–21°C. Too low temperatures will result in underdevelopment, and too high temperatures will result in overdevelopment (always check the label for accurate temperatures as they may vary).*
3. **Action:** Turn off all lights except the safelight.
   Rationale: *White light will fog the film. The safelight must have the correct filter for the type of film.*

4. **Action:** Lock the door to the darkroom.
   Rationale: *Accidental opening of the door will allow light into the room, with subsequent fogging of the film.*
5. **Action:** Unload the cassette and place the film in a hanger of a suitable design and size.
   Rationale: *Hangers minimize handling of the film during processing. There are two designs – channel and clip hangers. The size of the hanger must match that of the film.*
6. **Action:** Place the film in the developer tank, moving it gently to remove bubbles and to coat the emulsion evenly. Set the timer and leave in the developer for the recommended time.
   Rationale: *Uneven coating of the film will cause uneven development. The recommended time for development is usually 4 minutes. Removing the film too soon causes a pale or underdeveloped film; leaving it for too long causes a dark or overdeveloped film.*
7. **Action:** Take the film out of the developer tank, allowing any excess to drip back into the tank. Replace the lid of the developer tank.
   Rationale: *If developer is allowed to mix with the rinse water, the water will become contaminated over a period of time. The lid of the developer tank prevents oxidation of the chemicals by air when it is not in use.*
8. **Action:** Place the film in the rinse tank and agitate it gently.
   Rationale: *The water stops the action of the developer and rinses the film clean.*

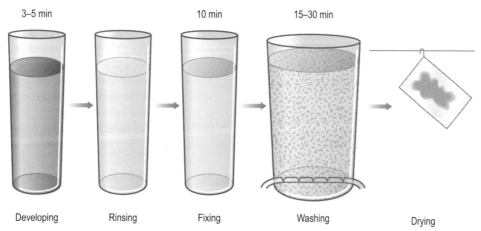

3–5 min   10 min   15–30 min

Developing   Rinsing   Fixing   Washing   Drying

Fig. 10.22 Routine for manual processing. (Redrawn from Lane and Cooper (2003), Butterworth-Heinemann.)

9. **Action:** Place the film in the fixer tank and leave for 10 minutes.
   Rationale: *Fixer hardens the emulsion and fixes the image so that it can be viewed in white light. You may look at the image after the milky appearance on the film has disappeared (clearing). It must be replaced in the tank for the full time. Timing is not critical but should be a minimum of 8 minutes. If the fixing process is not complete, the film will turn brown when stored.*

10. **Action:** Place the film in the wash tank for at least 30 minutes.
    Rationale: *The wash tank, which should be filled with running water, is used to remove any residual chemicals. If chemicals remain on the film, it will become yellow with time.*

11. **Action:** The room light can now be switched on.
    Rationale: *The film is no longer sensitive to white light after 30 seconds in the fixer but, if you can wait longer, there will be no risk of light fogging.*

12. **Action:** Hang the film up to dry or place it in a drying cabinet.
    Rationale: *The film must be thoroughly dried before storage. Viewing the radiograph for the final interpretation is best done using a dry radiograph as swelling of the emulsion during processing may cause distortion of the image.*

13. **Action:** Cassettes should always be reloaded after use in the dry area of the darkroom and stored ready for use. This may be done while you are waiting for the developing process to work.
    Rationale: *Loading must be done in the dark or under the safelight to prevent fogging. Avoid any splashing of chemicals in the wet area of the darkroom.*

Procedure: Starting up an automatic processor

1. **Action:** Check the levels of water and chemicals in the processor and in the replenisher tanks. Check the position of the rollers.
   Rationale: *The levels of the chemicals will fall with use. Other users may displace the rollers.*

2. **Action:** Turn on the water supply valve.
   Rationale: *Water is needed to wash the films and to maintain the constant temperature necessary for processing.*

3. **Action:** Turn on the mains supply to the machine and the processor's power switch.
   Rationale: *An electricity supply is essential.*

4. **Action:** Replace the lid of the processor.
   Rationale: *The lid should be removed when not in use but must be replaced to prevent leakage when in use.*

5. **Action:** Check the temperature of the processor.
   Rationale: *A low temperature will result in underdevelopment of the films. The machine may take about 20 minutes to reach its recommended temperature.*

6. **Action:** Feed two or three old clean films through the processor.
   Rationale: *These will remove dried chemicals from the rollers.*

7. **Action:** At the same time, check that the replenishment pumps are working.
   Rationale: *These work whenever a film is in the processor.*

Procedure: Automatic processing

1. **Action:** Switch the processor on in the prescribed way and check that the temperature is correct.
   Rationale: *If the temperature is too low, the films will be underdeveloped. If the recommended set-up procedure is not followed, vital stages may be missed, resulting in fogging of the film or a lack of water to the processor.*

2. **Action:** Lock the door of the darkroom and switch the lights off.
   Rationale: *Accidental opening of the door will allow light in, causing fogging of the film.*

3. **Action:** Remove the film from the cassette and place it on to the tray or entry roller of the processor.
   Rationale: *The film should be placed in the correct orientation for entry to prevent damage.*

4. **Action:** Allow the film to be taken into the processor.
   Rationale: *Impeding the movement of the film into the processor will cause scratching of the emulsion.*

5. **Action:** Wait for the audible or visible indicator before leaving the darkroom, inserting the next film or switching the light back on.
   Rationale: *If a second film is put in before the first film has moved into the processor, the two may stick together.*

6. **Action:** Reload the cassette and place it in the storage area ready for use.
   Rationale: *Loading must be done in the dark or under the safelight to prevent fogging. Avoid any splashing of chemicals or water.*

Procedure: Shutting down the automatic processor

1. **Action:** Make sure that there are no films in the processor.
   Rationale: If the processor is switched off with films still passing through, they may be irreparably damaged.
2. **Action:** Turn off the power switch on the processor and the mains isolator switch.
   Rationale: Power should never be left on when the processor is not in use.
3. **Action:** Turn off the water supply.
   Rationale: Water should never be left running unnecessarily.
4. **Action:** Remove the processor cover or lid.
   Rationale: The lid can be removed to give easy access.
5. **Action:** Remove any chemical residue from inside the processor.
   Rationale: Daily removal of any residue reduces damage that may occur if chemicals are left on the working parts for long periods of time.
6. **Action:** Place an antifungal tablet into the wash tank.
   Rationale: This reduces the build-up of fungi and algae in the wash water.
7. **Action:** Ensure that the lid or cover is left in a slightly raised position.
   Rationale: Air circulation through the processor reduces the build-up of condensation.

Procedure: Cleaning an automatic processor

1. **Action:** Put on a pair of rubber gloves and a plastic apron.
   Rationale: Processing chemicals can be irritant, and you should protect your hands and your clothes. Goggles will also protect your eyes from splashes.
2. **Action:** Switch off the electricity supply to the machine.
   Rationale: The combination of electricity and water could be fatal!
3. **Action:** Drain the water tank by opening the valve.
   Rationale: Draining the water allows proper cleaning to be carried out.
4. **Action:** Remove the cross-over rollers between the tanks and wash them in fresh water.
   Rationale: The cross-over rollers collect chemical residues, which dry on them. At most times these rollers are out of the liquids.
5. **Action:** Place a splashguard between the fixer and the developer tank.
   Rationale: This prevents cross-contamination between the tanks.
6. **Action:** Remove the rollers from the developer tank. Wash in fresh water, remove any residual chemicals and check their movement.
   Rationale: Dried developer on the rollers will scratch the emulsion, giving rise to roller marks, and prevent their free movement.
7. **Action:** Replace the developer racks after draining, taking care not to splash developer into the fixer.
   Rationale: This prevents cross-contamination between the tanks.
8. **Action:** Remove the rollers from the fixer tank. Wash in fresh water, remove any residual chemicals, and check their movement.
   Rationale: Dried fixer on the rollers will scratch the emulsion, giving rise to roller marks, and prevent their free movement.
9. **Action:** Replace the fixer racks after draining, taking care not to splash fixer into the developer.
   Rationale: This prevents cross-contamination between the tanks.
10. **Action:** Remove the rollers from the wash tank and clean in fresh water.
    Rationale: The effect of heat, emulsion residue and water creates a build-up of sludge and algae. This reduces the quality of the image produced and the function of the processor.
11. **Action:** Clean the empty tank with a sponge and fresh water.
    Rationale: Care should be taken to remove any algae that have built up on the tank sides.
12. **Action:** Replace the wash tank racks.
    Rationale: The racks should be replaced carefully and seated in their correct positions.
13. **Action:** Close the valve to the wash tank to allow refilling.
    Rationale: Without water, the processor will not wash the films and may overheat.
14. **Action:** Replace the cross-over racks.
    Rationale: These must be replaced last as they sit over all the other rollers.
15. **Action:** Replace the lid of the processor and switch the power back on.
    Rationale: The lid provides a light-tight seal to prevent fogging of the films.
16. **Action:** Pass a few old clean films through the processor.

Rationale: These will pick up any residue that has been dislodged during cleaning. It is also a means of checking for correct function before clinical radiographs are processed.

N.B.: Nowadays many practices use digital processors. The cassettes are specially designed but patient positioning is exactly the same as described above. The image is digital, is processed more quickly and can be enhanced post-processing.

MAINTENANCE OF RADIOGRAPHY EQUIPMENT

Procedure: Care of intensifying screens

1. **Action:** Moisten a soft cloth with a screen-cleaning detergent or a small amount of commercial detergent and water.
   Rationale: Intensifying screens are delicate and expensive pieces of equipment – any damage will appear on the radiograph, and the screen may be rendered useless. Avoid the use of any material that will scratch the screens. Do not use cotton wool as this leaves small pieces of lint on the screen.
2. **Action:** Wipe the screen gently.
   Rationale: The detergent should be used sparingly and only just touch the screen.
3. **Action:** Do not wet the screen and avoid spilling anything on the back of the screen.
   Rationale: Moisture damages the grains within the screen, affecting their efficiency, and will also cause the cardboard backing to disintegrate.
4. **Action:** Wipe the screen clean with a fresh dry cloth or piece of gauze.
   Rationale: All detergent and moisture must be removed to prevent damage to the screen.
5. **Action:** Stand the cassette upright and leave it slightly open to dry.
   Rationale: This prevents pooling of the detergent and allows air to circulate, reducing condensation.
6. **Action:** Record when the cleaning was done and by whom.
   Rationale: Regular cleaning of the screens improves image quality. Any damage can be traced.

Procedure: Checking safelight function

1. **Action:** Enter the darkroom and switch off the white light.

Rationale: White light will always fog the film.
2. **Action:** Do not switch on the safelight.
   Rationale: This film will be used to provide a baseline for your assessment.
3. **Action:** Select two films of the type commonly used in the practice but of the smallest size available.
   Rationale: Keep the cost of this assessment to a minimum.
4. **Action:** Take one film out of any protective covering and place your hand on it for 30 seconds.
   Rationale: If the darkroom is truly lightproof, there will be no image on this film.
5. **Action:** Repeat this process with the other film with the safelight switched on.
   Rationale: If the safelight is leaking light of the wrong wavelength, it will produce an image of the hand. If the safelight is in working order, there will be no image on the film.
6. **Action:** Process both films.
   Rationale: The image cannot be seen without processing.
7. **Action:** Compare the two films.
   Rationale: This technique can also be used to assess the degree of lightproofing of the darkroom.

Procedure: Checking for light leakage in a cassette

1. **Action:** Load the cassette to be investigated with a piece of new film and close it securely.
   Rationale: A new film is used to make sure that no fogging is present.
2. **Action:** Expose each edge of the cassette to high-intensity light (100 W) for about 15 minutes.
   Rationale: High-intensity light simulates the type of light to which the cassette may normally be exposed.
3. **Action:** Process the film and look at it on a viewer.
   Rationale: If the edges of the cassette are leaking light, the processed film will show a dark border. Any border greater than 3 mm wide should be assumed to have resulted from leakage of light.

Procedure: Checking the X-ray tube for leakage of X-rays

1. **Action:** Set up the X-ray machine for a low exposure.
   Rationale: The tube should be set up for normal use to make the test as realistic as possible.
2. **Action:** Close the light beam diaphragm.
   Rationale: This will reduce the exposure of the environment and the risk of scattered radiation.

3. **Action:** Place a series of non-screen films around the X-ray tube head. Make sure each one is labelled with its position in relation to the tube.
   Rationale: Non-screen film is flexible and can be used to cover the entire head.
4. **Action:** Make an exposure.
   Rationale: X-rays will barely escape as the primary beam, but if there is leakage from the head, it will affect the films around the head.
5. **Action:** Process the films and look at them on a viewer.
   Rationale: Signs of leakage appear as grey areas on the radiograph and may correspond to joints in the tube head. The machine should not be used until a further professional assessment has been made.

Procedure: Checking for the accuracy of the light beam diaphragm

1. **Action:** Place a loaded cassette on the table under the X-ray tube head, keeping the standard film focal distance.
   Rationale: Use a small piece of film to reduce costs.
2. **Action:** Switch on the light beam diaphragm and collimate it to produce an area of approximately 10 cm².
   Rationale: A small area prevents unnecessary contamination of the immediate environment and reduces the risk of scattered radiation.
3. **Action:** Place a row of paper clips along the perimeter of the illuminated square.
   Rationale: The paper clips mark the edges of the irradiated square once the light beam diaphragm is switched off.
4. **Action:** On each corner, place an unfolded paper clip with one end towards the corner.
   Rationale: The pointed end of the clip accurately delineates the corners.
5. **Action:** Using a low exposure, expose the film.
   Rationale: A low exposure reduces the risk of scattered radiation.
6. **Action:** Process and assess the radiograph.
   Rationale: If the light beam indicates the area exposed by the primary beam accurately, the border of paper clips will be on the edge of the exposed film, and the points of the unfolded clips will point to the corners. If the light beam diaphragm is inaccurate, an engineer should be called to correct the fault.

Procedure: Checking a cassette for poor film/screen contact

1. **Action:** Place a piece of zinc or copper netting or metallic material with small holes cut out of it on top of a small loaded cassette.
   Rationale: A specific test tool is available but any metal sheet with holes cut out will do as well. The holes must be present to provide a sharp edge as a means of assessment.
2. **Action:** Collimate the beam to cover most of the cassette, leaving a minimal border around the edge.
   Rationale: All radiographs should have at least a small border around the edge to indicate that the beam has been restricted to some degree.
3. **Action:** Expose the cassette using a low exposure.
   Rationale: A low exposure prevents unnecessary contamination of the immediate environment and reduces the risk of scattered radiation.
4. **Action:** Process and assess the radiograph.
   Rationale: Areas of poor film/screen contact will show as darker blurred areas. Even film/screen contact will produce a sharp uniform image. If the cassette is affected, it will be due to compression and ageing of the pressure pad underneath the back intensifying screen or warping of the screens. The cassette should be replaced.

DIAGNOSTIC ULTRASOUND

Procedure: Preparing the patient for an ultrasound examination

1. **Action:** Administer a sedative to the patient.
   Rationale: Ultrasonography is a non-invasive, painless procedure that is well-tolerated by most animals. In some cases, it may be easier to place a sedated patient in the correct position, and procedures such as biopsy or fine-needle aspiration may require deeper sedation or a general anaesthetic.
2. **Action:** Place the patient on an examination table in a position that provides sufficient access to the area under examination.
   Rationale: This may mean that the patient can remain standing or lie in lateral or dorsal recumbency. If the patient feels comfortable and secure, it will be unlikely to struggle. Avoid using areas where underlying bone and gas may block the movement of the ultrasound waves.

3. **Action:** Clip the area and apply spirit.
   Rationale: Fur must be removed to provide good contact between the skin and the transducer of the ultrasound machine. Spirit is used to remove any remaining dirt and grease on the skin surface.

4. **Action:** Apply coupling gel to the transducer and the skin.
   Rationale: Coupling gel ensures good contact between the skin and the transducer. Trapped air will create an artefact, which may affect the final diagnosis.

5. **Action:** Apply the transducer to the skin within the prepared area.
   Rationale: When the transducer is applied to the skin, high-frequency sound waves pass through the patient's soft tissues as pressure waves. At interfaces between organs or between different tissues, some sound waves are reflected and return to the transducer. Here they are detected by the ultrasound equipment, which produces a cross-sectional image of the internal structure of the tissues.

Procedure: Care of the ultrasound machine

1. **Action:** The ultrasound machine should be plugged into the mains and switched on just prior to use. It should be switched off immediately after use.
   Rationale: The machine may overheat if left on for long periods. Where the machine is only used occasionally, leaving it switched on wastes electricity.

2. **Action:** The transducers should be stored in a suitable holder.
   Rationale: All machines are equipped with a holder for the transducers, which will prevent damage. There are two types of transducer – linear array, which produces a rectangular field, and sector transducer, which produces a fan-shaped field.

3. **Action:** The transducer should be attached to the operator throughout the examination.
   Rationale: Transducers are very fragile and should not be dropped or banged. Using a wristband to attach the transducer to the user can prevent this.

4. **Action:** Select the correct mode prior to the examination.
   Rationale: This ensures that the procedure is carried out quickly and efficiently. There are three types of image display modes (Fig. 10.23). Most ultrasonography is performed using B-mode ('brightness' mode); M-mode shows movement of structures on the frozen image and is used in echocardiology;

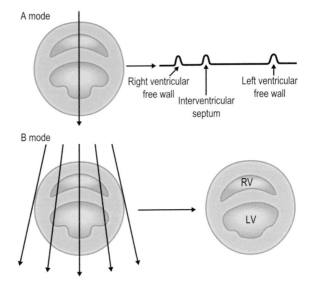

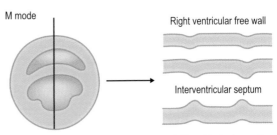

Fig. 10.23 Image display modes. LV, left ventricle, RV, right ventricle. (Taken from Aspinall and Aspinall (2013), Clinical Procedures in Small Animal Veterinary Practice, Saunders.)

A-mode was the first type developed and is rarely used.

5. **Action:** Clean the transducer thoroughly after use.
   Rationale: Gel and hair affect the function of the transducer and may be a source of cross-infection.

MAGNETIC RESONANCE IMAGING (MRI)

Procedure: Preparing the patient for an MRI examination

1. **Action:** Identify the patient and check records for implants and prostheses.
   Rationale: No patient with a prosthesis or implant can enter the scanning room as the magnetic field will interact with the metal and may cause tissue damage.

2. **Action:** Remove all collars, leads, catheters or cables.

Rationale: Nothing metallic should be used in the scanning room. Each room has its own assigned equipment, including non-ferrous equipment.

3. **Action:** Administer anaesthetic to the patient.

   Rationale: MRI scanning is a long procedure, and the patient must stay in position for long periods of time. The procedure is noisy, and the table moves continually throughout the examination. All of these would cause distress in a conscious animal.

4. **Action:** Place the patient on the scanner in the position identified within the scanning protocols.

   Rationale: Each examination has a set position into which the patient should be placed prior to examination.

5. **Action:** Place a radiofrequency (RF) coil over the area under examination, if required.

   Rationale: The RF coil enhances the image. It is required for some examinations. Type and position will be identified in the scanning protocols.

6. **Action:** Ensure the patient is settled.

   Rationale: The examination takes about 1 hour. During this time, it will be difficult to do anything more than monitor the patient.

7. **Action:** Check all cables and tubes will move freely at all times.

   Rationale: As the examination progresses, the patient will move on the table. Care should be taken to ensure that all cables have enough length to move with the patient.

8. **Action:** Once the examination is complete, collate the images and reports with the patient records.

   Rationale: A huge amount of information is produced from each scan. This needs to be recorded and filed as it becomes available. Some images will be sent for external reporting, and these will need to be detailed before sending and collating on return.

COMPUTERIZED TOMOGRAPHY (CT)

Procedure: Preparing the patient for a CT scan

1. **Action:** Administer anaesthetic to the patient.

   Rationale: CT scanning requires the patient to stay in position whilst the scanning table moves through the scanner.

2. **Action:** Place the patient on the scanner in the position identified within the scanning protocols.

   Rationale: Each examination has a set position into which the patient should be placed prior to examination.

3. **Action:** Ensure the patient is settled.

   Rationale: The examination takes about 15 minutes. During this time, it will be difficult to do anything more than monitor the patient.

4. **Action:** Check all cables and tubes will move freely at all times.

   Rationale: As the examination progresses, the patient will move on the table. Care should be taken to ensure that all cables have enough length to move with the patient.

5. **Action:** Ensure the safety of staff and leave the scanning room if possible.

   Rationale: CT scanning utilizes ionizing radiation. All safety procedures must be followed under the Ionising Radiations Regulations 2017.

6. **Action:** Once the examination is complete, collate the images and reports with the patient records.

   Rationale: A huge amount of information is produced from each scan. This needs to be recorded and filed as it becomes available. Some images will be sent for external reporting, and these will need to be detailed before sending and collating on return.

REFERENCES AND FURTHER READING

Ackerman, N., 2016. Aspinall's Complete Textbook of Veterinary Nursing. Elsevier, Oxford.

Cooper, B., Lane, D., 2000. Veterinary Nursing. Butterworth-Heinemann, Oxford.

Easton, S., 2012. Practical Veterinary Diagnostic Imaging. Wiley-Blackwell, Chichester.

Lane, D.R., Cooper, B. (Eds.), 2003. Veterinary Nursing, third ed. Butterworth-Heinemann, Oxford.

Lavin, L., 2007. Radiography in Veterinary Technology, fourth ed. Saunders, St Louis.

Masters, J., Bowden, C., 2001. Pre-Veterinary Nursing Textbook. Butterworth-Heinemann, Oxford.

11

Diagnostic laboratory techniques

Jennifer Davis

CHAPTER CONTENTS

INTRODUCTION

Laboratory tests are used to aid or confirm the diagnosis made by the veterinary surgeon. Many of these tests may be sent away to commercial laboratories, but most practices have some form of small laboratory of their own where a range of basic diagnostic tests may be carried out. It is often one of the veterinary nurses who is designated or volunteers to run the laboratory, and it is vital that this person is properly trained to produce consistent good-quality results in which the veterinary surgeon can have confidence. The methods described in this chapter have been in daily use in our practice laboratory. They are simple to carry out, require the minimum of equipment and are easily performed by both student and qualified veterinary nurses.

Biochemical analyses have been included in general terms only as most practices use wet or dry biochemical analysers, and it would be impossible to discuss all in detail. Although this 'push-button' technology is generally reliable, the author strongly recommends the regular throughput of quality control samples with known parameter values to ensure that the machine is reporting correctly.

Haematology analysers allow regular and accurate evaluation of single blood parameters, but for complete confidence, one should carry out a blood smear (see Differential white blood cell count procedure, later) to assess irregularities in cell morphology and to ascertain whether anaemias are regenerative or non-regenerative. I have described no specific methodologies for the range of haematology analysers currently available but it is appropriate to describe briefly the three types of technology employed:

1. The QBC Autoread (IDEXX): this utilizes qualitative buffy coat analysis. Cells have different densities and the QBC system employs a combination of an oversized haematocrit tube and a float to expand the buffy coat to quantify each type of white cell. In addition, the tube is coated with a fluorescent dye that stains cellular components when subjected to blue violet light.

2. Electronic impedance technology: the principle of this type of analyser is that cells are diluted with an isotonic solution, counted and sized by being passed through an aperture on the instrument. Each cell is identified and classified using its resistance to an electrical current.

3. Laser flow technology (Lasercyte/Procyte – IDEXX): this type uses lasers through which a stream of cells is passed. The system counts and identifies cells using the principle that individual types of cell reflect laser light differently depending on their size and granularity.

Enzyme-linked immunosorbent assay (ELISA) tests for feline leukaemia virus, feline immunodeficiency virus and *Giardia* for example, are now so commonly used and are so simple to perform that specific instructions have not been included. This type of test falls into two groups: the read-by-eye test, which is designed for practice use, and more complex plate ELISA methods, which require a photometer plate reader to assess optical densities and interpretation. The latter is more suited to commercial laboratories.

HEALTH AND SAFETY IN THE LABORATORY

Whilst undertaking laboratory procedures, observe the following guidelines:

- Wear a long-sleeved laboratory coat, gloves, mask (where necessary) and eye protection at all times
- Wear the minimum of jewellery
- The use of nail varnish is not acceptable, and nails must be kept short and clean
- Do not lick gummed labels or your fingers, or suck the ends of pencils or pens
- A wash basin reserved for hand washing and equipped with antibacterial soap and paper towels should be available
- Hands should be washed on entry to the laboratory and on leaving the room
- All work surfaces should be cleaned and disinfected daily and after every hazardous procedure

- As soon as you have finished with equipment, store it away tidily to avoid accidents
- Samples and contaminated equipment should be disposed of safely and correctly
- Sharps containers and clinical waste bags must be available in the laboratory at all times
- If hazardous chemicals/reagents are used, take note of warning labels and act accordingly
- Many bacteria are potential pathogens and should be handled in a contained environment such as a safety cabinet
- Avoid mouth pipetting
- Know where the first aid kit is stored, where the eye wash station is situated and what action to take in an emergency. You should be familiar with the accident book
- It is a good idea to list and describe all procedures in a laboratory manual so that all staff members use the same methodologies
- The use of external quality assurance or quality control schemes ensures confidence in your results.

CARE OF LABORATORY EQUIPMENT

Procedure: Care and use of autoclaves

1. **Action:** Autoclaving is the most reliable method for sterilizing culture media and laboratory equipment.
   Rationale: When water is boiled within a closed vessel and at increased pressure, steam is formed, and the temperature rises above 100°C. The high temperature will kill all microorganisms and bacterial spores. (Some spores may survive a 15-minute programme.)
2. **Action:** Before use, check that there is sufficient water to cover the element.
   Rationale: Autoclaves must not be allowed to boil dry.
3. **Action:** Load the items.
4. **Action:** Place an indicator strip near to the middle of the load.
   Rationale: These strips change colour to indicate when full sterilization has taken place.
5. **Action:** Do not overfill the chamber.
   Rationale: Items in the middle of the load may not be completely sterilized if the chamber is overloaded.
6. **Action:** Check that the steam discharge tap is open.
7. **Action:** Adjust the safety valve to the required pressure.

Rationale: Each type of object has a specific required temperature, e.g. culture media are usually autoclaved at 121°C for 15 minutes.
8. **Action:** Allow steam and air mixture to escape until all air has been eliminated from the chamber.
   Rationale: You will see the steam escaping.
9. **Action:** Close the discharge tap.
10. **Action:** When pressure reaches the required level, the safety valve will open – at this point, start to time the load.
    Rationale: A minute timer is useful.
11. **Action:** When the time is complete, turn off the heater and allow the autoclave to cool.
    Rationale: When cool, the gauge should read 0 lb/sq. inch (atmospheric pressure).
12. **Action:** Open the discharge tap.
13. **Action:** Unload the items.
14. **Action:** Pour out any water left in the chamber and wipe clean with a soft cloth.

Procedure: Care and use of the balance

1. **Action:** Always make sure that the balance is placed on an even and stable surface.
   Rationale: Balances are extremely delicate instruments and can be damaged by excessive vibration.
2. **Action:** Items placed on the top pan must be centred for accurate weight distribution.
   Rationale: Use forceps to place items carefully into the middle of the pan.
3. **Action:** Instrument accuracy can be checked using calibrated weights.
   Rationale: Use a suitable weight in the middle of the balance range to check the accuracy. This will depend on the number of decimal places to which your balance measures.
4. **Action:** Before weighing, zero the balance using the TARE button.
   Rationale: If using a balance boat, place the boat on the balance before zeroing the machine.
5. **Action:** Weigh the item under test.
6. **Action:** Record the result.
7. **Action:** Carefully remove the item from the pan.
   Rationale: Use forceps for small items.
8. **Action:** Turn off the power supply to the balance.
9. **Action:** Clean the pan using a damp soft cloth (if spillage has occurred) or a soft, clean lint-free tissue.
   Rationale: More detailed maintenance should be carried out by a trained engineer at an annual service.

Procedure: Care and cleaning of glassware

1. **Action:** Important – if the glassware contains hazardous material, autoclave the glassware with the contents intact at 121°C for 45 minutes prior to discarding the contents.
   Rationale: Health and safety precautions must be observed when pathogens are likely to be present. Spore-forming organisms may withstand 15 minutes in an autoclave.

2. **Action:** If autoclaving is not required, proceed as follows: rinse the glassware immediately after use and place in a solution of non-toxic commercial laboratory detergent.
   Rationale: Detergents designed for laboratory use are available – harsh detergents are too abrasive and will damage glass.

3. **Action:** Using disposable gloves and a soft brush, remove any material present on the glassware.
   Rationale: Use a test tube brush for narrow tubes – hard brushes scratch the surface of the glass.

4. **Action:** Transfer glassware to a fresh solution of detergent and leave to soak for 20–30 minutes.
   Rationale: Heavy soiling may require a longer soaking.

5. **Action:** Once the glassware is visibly clean, rinse in tap water two or three times.

6. **Action:** Transfer to a container of distilled/deionized water and rinse.
   Rationale: Two or three changes of distilled water are recommended.

7. **Action:** Allow to drain.
   Rationale: Water runs off clean glass evenly. If any dirt remains, areas with a greasy appearance will be visible.

8. **Action:** Dry in drying oven at 160°C for 1 hour or allow to dry in the air.
   Rationale: If air-drying, the atmosphere must be dust-free.

9. **Action:** If glassware is to be used for sterile procedures, sterilize in an autoclave at 121°C for 15 minutes.
   Rationale: Bottles should be autoclaved with the lids screwed loosely to allow for the escape of expanding hot air. Tighten the lids after autoclaving, which prevents contaminated air being sucked in by the cooling air. Plug test tubes with cotton wool.

10. **Action:** Always cool glassware slowly. Do not put hot glassware on a cold surface.
    Rationale: Glass will crack if it is subjected to sudden temperature changes.

11. **Action:** Check for cracks and chips, and store in a dust-free atmosphere until use.
    Rationale: Cracks or chips reduce thermal strength, leading to sudden breakage.

Procedure: Care and use of the centrifuge

1. **Action:** Always ensure that the centrifuge is placed on an even and stable surface.
   Rationale: Slight vibration occurs when the machine is in motion and an uneven surface may cause the machine to move around.

2. **Action:** Only use tubes recommended by the manufacturer.
   Rationale: Centrifuge tubes often have a tapered bottom and are designed to withstand centrifugal force.

3. **Action:** The top of the centrifuge tube must not protrude above the top of the bucket. When using a microhaematocrit centrifuge, ensure that the plasticine end of the capillary tube is against the outer ring of the instrument.
   Rationale: Centrifugal force pushes material outwards. The plasticine end prevents material escaping from the tube.

4. **Action:** Vacutainer tubes may be spun with their stoppers in place.
   Rationale: If the tube is opened or broken, aerosol contamination of the environment could occur.

5. **Action:** Lock the lid of the centrifuge securely.
   Rationale: Most machines will not allow you to use them without locking the lid first. If you do not, the lid may fly open during use.

6. **Action:** Set the spin speed as appropriate.
   Rationale: For example, urine requires a lower speed than heparinized blood for biochemistry.

7. **Action:** After use, turn off the power supply.

8. **Action:** Take out the buckets.

9. **Action:** Wipe the rotor and buckets with a soft cloth and a mild disinfectant solution.
   Rationale: To prevent contamination of the next sample.

10. **Action:** Replace the buckets and close the lid.

Procedure: Care and cleaning of the incubator

1. **Action:** Remove all media from the incubator.
   Rationale: If you take too long to clean out the incubator, the agar plates have to stand at room temperature, slowing the growth of the bacteria.

2. **Action:** It is sensible to clean the instrument when workload is low but it should be done at least once a week.

   Rationale: *Incubators are used to culture bacteria, so the risk of contamination of samples is high.*

3. **Action:** Remove all the shelves and racks.

   Rationale: *These are more easily cleaned when out of the incubator.*

4. **Action:** Using a mild detergent and soft cloth, wipe all the incubator surfaces and the shelves.

   Rationale: *Take care not to touch any electrical parts. If in doubt, switch off the power supply before cleaning.*

5. **Action:** Allow to dry.

6. **Action:** Using a disinfectant solution and fresh cloth, wipe all the incubator surfaces and shelves.

   Rationale: *The disinfectant used must be bactericidal and fungicidal to be effective.*

7. **Action:** Allow to dry.

8. **Action:** Replace the shelves.

9. **Action:** Place a thermometer in glycerol in the middle of the incubator. Check that the bulb is covered. Switch on the incubator.

   Rationale: *The temperature of the glycerol alters slowly and allows the thermometer to be read without rapid fluctuations.*

10. **Action:** Read the thermometer after 1 hour.

    Rationale: *Most incubators run at $37 \pm 1°C$. It is essential to check that the incubator reaches the correct temperature to ensure efficient incubation of the agar plates.*

11. **Action:** Every month check on the door seal, electrical wiring and thermostat.

    Rationale: *If in doubt about any component, inform the practice or laboratory manager.*

Procedure: Care and use of the microscope (Fig. 11.1)

1. **Action:** Always ensure that the microscope is placed on an even and stable surface.

   Rationale: *Slight vibration will make it difficult to view the object.*

2. **Action:** Before use, clean the eyepieces, condenser and objective lenses with lens tissue.

   Rationale: *Lens tissue is lint-free and prevents bits being left on the surfaces.*

3. **Action:** Clean the oil immersion lens with cleaning fluid.

   Rationale: *Isopropanol is most commonly used.*

4. **Action:** Turn the light control to a minimum.

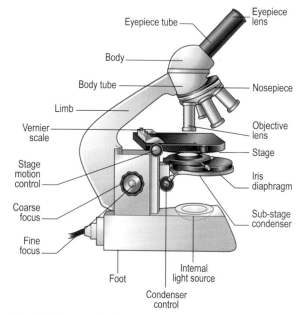

Fig. 11.1 A monocular light microscope. (Adapted, with permission, from Masters and Bowden (2001), Butterworth-Heinemann.)

   Rationale: *This prevents a sudden power surge, which may break the bulb when the microscope is switched on.*

5. **Action:** Turn on the instrument.

6. **Action:** Adjust the eyepieces.

   Rationale: *Use both eyepieces and position them so that both fields converge as one. Some microscopes have one eyepiece - monocular, some have two - binocular.*

7. **Action:** Place the slide on the stage. Some instruments have clips to hold the slide.

   Rationale: *The slide should remain firmly in place to avoid unintentional loss of a particular field.*

8. **Action:** Move the slide by using the knobs on the mechanical stage.

   Rationale: *This allows the whole slide to be examined smoothly and accurately without touching the slide with your fingers.*

9. **Action:** Examine the slide using the ×10 objective lens.

   Rationale: *At this stage the light can be adjusted using the light source knob or by repositioning the condenser.*

10. **Action:** Focus first with the coarse and then with the fine adjustment knobs.

    Rationale: *Always focus upwards from the slide to prevent accidental damage to the slide.*

11. **Action:** If using oil immersion, place a drop of oil on to the slide.
    Rationale: *Oil immersion provides increased magnification and is used for examination of bacteria and blood smears.*
12. **Action:** Rotate the nosepiece until the ×100 objective lens is above the slide.
13. **Action:** Drop the objective lens into the drop of oil. Always watch what you are doing – do not look at it through the eyepiece, as you will find it impossible to judge distances and may smash through the slide.
    Rationale: *The lens must be lying in the oil to avoid distortion of the image. Avoid contaminating the dry lenses.*
14. **Action:** Focus using the fine control.
    Rationale: *You may need to adjust the light to improve your view.*
15. **Action:** After use, remove the slide from the stage.
    Rationale: *Move the clips before trying to remove the slide.*

16. **Action:** Reduce the light and turn off the power.
17. **Action:** Turn the objective lenses on the nosepiece until the lowest power is in position above the stage.
    Rationale: *Ready for use next time.*
18. **Action:** Remove any oil from the objective lenses using lens tissue and, if necessary, lens-cleaning fluid.
    Rationale: *Ready for use next time.*
19. **Action:** Cover the instrument when not in use.
    Rationale: *This will prevent the build-up of dust on the objective and eyepiece lenses.*

Procedure: Use of the Vernier scale (Fig. 11.2)

1. **Action:** The Vernier scale is a graduated device attached to the stage of the microscope.
    Rationale: *It allows the position of an object on a slide to be accurately recorded so that you can find it again.*
2. **Action:** One scale lies along a vertical edge and another along a horizontal edge.

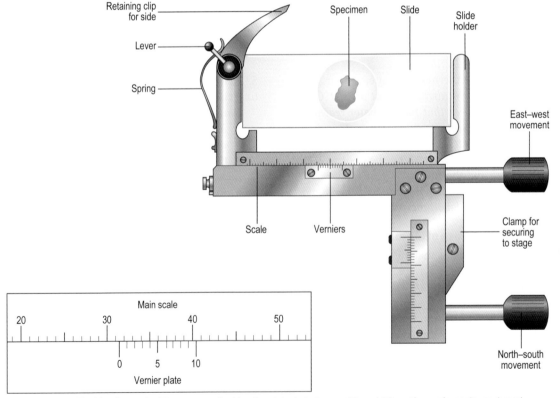

Fig. 11.2 The Vernier scale. The zero on the Vernier plate is between 31 and 32 on the main scale, and mark number 6 on the Vernier plate is exactly opposite a division on the main scale. The reading is therefore 31.6.

Rationale: Use both position numbers to give a grid reference similar to that on a map.

3. **Action:** Place the slide on the microscope stage and fix it with the clips, if present.
   Rationale: The slide must not move around as this will invalidate your scale references.

4. **Action:** Locate the object you wish to identify.

5. **Action:** Look at the scale on the vertical axis.
   Rationale: See Fig. 11.2.

6. **Action:** Record the number where the zero mark on the Vernier plate meets the main scale.
   Rationale: Record the lower number if it falls between two divisions. In Fig. 11.2, the zero mark falls between 31 and 32.

7. **Action:** Make a note of which of the marks on the Vernier plate is exactly opposite a division on the main scale.
   Rationale: In Fig. 11.2, mark number 6 is exactly opposite a division on the main scale.

8. **Action:** Record this reading, placing it after the decimal point.
   Rationale: In Fig. 11.2 this will give a reading of 31.6.

9. **Action:** Repeat steps 6–8 using the horizontal axis.
   Rationale: You now have two readings, e.g. 31.6 and 90.1.

10. **Action:** You now have a grid reference for that object on that slide, provided the slide is placed in the same position on the stage.
    Rationale: By tradition, slides are placed on the stage with the label to the right.

11. **Action:** Record your grid reference using the horizontal reading followed by the vertical reading.
    Rationale: In this example, the reference would be 90.1 × 31.6. You may now remove the slide and go back to the same location later on.

Procedure: Use of volumetric and automatic pipettes

1. **Action:** Using a soft cloth, clean the external parts of the pipette with a weak solution of commercial laboratory detergent.
   Rationale: This removes grime accumulated by daily handling.

2. **Action:** Allow to dry.

3. **Action:** Wipe the barrel end of the pipette (not the plunger) with isopropanol.
   Rationale: Wiping with spirit disinfects the part of the pipette that is attached to the tip.

4. **Action:** Some pipettes require the seals to be greased regularly – refer to the manufacturer's instructions.
   Rationale: Special grease is usually included in the maintenance kit supplied with the pipette.

5. **Action:** When needed for use, attach a disposable tip.

6. **Action:** Depress the plunger, place the tip in the solution and slowly release the plunger.
   Rationale: The fluid will be aspirated into the tip.

7. **Action:** Transfer the tip to your next vessel, e.g. a test tube, and place against the inner side of the vessel. Depress the plunger slowly.
   Rationale: The fluid will run down the side of the vessel.

8. **Action:** Discard the tip.
   Rationale: Tips should not be used more than once to avoid cross-contamination.

9. **Action:** The accuracy of your dispensing may be checked using a weight and balance.
   Rationale: Calibrate the pipette by weight, e.g. 1 ml of distilled water weighs 1 g.

10. **Action:** Pipettes should be stored in a pipette rack or in the box provided when not in use.
    Rationale: If pipettes are not stored properly, the dispensing end may be damaged.

Procedure: Decontamination and disposal of laboratory waste

1. **Action:** If possible, samples and contaminated agar plates should be placed in autoclave bags and autoclaved in a steam autoclave at 121°C for 45 minutes.
   Rationale: Some spore-forming bacteria will survive a 15-minute run. Make sure that the autoclave has enough water to last a prolonged run. Contaminated laboratory waste should not leave the laboratory in a potentially harmful form.

2. **Action:** It is good practice to include an indicator, e.g. TST strip, to confirm that complete sterilization has taken place.
   Rationale: If this device fails, the load is still unsafe and it must be reprocessed.

3. **Action:** Once sterilized, place the unopened autoclave bag into yellow hazardous waste bags and send away for incineration by a licensed waste disposal firm.
   Rationale: This further reduces the risk of contaminating the environment with the waste material.

4. **Action:** Sharps and other disposable items must be placed within a yellow commercial sharps bin, which is sealed and sent for incineration.
   Rationale: This ensures that objects such as needles or scalpel blades sticking through will not injure anyone handling the bin.
5. **Action:** Metal items may be cleaned using non-hypochlorite disinfectants.
   Rationale: Hypochlorite disinfectants will react with metal.
6. **Action:** Some equipment may need special cleaning and disinfection.
   Rationale: Always follow the manufacturer's instructions as there may be delicate parts that could be damaged by incorrect treatment.
7. **Action:** Clean all work surfaces with disinfectant after every procedure.
   Rationale: Disinfectants must contain a bactericide, a fungicide and a virucide to be fully effective.
8. **Action:** At the end of each working day, leave the laboratory clean and tidy.
   Rationale: Untidy work areas lead to accidents.

Procedure: Care of the water bath

1. **Action:** Turn off the power supply.
2. **Action:** Remove the thermometer and shelf.
   Rationale: The bath should have a thermometer to monitor the temperature – do not rely entirely on the dial.
3. **Action:** Pour away the water.
4. **Action:** Wipe all the surfaces with detergent.
   Rationale: If there are excessive deposits of calcium, soak the internal surfaces in a solution of Calgon for 2–3 hours.
5. **Action:** Replace the water.
   Rationale: The base tray must be covered – never run a water bath when it is empty.
6. **Action:** Replace the thermometer.
   Rationale: Holders sited on the side of the bath should hold thermometers in place.
7. **Action:** Switch on the power.
8. **Action:** Reduce heat loss by using a lid. This should not be used for open test tube work.
   Rationale: Condensation accumulates on the lid and drips into the fluid in the test tubes.
9. **Action:** Check that the correct temperature has been reached.
   Rationale: Allow 20–30 minutes for the bath to warm up.

10. **Action:** Put the items in a rack inside the bath and set the timer.
    Rationale: Always use the rack – bottles and tubes may float if free-standing.
11. **Action:** After the incubation time is complete, remove the items.
    Rationale: Always use tongs to remove very hot bottles and tubes.
12. **Action:** Turn off the water bath and allow to cool.

Procedure: Packaging a sample for posting to a referral laboratory

Materials required: postal box or padded envelope, specimen transport bag labelled with a hazard warning symbol, submission form, absorbent material such as cotton wool, laboratory address label that also has 'Pathological Specimen' written on it.

1. **Action** Always use first class post or a courier to ensure next day delivery.
   Rationale: Most samples deteriorate if not tested as soon as possible after sampling.
2. **Action:** Label all tubes, slide holders and sample pots with the patient's name, the client's name and the date the sample was taken.
   Rationale: The laboratory will check that the name on the tube is the same as that on the submission form to avoid muddling samples.
3. **Action:** Complete the submission form with all details required by the laboratory.
   Rationale: The laboratory will require the correct sample and a complete history to interpret the results.
4. **Action:** Wrap the samples in absorbent material and place in the sample bag with the submission form.
   Rationale: It is essential that samples do not leak in transit and are not crushed by the postal system.
5. **Action:** Some tests require the samples to be posted with frozen ice packs within a box or package that has been supplied by the reference laboratory.
   Rationale: Samples may deteriorate rapidly if not maintained at temperatures specified for transit.
6. **Action:** Attach the laboratory address label to the package. Write 'Pathological Specimen' on the package or use a gummed label with it prewritten. Write the sender's address on the back of the package.
   Rationale: The postal regulations require all this information to be on the outside of the package

in case it is damaged in transit. The label warns the postman to take care.

7. **Action:** All biological substances must be packaged in accordance with Royal Mail regulations using the International Air Transport Association (IATA) Guidance document.

   Rationale: These regulations may change from time to time. If there is any uncertainty, search Royal Mail website for more information. Most laboratories are unable to take category A specimens, i.e. those which pose a high risk to humans.

8. **Action**: Dispatch the parcel immediately or refrigerate until the samples can be taken to the post office.

   Rationale: Keeping samples cool helps to preserve components for analysis. Some samples may have to be frozen before transit.

PRACTICAL LABORATORY TECHNIQUES

CYTOLOGY

Procedure: Preparation of a smear using samples from fine-needle aspirate (FNA) biopsies and thoracic fluid

Equipment. Microscope slides (prepared and polished by the manufacturer or degreased in methanol and dried), centrifuge tubes, centrifuge, Pasteur pipette, stains as appropriate.

1. **Action:** Place the sample/fluid in a centrifuge tube and centrifuge at 1500 rpm for 2–3 minutes. Sediment can also be produced in the bottom of the tube by leaving it to stand for about 30 minutes.

   Rationale: Centrifugation is used to spin down the cells and concentrate them at the bottom of the tube. Some samples, such as thoracic fluid, may contain very few cells.

2. **Action:** A smear may be made by touching a slide against a lesion.

   Rationale: Cells stick to the slide and can be used for the examination. This is known as a 'touch prep'.

3. **Action:** FNAs may be prepared without centrifugation if sufficient cells have been harvested. Deposit cells on the slide by pushing the plunger of the syringe.

   Rationale: FNAs are usually rich in cells.

4. **Action:** Decant the supernatant liquid from the centrifuge tube and discard. This leaves the sediment in the bottom of the tube.

Rationale: The use of a conical tube helps in the separation of the sediment from the supernatant.

5. **Action:** Resuspend the cells by flicking the tube with your finger.

   Rationale: This remixes the cells with any remaining liquid and ensures a more even spread of cells on the slide.

6. **Action:** Using a pipette, place one or two drops on to the centre of a microscope slide.

7. **Action:** Make two smears using the 'squash' method (Fig. 11.3).

   Rationale: This is used when there are few cells present in the sample. A 'wedge' method will spread the cells too thinly.

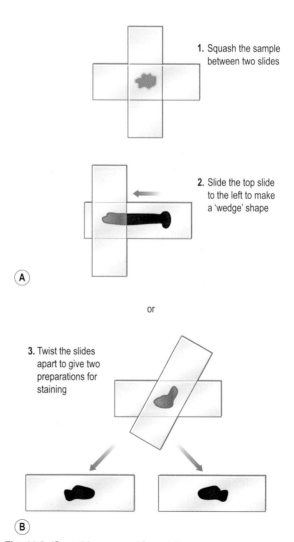

1. Squash the sample between two slides

2. Slide the top slide to the left to make a 'wedge' shape

Ⓐ

or

3. Twist the slides apart to give two preparations for staining

Ⓑ

Fig. 11.3 'Squash' prep used for cytology.

8. **Action:** Allow the smears to air-dry.
   Rationale: The use of artificial heat will damage the cells.
9. **Action:** Stain the smear with Leishman's or Diff-Quik stain, Gram stain or Sudan III stain as appropriate.
   Rationale: Gram stain is used for bacterial examination, Leishman's/Diff-Quik stain is used for blood cells, and Sudan III stain is used to stain fat in a lipoma.

FAECAL EXAMINATION

Procedure: Preparation and storage of faeces for examination

1. **Action:** Faeces may be collected from the ground immediately after defecation. Three samples collected by the owner over 3 days and stored in the fridge may yield more beneficial results.
   Rationale: Old samples may have deteriorated, parasite eggs may hatch and larvae may crawl away. Grass, soil or bacteria may contaminate the sample. Some organisms, e.g. Campylobacter spp., are excreted intermittently. The likelihood of isolating the organism increases if several samples are tested.
2. **Action:** Faeces may be collected using a gloved finger inserted through the anal sphincter into the rectum.
   Rationale: This ensures a fresh uncontaminated sample but care must be taken not to damage the rectal wall.
3. **Action:** Place the sample in a sterile container. There should be sufficient faeces to fill the container.
   Rationale: Too much air in the container encourages parasite eggs to hatch prior to examination.
4. **Action:** Store the faeces in the fridge before examination.
   Rationale: Bacterial growth is slowed down in a cool temperature, and the sample is preserved for longer.
5. **Action:** Bacterial tests must be carried out as soon as possible after collection.
   Rationale: More fastidious organisms such as Campylobacter spp. may be overgrown by more predominant species such as Escherichia coli and will be lost on culture.

Procedure: Worm egg count – modified McMaster method

Equipment. McMaster worm egg-counting chamber, measuring cylinder, saturated salt or sugar solution, Pasteur pipette, balance, balance boat, microscope, two glass beakers, tea strainer or sieve, spatula.

1. **Action:** Weigh 3 g of faeces into a beaker.
   Rationale: The faeces should be fresh and moist.
2. **Action:** Measure 45 ml of saturated salt or sugar solution using the measuring cylinder and pour it into the beaker.
3. **Action:** Mix the solution with a spatula.
4. **Action:** Pour the solution through the sieve into a second beaker.
   Rationale: This removes large particles but allows the eggs to go through.
5. **Action:** Discard the debris remaining in the sieve.
6. **Action:** Mix the solution in the beaker gently.
7. **Action:** Allow the solution to stand at room temperature for 5–10 minutes.
   Rationale: This allows the worm eggs to float to the top of the saturated sugar solution.
8. **Action:** If using a single-chamber type of McMaster slide, prepare it by placing the coverslip grid-side down.
   Rationale: Some slides have only one chamber and use a coverslip grid, while others have two chambers with integral grids (Fig. 11.4).
9. **Action:** Withdraw approximately 2 ml of the solution using a Pasteur pipette.

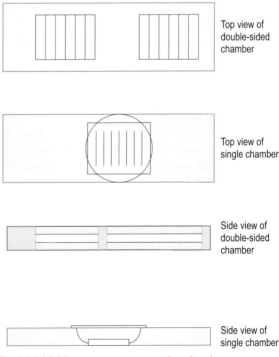

Top view of double-sided chamber

Top view of single chamber

Side view of double-sided chamber

Side view of single chamber

Fig. 11.4 McMaster worm egg-counting chambers.

Rationale: Make sure that you have enough liquid to fill the chamber of the slide completely. This stops bubbles forming over the grid.

10. **Action:** Fill the counting chamber and apply the coverslip (Fig. 11.4).

    Rationale: The coverslip must make contact with the solution to avoid inclusion of air bubbles and distortion of the image.

11. **Action:** Leave the counting chamber on the bench for 5–10 minutes.

    Rationale: This allows the worm eggs and Eimeria *oocysts time to float to the top of the chamber. They are then visible when you focus on the grid. N.B.: Tapeworm segments do not float – use a direct smear.*

12. **Action:** Examine the counting chamber using the ×10 objective on the microscope.

13. **Action:** Count all the eggs seen over the grid (Fig. 11.5).

    Rationale: Count those on the lines as well as those between the lines.

14. **Action:** Calculate the number of eggs as follows:
    * For a single counting chamber, multiply the number of eggs by 100
    * For double-chambered slide, multiply the total number of eggs on the slide by 50. This gives the number of eggs per gram of faeces.

    Rationale: This is a quantitative method and used to evaluate the severity of an infection. (A qualitative analysis tells you whether there are parasites present but does not indicate the severity of the infection.)

Procedure: Baermann sedimentation technique for the detection of lungworm larvae in faeces

Lungworms are nematodes, and several species are found in veterinary medicine.

Aelurostrongylus abstrusus is the main lungworm of cats, and *Oslerus (Filaroides) osleri* of dogs. This technique is also used to identify the larvae of *Angiostrongylus vasorum*, the French heartworm, cases of which are increasing in frequency in the UK. Diagnosis is confirmed by the presence of larvae in faeces or in bronchoalveolar lavage. Both use the Baermann technique; however, a simple, quick and easy blood test is now commercially available to detect canine angiostrongylosis. The presence of the antigen in canine blood indicates that the animal is actively infected with the parasite.

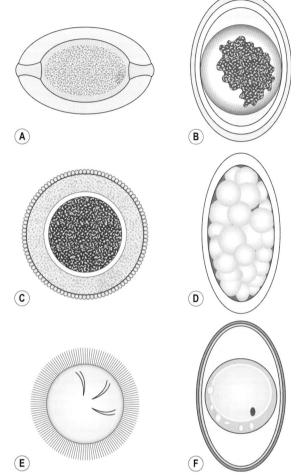

Fig. 11.5 Worm eggs and oocysts. A, *Trichuris* spp.; B, *Toxascaris* spp.; C, *Toxocara* spp.; D, *Uncinaria* spp.; E, *Taenia* spp.; F, *Isospora* spp. (Redrawn from Lane and Cooper (2003), Butterworth-Heinemann.)

Equipment. Faecal samples collected over a 3-day period, 500 ml glass funnel-shaped beaker, Pasteur pipette – extra-long, Petri dish or glass slides and coverslips, wooden tongue depressor, tea strainer or fine gauze/muslin (you may need more than one layer), stereo microscope or binocular microscope with ×10 objective.

1. **Action:** Over a 72-hour period, collect three separate, freshly passed faecal samples in sterile containers and store in the fridge prior to testing.

    Rationale: Old samples may have deteriorated, larvae may have crawled away, or many types of parasitic and non-parasitic larvae may be inadvertently collected. Lungworm larvae are excreted intermittently, so taking several samples increases the chance of finding them.

2. **Action:** Fill the flask almost up to the top with warm tap water.

    Rationale: Warm water stimulates larvae to move about and sink to the bottom of the flask.

3. **Action:** Using the tongue depressor, mix each sample well and take an aliquot of approximately 10 g from each to obtain one well-mixed 30 g sample.

    Rationale: Mixing ensures the likelihood of finding larvae in the test sample as they may be present in very low numbers.

4. **Action:** Place the sample into the tea strainer or the muslin and arrange it across the top of the beaker so that the faeces are partially submerged. If the faeces sample is very watery, more layers of muslin may be required.

    Rationale: The faecal material must be in contact with the water to allow the larvae to swim down through the water to the bottom of the beaker.

5. **Action:** Leave the beaker at room temperature for 18–24 hours.

    Rationale: This gives the larvae time to swim down to the bottom of the water, ready to be harvested for examination.

6. **Action**: Taking a long pipette, push the air out by squeezing the bulb and, while maintaining pressure, push down through the water to the bottom of the flask. Release the bulb and allow the faecal material at the *bottom* of the flask to flow back into the pipette.

    Rationale: You need to collect the material at the bottom of the flask as this is where you will find larvae. You can pour off the supernatant first but be careful not to disturb the sediment at the bottom of the flask.

7. **Action:** Place the contents of the pipette into a Petri dish or take one or two drops only and put them straight on to a glass slide and cover with a cover slip.

8. **Action:** Repeat actions 6 and 7 several times.

    Rationale: You need to collect sufficient faecal fluid to cover the bottom of the Petri dish or to allow examination of several slides.

9. **Action:** Examine the contents of the Petri dish using a low-power stereo microscope. Slides may be examined using ×10 objective and a standard binocular microscope.

    Rationale: Lungworm larvae are quite large and will move around if still alive. Low-power magnification is sufficient to spot them.

10. **Action:** Once you have seen a larva, it is vital that you identify it fully.

    Rationale: Free-living larvae of other nematode species may be present in faecal samples harvested from the ground and these can be mistaken for lungworm larvae.

11. **Action:** Lungworm larvae are short, thick larvae with granular contents and a hooked tail (Figs 11.6 and 11.7).

12. **Action:** A single larva is considered significant.

    Rationale: A normal healthy animal should not have any larvae in the faeces.

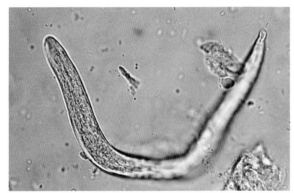

Fig. 11.6 Characteristic first-stage larva of *Aelurostrongylus abstrusus*, the feline lungworm. (Taken from Hendrix and Sirois (2007), Mosby.)

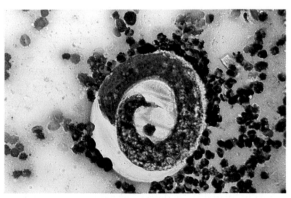

Fig. 11.7 Characteristic infective stage of *Filaroides osleri*, a canine lungworm. (Taken from Hendrix and Sirois (2007), Mosby.)

HAEMATOLOGY

For examples of all blood cells refer to Fig. 11.8.

Procedure: Packed cell volume (PCV)

Equipment. Blood sample in ethylene diamine tetra acetic acid (EDTA) tube, capillary tube (plain), microhaematocrit reader, microhaematocrit centrifuge, soft plasticine or Cristoseal.

1. **Action:** Collect a blood sample in an EDTA tube.
   Rationale: *Sodium EDTA is an anticoagulant that prevents the blood from clotting. It is used to preserve most blood samples used for haematology.*

2. **Action:** Gently invert the tube and roll the sample 10 to 20 times or use a blood roller (see Competency in using haematology analyser, later). Once thoroughly mixed (do not shake), take the sample and place the end of a capillary tube in the blood.

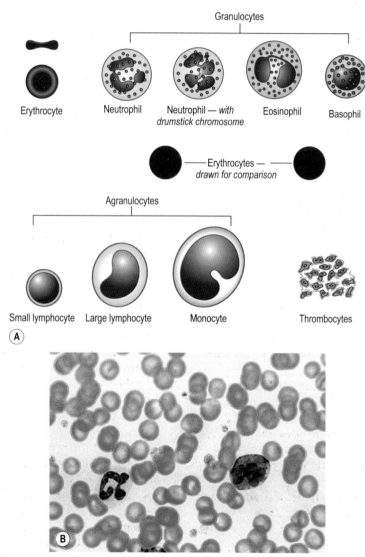

Fig. 11.8 A, The range of blood cells visible in a blood smear. B, Light micrograph of canine basophil *(left)* and nearby neutrophils *(right)*. (Taken from Aspinall V and Aspinall R (2013), Saunders.)

Rationale: Gentle movement mixes the blood with the anticoagulant. If you are too rough, the cells will be damaged and the red cells will rupture, causing haemolysis.

3. **Action:** Hold the tube at a 45° angle and allow the tube to fill until it is three-quarters full.
   Rationale: Blood will be drawn up the tube by capillary action.

4. **Action:** Place the opposite end of the tube into the plasticine pad.
   Rationale: If you use the end containing the blood, you will contaminate the plasticine.

5. **Action:** Twist the capillary tube two or three times and take it out of the plasticine.
   Rationale: This creates a plug that will prevent blood running out of the tube.

6. **Action:** Wipe the tube with soft tissue.
   Rationale: To remove excess blood, which could be a source of infection.

7. **Action:** Place the tube in one groove of the centrifuge with the plasticine plug facing outwards against the outer rim.
   Rationale: Centrifugal force causes the fluids to spin outwards. The sealed end prevents blood escaping as it is forced towards the perimeter.

8. **Action:** Place a similar tube on the opposite side of the centrifuge.
   Rationale: This balances the other tube and reduces vibration and subsequent damage to the centrifuge.

9. **Action:** Screw the safety plate down over the tubes and close the lid.
   Rationale: The safety plate prevents the tubes spinning out of position. Both plate and lid are essential for safety.

10. **Action:** Centrifuge for 5 minutes at 10,000 rpm.

11. **Action:** When the machine stops, remove the lid, safety plate and tube.
    Rationale: Never attempt to open the centrifuge while it is still running.

12. **Action:** Place the tube into the groove on the micro-haematocrit reader.
    Rationale: The blood will have separated into three layers (Fig. 11.9) – from the top downwards:
    - *Plasma*
    - *Buffy coat – white blood cells*
    - *Red blood cells.*

13. **Action:** Line up the top of the plasticine plug with the line on the bottom of the reader (Fig. 11.9).
    Rationale: The top of the plug marks the lowest point of the blood column.

14. **Action:** Line up the top of the plasma with the diagonal line at the top of the reader.
    Rationale: The bottom of the plasma meniscus is used as the measuring point.

15. **Action:** Move the slide so that the middle line is level with the top of the red cells (Fig. 11.9).

16. **Action:** Read the measurement from the scale on the right side of the reader.
    Rationale: The scale is marked 1 to 100 – the reading can be expressed as a percentage, i.e. 45 becomes 45%.

17. **Action:** The PCV is the percentage of whole blood that consists of red blood cells.
    Rationale: PCV can also be calculated by measuring the length of tube occupied by red cells (A) and the total length of the blood column (B) (Table 11.1).

$$PCV\% = A/B \times 100$$

Procedure: Total white blood cell count using a haemocytometer

This procedure is also useful for counting white blood cells in fluids such as synovial fluid, pleural effusions, etc.

Equipment. Blood sample in EDTA tube, haemocytometer and coverslip (Fig. 11.10), 2000 μl (2 ml) and 100 μl (0.1 ml) volumetric pipettes and tips, sterile container, tissue, white cell counting fluid (glacial acetic acid – Table 11.2), microscope.

1. **Action:** Using a 2 ml volumetric pipette, place 2 ml of white cell counting fluid (glacial acetic acid) in a sterile container.
   Rationale: Particles of dust from a dirty container may be mistaken for cells when counting.

2. **Action:** Mix the blood in an EDTA tube by gentle agitation. Add 0.1 ml of the blood to the white cell counting fluid and mix well.
   Rationale: This is a 1:20 dilution.

3. **Action:** Leave to stand at room temperature for 5–10 minutes.

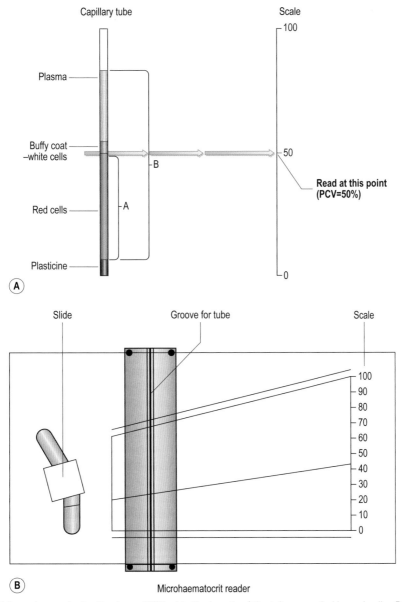

Fig. 11.9 Measuring packed cell volume (PCV). *A* is the length of the tube occupied by red cells; *B* is the total length of the column of blood.

Rationale: *The addition of glacial acetic acid to whole blood results in lysis of the red cells, leaving only the white cells to be counted.*

4. **Action:** Place the coverslip on the haemocytometer and press firmly until Newton's rings can be seen.
   Rationale: *Newton's rings appear as coloured rings and indicate that close contact has been made*

between the coverslip and the counting slide. Close contact ensures that the area filled with blood is an accurate volume.

5. **Action:** Using a capillary tube, draw up some of the treated blood and fill one side of the counting chamber. Do not allow fluid to flow into the well surrounding the plinth on which the grid is situated (Fig. 11.10).

Blood parameter	Dog	Cat
TABLE 11.1 Haematology ranges for dog and cat		
Red blood cells ($\times 10^{12}$/l)	5.0–8.5	5.5–10.0
Packed cell volume (% of whole blood)	37–57	27–50
Total white blood cells ($\times 10^9$/l)	6–15	4–15
Mature neutrophils ($\times 10^9$/l)	3.6–10.5	2.5–12.5
(% of all blood cells)	60–70	45–75
Band neutrophils ($\times 10^9$/l)	0–0.3	0–0.45
(% of all blood cells)	0–2	0–3
Eosinophils (% of all blood cells)	2–10	4–12
Basophils (% of all blood cells)	Rare	Rare
Monocytes (% of all blood cells)	3–10	0–4
Lymphocytes – small (% of all blood cells)	12–30	20–55
Lymphocytes – large (% of all blood cells)	Approx. 8%	Variable
Platelets ($\times 10^9$/l)	200–500	200–600

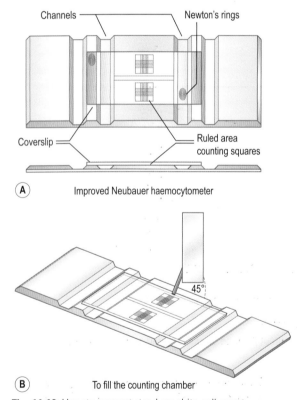

(A)   Improved Neubauer haemocytometer

(B)   To fill the counting chamber

Fig. 11.10 How to prepare a red or white cell count.

Rationale: If the end of the capillary tube is placed at the outside edge of the coverslip, fluid will run under the coverslip and across the grid. Removing the capillary tube just before the fluid reaches the end of the grid will halt the flow.

6. **Action:** Wait for 2 minutes.
   Rationale: At first, the white blood cells float around and are impossible to count. Wait for 2 minutes, and they will settle.
7. **Action:** Place the counting chamber on the microscope stage, being careful to keep it horizontal. Using the $\times 10$ objective lens, count the white cells in all four large corner squares (Fig. 11.11 – marked W).
   Rationale: Each large corner square is made of 16 smaller squares. You will count the white cells in 64 (16×4) small squares (Fig. 11.11).
8. **Action:** Count only the white cells in the spaces and those on the top and right-hand lines of each square.
   Rationale: If you count all the cells on all the lines, you will count some cells twice.
9. **Action:** To calculate the number of white cells:

Total number of white cells in all four large squares = A

Number of cells per litre of blood = A/20 $\times 10^9$

Procedure: Total red cell count using a haemocytometer

Equipment. Blood sample in EDTA tube, haemocytometer and coverslip (Fig. 11.10), 20 ml and 0.1 ml (100 µl) volumetric pipettes and tips, sterile container, tissue, red cell counting fluid (Gowers' solution – Table 11.2), microscope.

1. **Action:** Using a pipette, dispense 20 ml of red blood cell solution into a clean sterile container.

TABLE 11.2   Leucocyte and erythrocyte counting fluids

	Leucocyte counting fluid	Erythrocyte counting fluid (Gowers' solution)
Contents	2 ml glacial acetic acid 1 ml gentian violet (1% aqueous) 100 ml distilled water	12.5 g anhydrous sodium sulphate 33.3 g glacial acetic acid 200 ml distilled water
Method	Filter through filter paper before use and shake well until mixed. Store in a dark glass bottle	Filter through filter paper before use and shake well until mixed. Store in a dark glass bottle
Use	Destroys red cells, leaving only white cells in the blood sample. Used for total white cell count by means of a haemocytometer	Destroys white cells, leaving only red cells in the blood sample. Used for red cell count by means of a haemocytometer

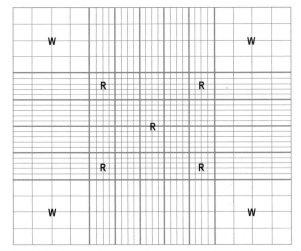

Fig. 11.11 Image of haemocytometer viewed under the microscope. Count the squares labelled R to calculate a red blood cell count. Count the squares labelled W to calculate a white blood cell count.

Rationale: Particles of dust in a dirty container may be mistaken for cells when counting.

2. **Action:** Mix the blood in an EDTA tube by gentle agitation. Add 0.1 ml of the blood to the red cell counting fluid and mix well.
   Rationale: This gives a dilution of 1:200.

3. **Action:** Leave to stand at room temperature for 5–10 minutes.
   Rationale: Red cell solution (Gowers' solution) destroys white cells so that only the red cells remain.

4. **Action:** Place the coverslip on the haemocytometer and press gently until Newton's rings appear.
   Rationale: Newton's rings appear as coloured rings and indicate that close contact has been made between the coverslip and the counting slide. Close

contact ensures that the area filled with blood is an accurate volume.

5. **Action:** Using a capillary tube, draw up some of the treated blood and fill one side of the counting chamber. Do not allow fluid to flow into the well surrounding the plinth on which the grid is situated (Fig. 11.10).
   Rationale: If the end of the capillary tube is placed at the outside edge of the coverslip, fluid will run under the coverslip and across the grid. Removing the capillary tube just before the fluid reaches the end of the grid will halt the flow.

6. **Action:** Wait for 2 minutes.
   Rationale: At first, the red blood cells float around and are impossible to count. Wait for 2 minutes, and they will settle.

7. **Action:** Place the counting chamber on the microscope stage, being careful to keep it horizontal. Using the ×10 objective lens, locate the central square of the nine large squares (Fig. 11.11).

8. **Action:** Change to the ×40 objective lens.

9. **Action:** Count all the cells in five of the 25 small squares in the central area (Fig. 11.11 – marked R).
   Rationale: Each small square is divided into 16 smaller squares – a total of 80 (16 × 5) small squares are counted.

10. **Action:** Count only the cells in the spaces and those resting on the top and the right-hand lines of each square.
    Rationale: If you count the cells on all the lines you will count some cells twice.

11. **Action:** To calculate the number of red cells:

Total number of cells $= A$

$A/100 =$ no. of red cells $\times 10^{12}$/litre

Procedure: Preparation of a blood smear

Equipment. Blood sample in EDTA tube, microscope slides commercially prepared and polished or previously soaked in methanol and dried, capillary tube, glass cutter, marker pen.

1. **Action:** Keep EDTA blood sample at room temperature. If it has been previously refrigerated, allow time for it to warm up.
2. **Action:** Mix the sample thoroughly by gently rolling it between your hands for at least 2 minutes and then inverting the tube 10–20 times. If a blood sample roller is available, roll for 10 minutes.
   Rationale: This suspends the cells evenly. Over-vigorous mixing will damage the cells.
3. **Action:** Prepare a spreader by chipping one corner off a glass slide. If necessary, use a glass cutter.
   Rationale: The use of a spreader stops the smear overlapping the edges of the slide.
4. **Action:** Take a microscope slide which has been soaked in methanol and dried.
   Rationale: Methanol removes grease from the slide and stops gaps appearing.
5. **Action:** Using a capillary tube, place a small drop of blood on the right-hand end of the slide.
   Rationale: Too large a drop makes the smear too thick; too small a drop gives too short a smear and/or hesitation lines.
6. **Action:** Place the spreader to the left of the blood drop at an angle of 45° to the horizontal and draw backwards to 'pick up' the blood.
   Rationale: The blood will run along the spreader as it makes contact.
7. **Action:** Push the spreader forward with even pressure towards the left-hand end of the slide. The sides of the smear should be parallel, and there should be a 'feathery tail' (Fig. 11.12).

Rationale: The smear should take up two-thirds of the slide and should be bullet-shaped. Straight edges are needed for the 'battlement' technique of counting cells.

8. **Action:** Label the slide with a marker pen.
   Rationale: This is important because, if you make several slides at once, they will all look the same.
9. **Action:** Allow the smear to air-dry.
   Rationale: The use of heat will damage the cells.
10. **Action:** Stain the smear with an appropriate stain.

Procedure: Reticulocyte count (Fig. 11.13)

Equipment. Blood sample in EDTA tube, new methylene blue stain, 5 ml test tube, Pasteur pipettes or volumetric pipette, incubator at 37°C, microscope with ×10 and ×40 objectives.

1. **Action:** Using a pipette, dispense 2 ml of methylene blue stain into the test tube.
   Rationale: Check that the stain is new methylene blue – you should not use McFadyean's methylene blue as this is used for identification of anthrax bacilli. New methylene blue stain often needs filtering to avoid precipitate build-up.
2. **Action:** Using a pipette, add 4–5 drops of well-mixed EDTA-treated blood to the test tube.
   Rationale: A heparinized sample is not suitable for haematology.
3. **Action:** Mix gently and place in the incubator at 37°C for 30 minutes.
   Rationale: The sample can be incubated at room temperature if no incubator is available.
4. **Action:** Remove the test tube from the incubator.
5. **Action:** Gently flick the tube with your fingers.
   Rationale: This resuspends the cells in any remaining fluid.
6. **Action:** Use this material to prepare a blood smear as previously described.
7. **Action:** Place the slide under the microscope and using first the ×10 and then ×40 objective lens, look

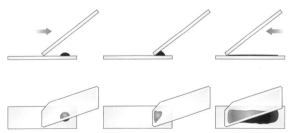

Fig. 11.12 Preparing a blood smear. (Redrawn from (Aspinall (2006), The Complete Textbook of Veterinary Nursing. Elsevier.)

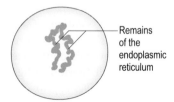

Remains of the endoplasmic reticulum

Fig. 11.13 A reticulocyte. As an immature circulating red cell, it can be stained with a supravital stain, e.g. new methylene blue.

for red blood cells with dark blue-stained strands in them.

> **Rationale:** *These cells are the immature red blood cells, known as reticulocytes (Fig. 11.13). The dark blue strands are remains of the endoplasmic reticulum in the cytoplasm. The presence of reticulocytes indicates that new red blood cells are being formed by the bone marrow to replace those lost, e.g. by old age or haemorrhage.*

8. **Action:** Count a total of 500 cells, noting the number of reticulocytes.

> **Rationale:** *Select an area where individual cells can be seen – this indicates that the smear is one cell thick – known as a monolayer.*

9. **Action:** Calculate the number of reticulocytes as follows:

$$\text{Reticulocyte count} = \frac{\text{No. of reticulocytes} \times 100\%}{\text{Total no. of cells counted}}$$

10. **Action:** A correction factor is now applied to this number.

> **Rationale:** *To accurately measure the responsiveness of the bone marrow, the count takes the PCV of the patient into consideration.*

11. **Action:** To calculate:

$$\text{Corrected reticulocyte count} = \frac{\text{Reticulocyte count} \times \text{patient's PCV}}{\text{Normal PCV for the species}}$$

Most practices have haematology and biochemical analysers in their labs, which perform many of the tests described above more quickly and more accurately. It is important that the student veterinary nurse is able to understand and perform the tests in the 'old-fashioned' way, as they may appear in practical exams, which is why they are included in this book. Chemical analysers are now considered essential pieces of equipment but, if they are to produce accurate and consistent results, they must be used correctly.

Procedure: Competence in using haematology and biochemical analysers

Select the correct sample tube for analysis, for example:
- EDTA for haematology (CBC, etc.)
- Heparin (liver enzymes, etc.)
- Oxalate fluoride (glucose) for biochemistry and electrolytes

- Clotted sample for endocrine analyses (ACTH stim, etc.)
- Citrate for clotting factors.

This is not a comprehensive list. It is wise to consult the laboratory sampling guidelines, as advice may vary between laboratories. Sending an incorrect sample will yield limited results or none at all and you may have to recall the patient.

A. Haematology
1. **Action:** Whole EDTA-treated blood is required for haematology, as well as a freshly prepared blood smear (see Preparation of a blood smear, earlier).

> **Rationale:** *EDTA helps to preserve cell morphology, enabling you to see cellular details microscopically. It also stops cells clumping together, allowing the analyser to count them more accurately. Clots will block the analyser probe and also give an inaccurate result.*

2. **Action:** EDTA sample tubes containing blood should be allowed to roll on a blood roller for 10 minutes prior to testing.

> **Rationale:** *This ensures each cell in is evenly suspended in the sample rather than sinking to the bottom of the tube, potentially leading to an error in counting.*

3. **Action:** Run the sample through the analyser according to the manufacturer's guidelines.

> **Rationale:** *Each analyser is different. Make sure you are familiar with how to use the instrument in your practice laboratory.*

B. Biochemistry and Electrolytes
1. **Action:** Heparinized plasma is generally used for biochemistry and electrolytes. Serum may be used but may give results slightly outside the reference ranges for the analyser in use.

> **Rationale:** *Most analysers work using reference ranges that have been set by the manufacturer to assess whether a result is outside the range and therefore abnormal. This research is most commonly carried out on heparinized plasma.*

2. **Action:** Prepare the plasma by centrifuging the sample at 1200 rpm for 2 minutes.

> **Rationale:** *Spinning the sample at high speed will force the red and white cells to the bottom of the tube, allowing the plasma to be harvested from the top using a Pasteur pipette. Blood samples will separate on the bench over time, but this is time-consuming and can lead to lysis of the red cells.*

3. **Action:** Dispense the plasma into another tube or cassette according to the manufacturer's instructions.
   Rationale: *Some analysers use dry chemistry (cassettes or rotors), whilst others use wet chemistry (test tubes or disposable wells).*

4. **Action:** Select the tests required and run the sample.
   Rationale: *Clinical conditions will require specific tests to evaluate the patient's condition. Often a series of results is needed as an aid to diagnosis.*

5. **Action:** Save and record all results.
   Rationale: *You may need to refer to the results more than once.*

6. **Action:** Alert the vet to any abnormal or spurious results immediately.
   Rationale: *You may have to repeat some tests if there is any doubt.*

Procedure: Giemsa stain – used to demonstrate blood parasites

Equipment. Prepared blood smear, Coplin staining jar, Giemsa stain – neat, Giemsa stain – diluted 1:3 with buffered water (pH 6.8), filter paper, distilled water (pH 6.8), Pasteur pipettes, staining rack, methanol, forceps, microscope, microscope oil.

1. **Action:** Prepare a blood smear as previously described and air-dry. Place on the staining rack.
   Rationale: *Do not use heat to dry the smear, as this will damage the cells.*

2. **Action:** Using a pipette, flood the smear with methanol.

3. **Action:** Leave for 3–5 minutes.
   Rationale: *This fixes the smear.*

4. **Action:** Drain off the methanol and allow the slide to dry in the air.

5. **Action:** Flood the slide with neat Giemsa stain, pouring it through filter paper onto the slide. Leave it for 30 seconds.
   Rationale: *Filtering the stain removes sediment, which may be mistaken for blood parasites.*

6. **Action:** Using forceps, transfer the slide to the Coplin jar containing Giemsa stain diluted 1:3 with buffered water (pH 6.8). Leave for 15–20 minutes.
   Rationale: *The slide is held vertically in the Coplin jar to prevent a build-up of stain sediment on the smear.*

7. **Action:** Remove the slide from the Coplin jar with forceps and rinse with buffered water.
   Rationale: *Avoid using tap water – an incorrect pH will alter the staining characteristics of the cells.*

8. **Action:** Wipe the underside of the slide and allow to dry.
   Rationale: *Do not touch the top of the slide – you will remove the blood smear!*

9. **Action:** Place the smear on the microscope stage and examine under oil immersion (×100).
   Rationale: *This stain is used to identify the presence of blood parasites such as the three Haemoplasma species that have been identified as the cause of feline infectious anaemia. It is also useful for differential white cell counts. Giemsa is a Romanowsky stain – one that uses a combination of two dyes, eosin and oxidized methylene blue.*

Procedure: Leishman's stain

Equipment. Prepared blood smear, Leishman's stain – neat, Leishman's stain – diluted 1:3 with buffered water (pH 6.8), buffered distilled water pH 6.8, Coplin jar, tissues or blotting paper, staining rack, filter paper, forceps, microscope, microscope oil.

1. **Action:** Prepare a blood smear as previously described and air-dry. Place on the staining rack.
   Rationale: *Do not use heat to dry the smear, as this will damage the cells.*

2. **Action:** Flood the slide with neat Leishman's stain, pouring it through a piece of filter paper. Leave for 1 minute.
   Rationale: *Filtering the stain removes sediment, which may be mistaken for blood parasites.*

3. **Action:** Using forceps, transfer the slide to the Coplin jar containing Leishman's stain diluted with buffered distilled water to a pH of 6.8. A gold film should be visible on the top of the liquid. Leave for 5 minutes.
   Rationale: *The Coplin jar holds the slide in a vertical position to prevent the build-up of sediment. The gold film indicates that the stain is at the correct pH.*

4. **Action:** Using forceps, remove the slide and rinse with buffered water.
   Rationale: *Do not use tap water – if the pH is incorrect, it may change the staining characteristics of the cells.*

5. **Action:** Wipe the underside of the slide and air-dry.
   Rationale: *Do not touch the top of the slide – you will remove the blood smear!*

6. **Action:** Examine under the microscope using oil immersion (×100).

Rationale: Leishman's is the stain most commonly used for differential white cell counts because it provides good cellular definition. Leishman's stain is a Romanowsky stain – one that uses a combination of two dyes, eosin and oxidized methylene blue.

Procedure: Diff-Quik stain

Equipment. Prepared blood smear, Diff-Quik kit, which consists of three solutions - fixative, stain 1 and stain 2, Coplin jars, forceps, distilled water buffered to pH 7.2, tissue, microscope, immersion oil.

1. **Action:** Prepare a blood smear as previously described and air-dry.
   Rationale: Do not use heat to dry the smear, as this will damage the cells.
2. **Action:** Dispense the staining solutions into Coplin jars.
   Rationale: These glass jars with lids will prevent dust from falling into the stains.
3. **Action:** Dip the slide into the fixative solution for 1 second, five times. Allow excess to drip back into the jar.
   Rationale: Leaving the slide in the fixative for too long results in unsatisfactory staining.
4. **Action:** Dip the slide into stain solution 1 for 1 second, five times. Allow excess to drip back into the jar.
   Rationale: This solution stains the cellular components red.
5. **Action:** Dip the slide into stain solution 2 for 1 second, five times. Allow excess to drip back into the jar.
   Rationale: This solution stains the cellular components blue.
6. **Action:** Rinse the slide with buffered water.
7. **Action:** Wipe the underside of the slide.
   Rationale: If you always keep the smear side facing towards you while staining, you will not be tempted to wipe the wrong side and lose your smear.
8. **Action:** Allow the smear to air-dry.
   Rationale: Do not use heat to dry the smear as this will damage the cells.
9. **Action:** Place the slide on the microscope stage and examine using oil immersion (×100).
   Rationale: Stains must be renewed once a week to maintain their effectiveness. Diff-Quik is a Romanowsky stain – one which uses a combination of two dyes. Although it is quick and easy to use, it gives poor cellular definition.

Procedure: Differential white blood cell count

Equipment. Prepared blood smear, Leishman's, Diff-Quik kit or Giemsa stain, microscope, immersion oil.

1. **Action:** Prepare a blood smear and air-dry as described previously.
2. **Action:** Stain using Leishman's, Diff-Quik or Giemsa stain as described previously.
   Rationale: Leishman's or Diff-Quik kit provides good cellular definition and is quicker to do than Giemsa.
3. **Action:** Place the slide on the microscope stage and examine under the ×10 objective lens.
   Rationale: This enables you to select an area at least one-third from the end of the smear on the side edge.
4. **Action:** Move out the ×10 objective and place a drop of oil on the slide. Move the ×100 objective into position, making contact with the drop of oil.
   Rationale: Watch what you are doing from the side, not through the lens – this may damage the slide. The use of oil immersion provides increased magnification.
5. **Action:** Carefully focus on the selected field using the fine adjustment knob.
   Rationale: Do not use the coarse focus as the incremental movements mean your view goes out of focus very quickly.
6. **Action:** Move the slide following the line of a 'battlement' (Fig. 11.14) as follows: move two fields along the edge of the smear, two fields up, two fields along, two fields down. While you are doing this, count 100 white blood cells.
   Rationale: This enables you to cover a reasonable area of the smear and overcomes biased cell distribution on the slide. You may count more than 100 – the greater the number of cells counted, the greater the accuracy of the sample.
7. **Action:** As you count, record the numbers of each cell type (Fig. 11.14).
   Rationale: You may record your results manually on paper or using some form of commercial differential counter.
8. **Action:** Calculate the percentage of each cell type using these figures (Table 11.1).
   Rationale: For example, suppose you have counted 72 neutrophils among your 100 cells, then the percentage of neutrophils in the blood is 72/100 = 72%.

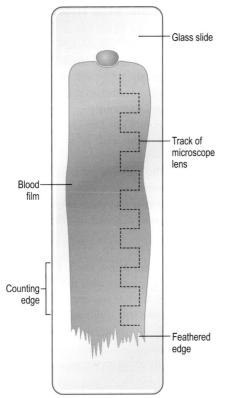

Fig. 11.14 The battlement technique for differential blood films. (Redrawn from (Lane and Cooper (2003), Butterworth-Heinemann.)

HISTOPATHOLOGY

Procedure: Preparation of tissue for histological examination

Equipment. Formol saline, wide-mouthed sample container, scissors or scalpel.

1. **Action:** Make up a 10% formol saline by diluting one part of formalin with nine parts of normal saline.
   Rationale: 10% formol saline is the most commonly used fixative.
2. **Action:** Select a wide-mouthed container.
   Rationale: Tissue is soft when taken from a patient and hardens as it becomes fixed. Removing hardened tissue from a narrow-mouthed container is very difficult.
3. **Action:** Select a piece of tissue no more than 1–2 cm thick. If the tissue sample is large, slice it into two or three pieces.
   Rationale: Diffusion through the tissue takes too long if the tissue is too thick.

4. **Action:** Add approximately 10 times the volume of the sample of formol saline.
   Rationale: The sample must be completely submerged in the formol saline.
5. **Action:** If the sample is to be posted, avoid using any more than 60 ml of formol saline. If the sample will not be adequately fixed in 60 ml, fix it in a large pot, remove it and wrap it in formalin-soaked gauze and post in a plastic bag.
   Rationale: Always check the postal regulations before sending samples through the post. Formalin is toxic and must not be allowed to leak out of the package. Formalin fumes may also have a detrimental effect on cytology smears. Allow good separation between slide containers and tissue in pots when packing parcels.
6. **Action:** Wrap the sample in absorbent material and place in a leak-proof polypropylene transport box.
   Rationale: Glass bottles should not be sent through the post.
7. **Action:** Send it to the laboratory using next day delivery.
   Rationale: Samples may deteriorate if left too long.

MICROBIOLOGY

Nowadays most practices will use disposable loops to transfer and spread bacterial cultures. These are supplied in individual sterile packs and therefore do not require heat sterilization in the flame of the Bunsen burner. Each disposable loop will allow *one action*, after which it must be discarded into clinical waste.

Procedure: Preparation of bacterial smears

Equipment. Platinum loop (may use a single-use/disposable loop), Bunsen burner, glass microscope slide, sterile normal saline, agar plate containing bacterial growth.

1. **Action:** Heat the platinum loop in the flame of a Bunsen burner. Allow it to cool.
   Rationale: Flaming the platinum loop will sterilize it. Cooling prevents damaging the bacteria.
2. **Action:** Using the loop, place 2–3 drops of saline onto the centre of the microscope slide.
   Rationale: This is used to dilute and spread the bacterial colony.
3. **Action:** Flame and cool the loop again.
4. **Action:** Using the loop, select an isolated bacterial colony and carefully remove it from the agar plate.

Rationale: If there is more than one type of organism on the plate, you will need to make a smear for each type.

5. **Action:** Mix the colony with the saline on the slide, spreading out the fluid to cover 1–2 cm².
   Rationale: Mixing with saline results in a single layer of cells, allowing you to identify the shape of the cells.
6. **Action:** Flame and cool the loop. Discard in the appropriate way.
   Rationale: The loop has been contaminated and must be sterilized before it is discarded to prevent the spread of disease.
7. **Action:** Pass the smear gently over the Bunsen burner flame until it is dry.
   Rationale: This fixes the slide. If the smear is still wet when it is stained, some bacteria may float off, contaminating the stain and causing the loss of some areas of the smear.
8. **Action:** Stain the smear using Gram stain or methylene blue.

Procedure: Gram stain – rapid method

Equipment. Prepared bacterial smear, crystal violet stain, Gram stain or Lugol's iodine, acetone, carbol fuchsin (dilute) or safranine, staining rack, wash bottle containing tap water, blotting paper or tissue, microscope, timer, Pasteur pipettes.

1. **Action:** Place the prepared smear on the staining rack with the smear facing upwards.
   Rationale: You can also stain smears in Coplin jars.
2. **Action:** Using a pipette, flood the slide with crystal violet for 30 seconds.
   Rationale: At this stage the cell walls of Gram-positive organisms absorb the stain and become purple.
3. **Action:** Wash the slide with tap water.
   Rationale: To remove the crystal violet stain.
4. **Action:** Flood the slide with iodine for 60 seconds.
   Rationale: This fixes the smear.
5. **Action:** Flood the slide with acetone for 2–3 seconds.
   Rationale: This decolorizes the smear rapidly.
6. **Action:** Wash the slide with water.
   Rationale: To remove the stain.
7. **Action:** Flood the slide with carbol fuchsin for 30 seconds.
   Rationale: This counterstains the bacteria – Gram-negative bacteria stain pink at this stage.
8. **Action:** Wash the slide with tap water.
   Rationale: To remove the stain.
9. **Action:** Wipe the back of the slide.

Rationale: Do not wipe the front of the slide and lose the smear.

10. **Action:** Pass the slide rapidly over the flame of the Bunsen burner to dry it.
    Rationale: Do not overheat, as the slide may shatter.
11. **Action:** Place the slide under the microscope and examine using oil immersion ($\times 100$).
    Rationale: Bacteria range in size from 0.5 to 5 μm in length and are best viewed under high magnification. Gram-positive bacteria, e.g. Clostridium *spp.*, Staphylococcus *spp.* and Streptococcus *spp.*, stain purple; Gram-negative bacteria, e.g. Escherichia coli and Salmonella *spp.*, stain pink. Gram stain is used to identify the shape of bacteria and to classify them into Gram-positive or Gram-negative groups.

Procedure: Methylene blue stain

Equipment. Prepared bacterial smear, staining rack, Löffler's methylene blue, tissue or blotting paper, Pasteur pipette, wash bottle containing tap water, microscope.

1. **Action:** Place the prepared smear on the staining rack with the smear facing upwards.
   Rationale: You can also stain in Coplin jars.
2. **Action:** Using a pipette, flood the slide with methylene blue stain and leave for 3 minutes.
   Rationale: This stains the bacterial cells.
3. **Action:** Wash the slide with tap water.
   Rationale: To remove the stain.
4. **Action:** Pass the slide rapidly over the flame of the Bunsen burner to dry it.
   Rationale: Do not overheat, as the slide may shatter.
5. **Action:** Place the slide under the microscope and examine using oil immersion ($\times 100$).
   Rationale: Bacteria range in size from 0.5 to 5 μm in length and are best viewed under high magnification. The bacteria stain blue. Methylene blue stain is used to identify the shape of the bacteria.

Procedure: Bacterial culture

Equipment. Sample material, Petri dish containing agar gel, platinum loop (may use a single-use/disposable loop), Bunsen burner, incubator, marker pen.

Nowadays most practices use disposable loops, which are supplied in individual sterile packs and therefore do not require heat sterilization. Each disposable loop will allow *one action*, after which it must be discarded into clinical waste.

1. **Action:** Label the Petri dish with an appropriate laboratory code.

Rationale: Use the client's name, a number or the animal's name – develop your own system. It is important not to mix up samples – all agar plates look alike in the incubator.

2. **Action:** Flame the platinum loop in the Bunsen flame – heat until red hot from the handle end towards the loop and then bring up through the flame.
   Rationale: This sterilizes the loop and kills all bacteria, making it safe to use.

3. **Action:** Cool the loop by waving it in the air for a few seconds.
   Rationale: If the loop is too hot, it will kill bacterial cells and produce no growth on the plate.

4. **Action:** Dip the loop into the sample.
   Rationale: If it sizzles, it is too hot!

5. **Action:** Pick up the half of the Petri dish containing the agar and turn it over so that the surface of the agar is uppermost.
   Rationale: Petri dishes have a base into which the agar is poured and allowed to set, and a lid – they look similar.

6. **Action:** Smear the material on the loop over a small area on the left of the agar (Fig. 11.15).
   Rationale: This is known as the 'well' and is the start of your inoculation area.

7. **Action:** Replace the Petri dish into its lid.
   Rationale: Do not leave agar plates open to the air for too long as they may become contaminated.

8. **Action:** Flame and cool the loop as before. Remove the lid of the dish and check that the loop has cooled by placing it on a piece of the agar on one side of the plate.
   Rationale: If it sizzles, it is too hot.

9. **Action:** Pick up the Petri dish and, using the loop, make 3–4 short streaks all in the same direction from the 'edge' of the well (Fig. 11.15). Take care not to tear the agar.
   Rationale: This action begins to spread the contents of the sample evenly over the plate.

10. **Action:** Continue to spread the sample over the plate as shown in Fig. 11.15.
    Rationale: The aim is to dilute the sample and so form single colonies of bacteria on the final stroke.

11. **Action:** Place the lid on the dish and put it in the incubator with the agar side on top.
    Rationale: If the lid is uppermost, condensation will occur. The water droplets will drip down on to the

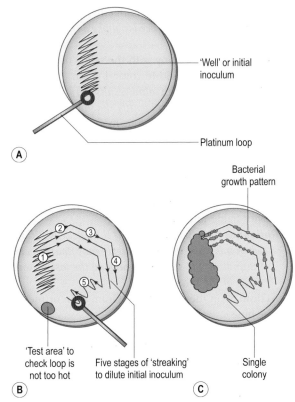

'Well' or initial inoculum

Platinum loop

A

Bacterial growth pattern

'Test area' to check loop is not too hot

Five stages of 'streaking' to dilute initial inoculum

Single colony

B   **C**

Fig. 11.15 Technique for the inoculation of an agar plate.

surface of the agar, causing the bacterial colonies to spread.

12. **Action:** Do not stack plates more than two or three high inside the incubator.
    Rationale: Air must be able to circulate freely, and overcrowding will prevent this.

13. **Action:** Incubate at 37°C for 18–24 hours.
    Rationale: Most pathogenic bacteria are normothermic and will grow at normal body temperature.

14. **Action:** Remove from the incubator and examine for signs of bacterial growth.
    Rationale: Colonies of bacteria appear as round, often slightly raised 'lumps' – the colour may be characteristic of the species. They are distributed along the streak lines.

15. **Action:** If there is no visible growth, incubate the plate for another 18–24 hours.
    Rationale: Some bacteria take longer to grow than others.

PARASITOLOGY

Procedure: Culture for ringworm fungus

Equipment. Sabouraud's agar or commercial ringworm agar, e.g. Dermafyt, forceps, Bunsen burner, marker pen, microscope slide, coverslip, inoculation loop, lactophenol cotton blue stain, Pasteur pipette

Remember, ringworm fungi are zoonotic – always wear gloves when handling samples!

1. **Action:** Place the forceps in the flame of the Bunsen burner for a few seconds. Remove and allow to cool to room temperature.
   Rationale: The forceps must be sterilized before use to reduce the risk of bacterial contamination.
2. **Action:** Remove the lid of the Petri dish containing the Sabouraud's agar or peel off the cover of the commercial agar.
   Rationale: Avoid contaminating the agar with your fingers.
3. **Action:** Using the forceps, take six to eight hairs from the sample to be examined and place them in the centre of the agar. Replace the lid or seal the cover of the commercial agar.
   Rationale: Avoid contamination by microorganisms in the atmosphere.
4. **Action:** Incubate at room temperature for up to 28 days.
   Rationale: Ringworm fungus grows very slowly, although some species may grow within 4 days.
5. **Action:** When fungal growth is visible, examine and identify.
   Rationale: On Sabouraud's medium, growth appears as a white fluffy colony. On a commercial agar, an indicator placed in the agar results in a red coloration. Some contaminants may also create a colour change – it is important to identify the fungus under the microscope.
6. **Action:** To make a smear of the fungus, use a pipette to place 2–3 drops of lactophenol cotton blue stain in the centre of a glass microscope slide.
   Rationale: The stain helps to spread the colony over the slide. The phenol in the stain inactivates spores and the blue stain aids visualization of the fungal spores and mycelia.
7. **Action:** Sterilize a platinum loop by passing it through the flame of the Bunsen burner and allow to cool. If using a presterilized disposable loop, there is no need to do this.
   Rationale: To prevent contamination of the fungus.
8. **Action:** Using the loop, pick up a small amount of the fungal colony and mix with the stain on the slide. Sterilize and discard the platinum loop. Disposable loops are disposed of in the clinical waste.
   Rationale: To prevent contamination by any remaining fungus on the loop.
9. **Action:** Place a coverslip over the material.
   Rationale: The use of a coverslip provides a uniform layer for examination.
10. **Action:** Place the slide under the microscope and examine using the ×10 objective and then the ×40 objective lenses.
    Rationale: Ringworm is caused by dermatophytes such as Trichophyton *and Microsporum* spp. *Look for the typical micro- and macroconidia (Fig. 11.16). Lactophenol cotton blue is used to stain the background and the spores to aid visualization of the fungus.*

Procedure: Use of a Wood's lamp – to detect *Microsporum canis*

Equipment. Wood's lamp, eye protection.

Remember, ringworm fungi are zoonotic – always wear gloves when handling samples or suspected cases!

1. **Action:** This is best performed in a darkened room.
   Rationale: A darkened room will intensify the fluorescent effect.
2. **Action:** Put on the eye protectors.
   Rationale: Ultraviolet light is potentially dangerous and can damage the conjunctiva and the retina.
3. **Action:** Switch on the lamp and allow it to warm up for 5 minutes.
4. **Action:** Ask an assistant (also wearing eye protectors) to restrain the patient on a non-slip examination table.
   Rationale: If the animal feels secure, it will be less likely to try to escape.
5. **Action:** Hold the lamp over the affected areas and look for signs of apple green fluorescence.
   Rationale: Only 60% of cases of Microsporum canis *infection show this fluorescence. Lack of fluorescent areas does not rule out ringworm infection. Other particles in the coat, e.g. skin flakes, dirt, detergent and paraffin oil, may fluoresce a non-specific blue–white.*
6. **Action:** Turn off the lamp immediately after use.
   Rationale: Long exposure to ultraviolet rays will burn the skin.

3. **Action:** If the presence of fleas is suspected, take a sample of hair containing black specks and cover with a few drops of water.

    Rationale: *Flea dirt appears as gritty black specks in the coat. These are made of partially digested blood, which forms a pink-stained solution when dissolved in water.*

Procedure: Collection of a skin scraping – to demonstrate the presence of burrowing ectoparasites

Equipment. Sterile sharp scalpel blade, clippers, clean collecting pot, suitable antiseptic powder or ointment.

1. **Action:** Select a suitable area of the patient for sampling and gently clip. If many areas are affected, take samples from several of them.

    Rationale: *This reduces the amount of hair in the sample. The technique is used to demonstrate the presence of burrowing mites such as* Sarcoptes *and* Demodex, *which will not be present on superficial hair (Fig. 11.17).*

2. **Action:** Hold a sharp, sterile scalpel blade at right angles to the skin and draw repeatedly across the area until it bleeds.

    Rationale: *The presence of blood indicates that the deeper layers of the skin have been reached. Use of a sharp blade makes the whole procedure easier and less painful for the patient.*

3. **Action:** Place the scalpel blade and all the skin debris into a clean collecting pot.

    Rationale: *This need not be sterile as identification of mites will not be confused with the appearance of contaminating microorganisms.*

4. **Action:** Dress the scraped area with a suitable antiseptic.

    Rationale: *This prevents the development of secondary bacterial infection.*

Procedure: Preparation of a smear to identify the presence of mites

Equipment. Scraped skin sample, 10% potassium hydroxide, glass slide, coverslip, Pasteur pipette, microscope, Bunsen burner, forceps.

1. **Action:** Place some of the material collected by skin scraping on to the centre of a microscope slide.

    Rationale: *Do not use too much material as the parasites may be masked by skin debris.*

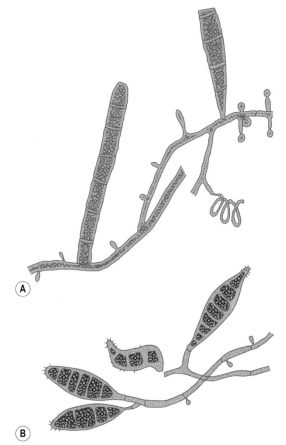

Fig. 11.16 Microscopic appearance of ringworm fungus. A, *Trichophyton* spp.: look for septate hyphae, micro- and macroconidia; the latter are thin-walled and cylindrical. B, *Microsporum* spp.: look for septate hyphae, micro- and macroconidia; the latter are thick-walled, long, spindle-shaped or distorted. (Redrawn from Lane and Cooper (1994), Butterworth-Heinemann.)

Procedure: Collection and examination of coat brushings – to demonstrate the presence of surface-living ectoparasites

Equipment. Toothbrush, flea or nit comb, Petri dish.

1. **Action:** Comb or brush through the patient's fur and collect the superficial debris and hairs in a Petri dish.

    Rationale: *The fur may contain parasites, eggs and faeces, as well as skin scales and dirt.*

2. **Action:** Examine with a hand lens or low-powered microscope.

    Rationale: *This is used to demonstrate the presence of surface-living ectoparasites such as* Cheyletiella spp., *fleas and lice (Fig. 11.17).*

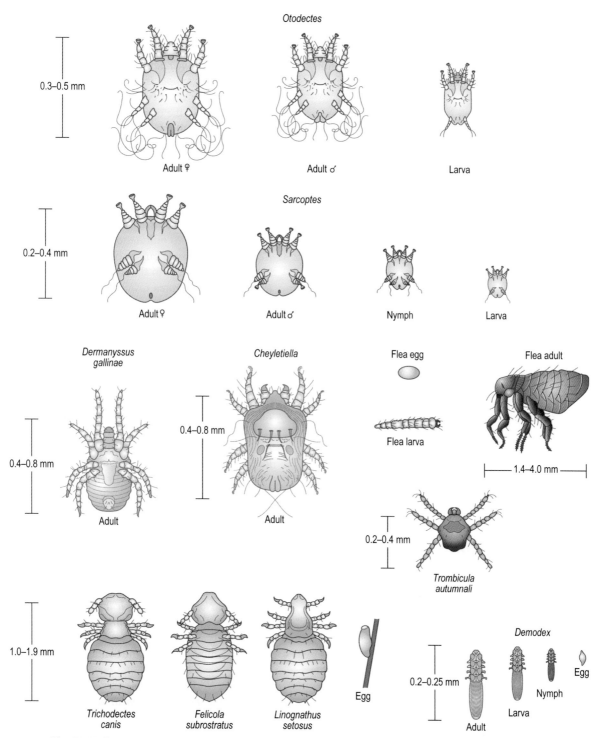

Fig. 11.17 Common ectoparasites of companion animals.

2. **Action:** With a pipette, add 2–3 drops of 10% potassium hydroxide. (N.B.: Some vets use liquid paraffin as an aid to obtaining a diagnostic sample. Do not mix liquid paraffin with potassium hydroxide – simply examine the smears using a coverslip and liquid paraffin.)

   Rationale: *This solution is caustic – take care!*

3. **Action:** Place a coverslip over the sample.

   Rationale: *This provides a uniform layer to examine and prevents the lens from becoming contaminated.*

4. **Action:** Holding the slide with forceps, warm it gently over a Bunsen burner – do not boil it.

   Rationale: *Warming breaks down and clears the debris, making the parasites easier to see.*

5. **Action:** Allow the slide to cool.

6. **Action:** Place the slide under the microscope and examine under the ×4 objective and then the ×10 objective.

   Rationale: *Larger parasites such as* Sarcoptes *may be seen under ×4 magnification, but* Demodex *will only be seen under a higher magnification (Fig. 11.17).*

7. **Action:** You may have to prepare several slides from your sample to be certain of the result.

   Rationale: *Parasites may only be present in low numbers and may easily be missed if only one smear is made.*

This technique may be used to demonstrate the presence of ear mites – *Otodectes cynotis* (Fig. 11.17). Brown-coloured discharge is collected from the ear and treated in the same way before microscopic examination.

URINE EXAMINATION

Procedure: Urine preservation

Equipment. Collecting containers.

1. **Action:** Samples may be collected by catheterization, capturing free-flowing urine midstream or cystocentesis. (For catheterization techniques, see Chapter 3.)

   Rationale: *Free-flow samples can be collected by the owner and are the most commonly used. A midstream sample is more representative of the bladder contents as the first part of the stream may contain contaminants from the urethra. A sample taken by cystocentesis is more reliable for bacteriology.*

2. **Action:** Collect the sample into a clean, preferably sterile, container.

   Rationale: *Owners may use clean jam jars, plastic containers or commercially designed collecting equipment. Cats may use any empty, clean litter tray or commercially prepared urine-collecting litter. If the sample is to be used for bacteriology, the container must be sterile.*

3. **Action:** Transfer the urine into a boric acid tube and a plain sample tube.

   Rationale: *Boric acid is used to preserve samples for bacteriology. The bacterial numbers remain unchanged in the boric acid solution until it is tested. Plain tubes are used for specific gravity estimation, dipstick tests and sediment examination. They may also be used for bacterial examination if used within 20 minutes of collection.*

4. **Action:** If the sample cannot be despatched or tested immediately, store it in the fridge.

   Rationale: *Refrigerated urine should be tested within 24 hours of collection.*

Procedure: Gross examination of urine

Equipment. Urine sample in clean sample pot.

1. **Action:** Collect sample in a clean transparent pot as described previously.

   Rationale: *You must be able to examine the urine easily.*

2. **Action:** Look at the colour of the sample.

   Rationale: *Normal urine is yellow but it may vary in intensity. Deep yellow urine is more concentrated than pale yellow urine; a brown-yellow colour may indicate the presence of bilirubin; a red colour may indicate the presence of blood or haemoglobin. Some drugs may change the colour of urine.*

3. **Action:** Hold the sample up to the light and examine its clarity.

   Rationale: *Normal urine is clear. Increased turbidity indicates the presence of sediment, e.g. crystals, bacteria, pus or blood cells.*

4. **Action:** Remove the lid of the container and smell the sample.

   Rationale: *Normal urine has a smell that is characteristic of the species, e.g. tomcat urine is instantly recognizable and is different from that of the queen. The smell of ammonia may be caused by stale urine; the smell of pear drops is due to the presence of ketones.*

Procedure: To test the specific gravity of urine by refractometer

Equipment. Urine sample, refractometer, Pasteur pipettes, distilled water, lint-free tissue.

1. **Action:** To calibrate the refractometer, wipe the glass prism (Fig. 11.18) with a piece of lint-free tissue and, using a pipette, place two drops of distilled water on to the prism. Place the plastic cover over the prism.
   Rationale: The refractometer must be calibrated before use to ensure that it measures accurately.
2. **Action:** Hold the refractometer up to the light and look at the scale through the eyepiece. Note the point on the scale that marks the boundary between the light and dark areas.
   Rationale: For distilled water, this should read 1.000.
3. **Action:** If the reading is not exactly 1.000, adjust the refractometer using the screw on the top of the instrument until the reading is 1.000. N.B.: Some refractometers may have a different method of adjustment – check the instructions.
   Rationale: The refractometer will now read accurately.
4. **Action:** Wipe off the distilled water with a piece of dry tissue.
5. **Action:** Using a fresh pipette, place two drops of the test urine on to the prism. Close the plastic cover.

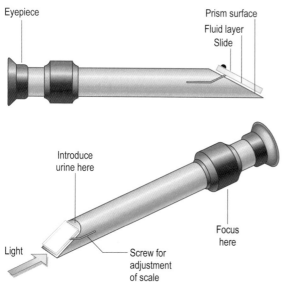

Eyepiece

Prism surface
Fluid layer
Slide

Introduce urine here

Focus here

Light

Screw for adjustment of scale

Fig. 11.18 Refractometer – for measuring the specific gravity of urine.

Rationale: If you use the same pipette, you may dilute the urine sample with water remaining in the pipette.

6. **Action:** Hold the refractometer up to the light and read the scale as before. Record your result.
   Rationale: The normal specific gravity of dog urine is 1.018–1.045. The normal specific gravity of cat urine is 1.020–1.040. Urine shows a higher specific gravity in cases of dehydration, reduced water intake and shock, and a lower specific gravity where water intake is increased, as is seen in cases of pyometra and chronic renal failure.
7. **Action:** Rinse off the urine with distilled water and wipe the refractometer with lint-free tissue.
   Rationale: Do not leave the urine sample to dry on the prism.
8. **Action:** Replace in the case.
   Rationale: The refractometer must be stored in its case to prevent accidental damage and keep it dust-free.

Procedure: To test urine for various parameters using a dipstick

Equipment. Fresh urine sample, minute timer, dipstick test.

1. **Action:** Select the correct type of dipstick test. The sticks are presented in a screw-top container containing large numbers of sticks. The instructions are printed on the label.
   Rationale: Commercial reagent dipsticks consist of a series of test reagent pads mounted on a plastic strip. The tests vary in number and in type, e.g. some may test only glucose, whereas others may have as many as ten tests, including those for pH, protein, blood and bilirubin. Make sure that the tests you need are included on the stick and that the tests are validated for animals – some are validated for humans and may give irrelevant results.
2. **Action:** Check the expiry date.
   Rationale: Out-of-date dipsticks may give unreliable results.
3. **Action:** Remove the lid of the dipstick container and take out one stick. Replace the lid.
   Rationale: Do not contaminate the remaining dipsticks with urine.
4. **Action:** Dip the stick in the fresh urine sample until all the pads are wet.

Rationale: *Results are more accurate if the sample is fresh. Never use on a preserved sample. Stale samples may have bacterial growth or be contaminated by faeces or blood, which may affect the results.*

5. **Action:** Remove the stick from the urine and tap gently on the inside of the sample pot.
   Rationale: *To remove any surplus urine.*

6. **Action:** Using the timer, make sure that you keep to the time intervals stated on the side of the bottle.
   Rationale: *Each test pad requires a specific time in contact with the urine before it reacts appropriately.*

7. **Action:** Check that you read the results from the correct end of the stick.
   Rationale: *If you read from the wrong end, you will get results that are incorrect for that test pad.*

8. **Action:** Hold the dipstick container in one hand and the dipstick in the other and compare the colour of each pad with the correct one on the side of the container.
   Rationale: *Each reagent pad will change colour. The range of colour changes is illustrated on the label, accompanied by the appropriate result.*

9. **Action:** Record your results.
   Rationale: *Do not rely on your memory – the results may need to be kept for some time.*

10. **Action:** Dispose of the dipstick in the clinical waste.
    Rationale: *Pathogens may be present on the stick.*

Procedure: Urine sediment examination

Equipment. Fresh urine sample, microscope, glass slide, coverslip, Pasteur pipettes, urine centrifuge tube, centrifuge, Sedi-Stain (optional).

N.B.: Samples that have been stored in a refrigerator should be brought to room temperature prior to testing. This action will allow any crystals that may have formed at low temperatures to disappear and avoids errors in interpretation.

1. **Action:** Using a pipette, place 3–5 ml of urine in a centrifuge tube.
   Rationale: *A conical tube helps to separate the sediment from the supernatant.*

2. **Action:** Place the tube in the centrifuge.

3. **Action:** Place a similar tube on the opposite side of the centrifuge.
   Rationale: *The machine must be balanced to prevent vibration and damage.*

4. **Action:** Spin at 1000–2000 rpm for 2–3 minutes.
   Rationale: *Spinning for a longer time will damage any cells present in the urine.*

5. **Action:** Using a pipette, remove and discard most of the supernatant, being careful not to disturb the sediment.
   Rationale: *Only the sediment is required for this procedure.*

6. **Action:** Flick the test tube with your fingers.
   Rationale: *This resuspends the sediment in any remaining liquid and makes a more even smear on the slide.*

7. **Action:** If you wish, add 1–2 drops of Sedi-Stain to the sediment in the tube, but this is optional.
   Rationale: *Sedi-Stain may make the material in the sediment easier to identify. Follow manufacturer's instructions for identification of cells.*

8. **Action:** Using a pipette, place 1–2 drops of the sediment on to the centre of a glass slide and add a coverslip.
   Rationale: *This provides a uniform layer for examination and protects the lens from contamination.*

9. **Action:** Place the slide under the microscope and examine using the ×10 and ×40 objective lenses.
   Rationale: *Look for evidence of casts, red and white blood cells, epithelial cells, spermatozoa, mucin threads, bacteria and crystals (Fig. 11.19).*

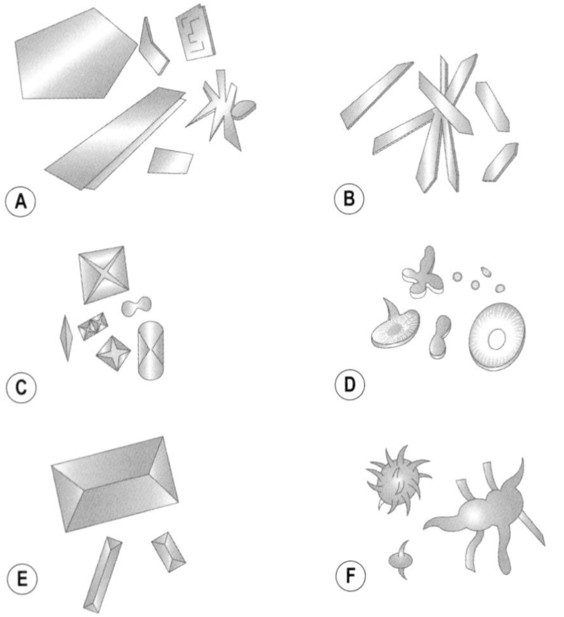

Fig. 11.19 Urine crystals: A, urates; B, hippuric acid; C, calcium oxalate; D, calcium carbonate; E, struvite; F, ammonium urate. (Redrawn from Lane and Cooper (2003), Butterworth-Heinemann.)

REFERENCES AND FURTHER READING

Ackerman, N., 2016. Aspinall's Complete Textbook of Veterinary Nursing, third ed. Elsevier, Oxford.

Aspinall, V., 2006. The Complete Textbook of Veterinary Nursing, 1st ed. Elsevier, Oxford.

Aspinall, V., 2011. The Complete Textbook of Veterinary Nursing, second ed. Elsevier, Oxford.

Aspinall, V., Aspinall, R., 2013. Clinical Procedures in Small Animal Veterinary Practice. Saunders, London.

Benjamin, M., 1974. Outline of Veterinary Clinical Pathology, second ed. Iowa State University Press, Iowa.

Cooper, B., Mullineaux, E., Turner, L., 2011. Textbook of Veterinary Nursing, fifth ed. BSAVA Gloucester.

Davidson, M., Else, R., Lumsden, J., 1998. Manual of Laboratory Techniques. BSAVA, Gloucester.

Hendrix, C.M., Sirois, M., 2006. Laboratory Procedures for Veterinary Technicians, fifth ed. Mosby, Missouri.

Kerr, M., 2002. Veterinary Laboratory Medicine, second ed. Blackwell Science, Oxford.

Lane, D., Cooper, B., 2003. Veterinary Nursing. BSAVA, Gloucester.

Masters, J., Bowden, C., 2001. Pre-Veterinary Nursing Textbook. Butterworth-Heinemann, Oxford.

Pinches, M., 2006. Getting results in clinical pathology 2. Pros and cons of in-clinic haematological testing. Pract. 28, 144–146.

REFERENCES AND FURTHER READING

12

Minor surgical procedures

Julian Hoad

CHAPTER CONTENTS

INTRODUCTION: REVIEW OF SCHEDULE 3 OF VETERINARY SURGEONS ACT 1966

The Veterinary Surgeons Act 1966 was created to prevent harm to animals by stopping anyone other than a qualified veterinary surgeon from performing any acts of surgery or medicine on an animal. Clearly, a blanket ban would make it difficult for owners to administer certain medications, or for farmers to carry out many husbandry procedures, so certain amendments were made to the Act (Schedule 3 Amendments 2002, updated February 2015), allowing laypersons to perform some procedures such as the removal of the hind dewclaws of puppies at less than 1 week of age. Importantly, the Schedule 3 amendments also allow qualified (and registered) veterinary nurses to perform any medical treatment or any minor surgery not including entry into a body cavity. Student veterinary nurses are also allowed to perform such acts provided certain criteria are met and that they are continuously, directly and personally monitored.

Unfortunately, there is no clear list of procedures allowable under Schedule 3, although there are plans to make further amendments to expand the role of the veterinary nurse in performing minor surgery. The Royal College of Veterinary Surgeons (RCVS) stipulates that the vet must decide whether or not the technique is too complex or likely to be too risky in a particular circumstance and whether the nurse is competent to do the procedure. An important aspect of competence is the ability to recognize that something is beyond one's capabilities or that help is needed, and to do this, there has to be a clear progression of training. Textbooks such as this, in-practice training and workshops are an excellent way of building these skills, and cadaver surgery (having gained the owner's permission) is even better. I would recommend any nurses wanting to progress with minor surgery to seek out any opportunity to scrub in to surgical procedures. This will give them experience in tissue handling and will also ensure that if an opportunity comes up to suture a wound, then they will already be surgically prepped and ready.

When starting to perform any minor surgical procedure, the nurse should ensure that the vet is immediately available, should any unforeseen problems occur, and the nurse should be able to react appropriately to any predicament. For example, he/she should know what to do if cardiorespiratory arrest occurs or if there is any haemorrhage.

Once competency has been gained, then making clients aware that a nurse has achieved that level of skill by having posters in the practice or announcements on social media will help educate clients that nurses are capable of performing these procedures. It is only by actively informing owners that nurses can undertake minor surgery that the perception of nurses' abilities will change.

Registered veterinary nurses are now accountable for their actions, so if a nurse is negligent, there is a chance that he/she will be found liable by the RCVS. The directing veterinary surgeon may also be found liable, depending on the circumstances, so it follows that, for both legal and animal welfare reasons, the practice team must make every effort to ensure that any surgical procedure is carried out to the best of that practice's capabilities.

Finally, despite the legal dispensation allowing veterinary nurses to perform minor surgery, the number of nurses doing such procedures remains very low. However, at present, there is a shortage of qualified vets in the UK, and this is likely to worsen after Brexit. Using nurses to their full potential surgically would free up a lot of 'vet hours' spent doing minor surgery. At a very basic level, the nurse may be asked to close a skin wound following major surgery, while a highly trained and experienced nurse could perform the more routine 'lumpectomies' and skin biopsies.

This chapter describes a few selected minor surgical procedures that should fall within the remit of Schedule 3 allowable operations. This is not an exhaustive list; rather, it is a selection of the most common ones, or those that provide a good basic surgical example, which may be adapted to other clinical situations.

USE OF INSTRUMENTS

Scalpels, scissors, tissue forceps, haemostatic forceps and needle holders are the main instruments required for minor surgery. Their use is generally self-explanatory, but some tips may prove useful. Whatever method is followed for a particular technique, it is always important to follow some basic rules of surgery, to increase the likelihood of a successful outcome. Halstead's seven principles of good surgical technique are outlined in Box 12.1. Close adherence to these is the key to successful surgery.

Several procedures refer to 'palming' an instrument, which is a useful technique when using looped instruments such as scissors, artery forceps and needle holders. These may be held by the third finger in the palm of the hand when not in use (Fig. 12.1). Palming an instrument allows the surgeon to use one instrument whilst holding one or more additional instruments in the same hand. The saved instrument may be swung into action when needed. This means that the instrument is readily available for use, and no time is wasted trying to locate it.

Procedure: Handling a scalpel

1. **Action**: A blade should always be placed on (and removed from) a blade holder using needle holders.
   Rationale: This reduces the risk of cutting yourself. Artery forceps and other jawed instruments should not be used as the hard blade will damage the jaws.

> **BOX 12.1   Halsted's seven principles of good surgical technique**
>
> 1. Gentle tissue handling
> 2. Accurate haemostasis
> 3. Preservation of blood supply
> 4. Strict aseptic technique
> 5. Tension-free wounds
> 6. Accurate reconstruction
> 7. Elimination of dead space

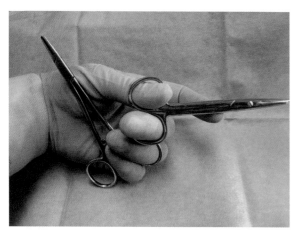

Fig. 12.1 Palming surgical instruments.

2. **Action**: The pencil grip is generally used for handling a scalpel (Fig. 12.2).
   Rationale: This grip gives fine control over the blade.
3. **Action**: The scalpel blade should be drawn backwards along the tissue, using enough pressure to make a single clean cut through the skin.
   Rationale: A sawing motion will produce an untidy wound and is more likely to damage blood vessels, slowing the rate of healing.
4. **Action**: Your free hand may be used to steady the skin and to provide a little tension to the wound edges.
   Rationale: This moves the edges away from the scalpel and improves visibility. It also helps to reduce the incision effort and results in a neater wound.

Procedure: Handling needle holders

There are various types of needle holders:
- **Gillies** – has a scissor action for cutting suture ends but does not have a ratchet
- **Olsen-Hegar** – has a cutting edge and a ratchet to hold the needle securely
- **Mayo-Hegar** – similar to long-handled artery forceps; has a ratchet for holding the needle but no cutting edge
- **McPhail's** – has a spring ratchet so that squeezing the jaws together opens the holder and releases the needle.

In general, the easier ones to use are locking (ratcheted) needle holders without scissors. This is because the scissors may cut the suture material inadvertently.

1. **Action**: Mayo-Hegar needle holders should be held in the tripod manner (see Handling surgical scissors, later).
   Rationale: This allows for precise placement of the needle and also allows palming of the needle holders.
2. **Action**: The needle is held about one-third of the way along its curve (Fig. 12.3) within the jaws of the needle holders.
   Rationale: Holding the needle too close to the suture end ('swaged on' area) will result in bending of the needle as it is weak at this point.
3. **Action**: The wrist is used to rotate the needle, pushing it through the tissue in a curve.
   Rationale: It is easier and less traumatic to allow the needle to follow its own curve through tissue.

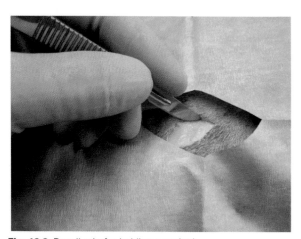

Fig. 12.2 Pencil grip for holding a scalpel.

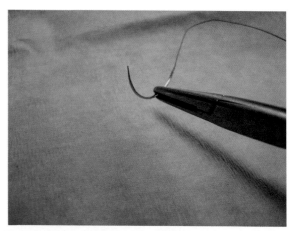

Fig. 12.3 Using needle holders. The needle is held approximately one-third of the way along its length.

Procedure: Handling surgical scissors

1. **Action:** The tripod hold is most commonly used for scissors (Fig. 12.4).

   Rationale: The tripod hold allows a more precise placement of the scissors and provides a strong shearing force. It also allows the scissors to be palmed if desired.

2. **Action:** The tips of the thumb and third finger are placed in the scissors loops, and the index finger is used to direct the tip of the scissors.

   Rationale: The second finger helps to steady the scissors.

3. **Action:** For cutting fine tissue, use the tips of the scissors; for cutting thicker tissues, the base of the scissors may be better.

   Rationale: The shearing forces are greater at the base of the scissors, but there is greater control at the tip, ensuring a more precise cut.

4. **Action:** Blunt dissection involves inserting the tip of the closed scissors into tissue and opening them whilst they are inserted.

   Rationale: Blunt dissection reduces the risk of inadvertently cutting through blood vessels or nerves. Fine scissors such as Metzenbaums are more suitable for this technique.

5. **Action:** Scalpel blades should be used to cut skin and scissors should be used to cut subcutaneous tissue.

   Rationale: The shearing action of scissors crushes minute blood vessels in the skin and can delay healing or increase scar formation.

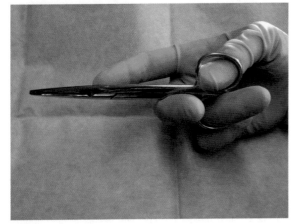

Fig. 12.4 Tripod hold for scissors.

6. **Action:** Surgical scissors should not be used to cut suture material.

   Rationale: This will blunt the scissors. Suture scissors should always be used for this purpose.

SURGICAL PROCEDURES

Procedure: Surgical treatment of abscesses

1. **Action:** Assess the patient for dehydration and commence intravenous fluids if required.

   Rationale: Animals with abscesses are typically pyretic and may not have eaten or drunk for several days.

2. **Action:** Administer a premedication (premed) to the patient as directed by the veterinary surgeon.

   Rationale: A premed will contain an analgesic and will also reduce the total amount of anaesthetic agent required.

3. **Action:** Stabilize the patient under sedation or general anaesthetic.

   Rationale: This will reduce any pain and prevent unwanted movement from the patient.

4. **Action:** Clip the skin surrounding the abscess and prep for aseptic surgery (see Chapter 7).

   Rationale: This reduces the risk of introducing new bacteria into the abscess. It also makes it easier to keep the wound clean during the healing process.

5. **Action:** Drape the surgical site (see Chapter 7).

   Rationale: This reduces the risk of new bacteria getting into the wound. Waterproof drapes prevent the patient becoming wet when the abscess is flushed.

6. **Action:** Observe strict aseptic technique: wear gloves, gown and mask.

   Rationale: This will reduce the risk of introducing new bacteria into the wound, such as methicillin-resistant Staphylococcus aureus (MRSA) and will protect you from acquiring infection from the patient.

7. **Action:** Make a stab incision into the abscess, preferably at the most dependent area. A no. 11 scalpel blade is most useful for this.

   Rationale: Making the opening at the most dependent part will help gravity to drain the abscess.

8. **Action:** Ensure exudate is emerging from the incision. If none is seen, try going a little deeper with the blade, ensuring that no damage is done to the deeper tissues.

Rationale: If none is seen, it may be that the incision is not deep enough.

9. **Action:** Using the blade, make an X-shaped incision about 1 cm in size. Alternatively, a small triangle of skin may be cut out.

   Rationale: A stab incision may heal too quickly to allow adequate drainage.

10. **Action:** Gently squeeze the area surrounding the incision to release the purulent material.

    Rationale: The pus may be quite viscous and require encouragement to leave the wound.

11. **Action:** Using a 20 ml syringe, three-way tap, 19G needle and giving set, flush the wound with at least 500 ml of warmed sterile saline (Fig. 12.5A, B). If any necrotic tissue remains, scrape the cavity with a sterile Volkmann curette or a no. 10 scalpel blade.

    Rationale: Flushing the wound removes much of the bacteria and necrotic tissue. Scraping will remove further necrotic material which, if left, could delay the healing process.

12. **Action**: The wound is left open to drain.

    Rationale: Suturing the wound may result in wound breakdown, as bacterial infection will still be present within the abscess cavity.

13. **Action:** Antibiotics and suitable analgesics are prescribed for an appropriate length of time.

    Rationale: To kill off any infection and to prevent recurrence.

14. **Action:** The owner may be instructed to bathe the wound in salty water for a few days.

Rationale: The combination of bathing and the use of antibiotics should result in healing of the wound within 7–10 days.

SKIN BIOPSY TECHNIQUES

Biopsies are samples of tissue that may help us to gain insight into a particular disease process. The collection of a biopsy may be carried out to investigate a skin disease (dermatopathy) or an abnormal mass, and the results may provide valuable information as to the presence of a disease and an indication of what the treatment should be. A biopsy procedure should ideally give maximum information for minimal patient morbidity. When neoplasia is suspected, it is preferable to perform a biopsy prior to considering surgery to assess whether it is possible to remove just the mass (local excision), or whether a large area of normal tissue surrounding the growth must be removed to ensure that any stray neoplastic cells are also removed (wide margin of excision). Table 12.1 lists common skin and subcutaneous tumours of the cat and dog.

The main types of biopsy are:

- **Surgical** – either taken with a scalpel or with a biopsy punch. This type provides the greater amount of tissue and enables the pathology laboratory to view the cells and any associated disruption of the architecture of the tissue. Patient must be anaesthetized.
- **Fine-needle aspirates** – these only allow cells to be assessed as the tissue is disrupted. This limits the

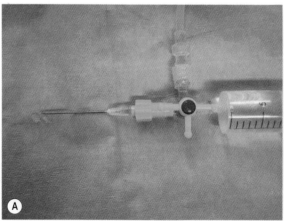
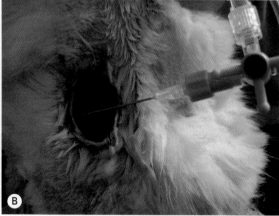

Fig. 12.5 A, Using a three-way tap, needle and syringe to flush wounds such as an abscess. B, Flushing an abscess with saline. (Hoad (2006), Elsevier.)

TABLE 12.1 Common skin and subcutaneous tumours of the dog and cat

Skin tumours	Subcutaneous tumours
Mast cell tumour (M)	Lipoma (B, M – rarely (liposarcoma), but may be infiltrative)
Squamous cell carcinoma (M)	Haemangioma (B)
Histiocytoma (B)	Haemangiosarcoma (M)
Lymphoma (M)	Soft-tissue sarcoma (M, but slow metastatic rate – these tumours tend to recur)
Melanoma (B, M)	Lymphoma (M)
Basal cell tumour (B)	Mast cell tumour (M)
Sebaceous adenoma (B)	
Sebaceous adenocarcinoma (M)	
Trichoepithelioma (B)	
Papilloma (B)	

M, malignant; B, benign.

amount of information that the pathologist can obtain and sometimes results in a lack of diagnosis. Patient may be conscious or sedated.

- **Tissue core biopsy** – requires much less tissue but still allows the layout of the tissue to be evaluated.

Procedure: Surgical biopsy

1. **Action:** Administer a premed to the patient as directed by the veterinary surgeon.
   Rationale: A premed will contain an analgesic and will also reduce the total amount of anaesthetic agent required.
2. **Action:** Stabilize the patient under sedation or general anaesthetic.
   Rationale: This will reduce any pain and prevent unwanted movement from the patient.
3. **Action:** Clip the skin surrounding the biopsy area and prep for aseptic surgery (see Chapter 7).
   Rationale: This reduces infection and wound-healing complications. Note that in some skin investigations this step is missed out as it can destroy subtle pathological changes.
4. **Action:** Drape the surgical site.
   Rationale: This reduces contamination of the wound.
5. **Action:** Observe strict aseptic technique: wear gloves, gown and mask.
   Rationale: This reduces contamination of the wound.

6. **Action:** Using a no. 10 or 15 scalpel blade on a holder, make an elliptical incision through the skin at one edge of the biopsy site, aiming to remove a piece of tissue of about 1 × 0.5 cm.
   Rationale: This allows the wound to be closed more easily than a circular incision. The edge of a mass affords the best biopsy as the central area may have tissue necrosis, which will obscure the diagnosis.
7. **Action:** The biopsy should include all skin layers and some normal tissue at the edge.
   Rationale: This will allow the pathologist to examine the normal tissue for evidence of invasion, which is one sign of malignancy.
8. **Action:** Close the skin wound using simple interrupted sutures of non-absorbable suture material, e.g. Ethilon. (See Fig. 8.10 and Table 8.6.)
   Rationale: Absorbable sutures may not absorb well in abnormal tissue.
9. **Action:** Place the biopsy in a 10% solution of formol saline.
   Rationale: This fixes the tissue and delays decomposition, preserving the histological features.
10. **Action:** Seal the biopsy container appropriately and label it with the patient's details.
   Rationale: Control of Substances Hazardous to Health (COSHH) regulations apply to all biological samples.
11. **Action:** Send the sample to the pathology laboratory with a completed histopathology request form (see Chapter 11) that includes the following information:
    - The patient's details
    - A brief description of the appearance and position of the biopsied tissue
    - How long it has been present
    - Any previous or concurrent treatment
    - Whether margins have been included in the biopsy.
    Rationale: The pathologist will be able to take all this information into consideration when considering the prognosis.
12. **Action:** The patient should be discharged with instructions to the owner on wound care and when to expect the biopsy results.
    Rationale: Antibiotics are generally not required following a biopsy.

Procedure: Punch biopsy

1. **Action:** Follow steps 1–5 as above.
   Rationale: This is a surgical biopsy and so will require the same aseptic technique.
2. **Action:** Select a sterile biopsy punch of suitable size and place it perpendicular to the skin surface over the area to be biopsied.
   Rationale: A larger punch will give a better chance of a useful biopsy.
3. **Action:** Using slight downward pressure, rotate the punch backwards and forwards, cutting through the skin as evenly as possible (Fig. 12.6A).
   Rationale: Ensure that the punch has gone all the way through the skin and has not damaged underlying tissue, i.e. muscles, nerves or blood vessels.
4. **Action:** Lift the punch away from the skin at a slight angle: this should remove the circle of tissue. If the tissue remains in situ, use a hypodermic needle to lift one edge and then cut the attachments with scissors (Fig. 12.6B).
   Rationale: Using forceps to lift the tissue may damage the biopsy.
5. **Action:** Follow steps 7–12 as above
   Rationale: The product of this procedure is dealt with in exactly the same way as the surgical biopsy.

Procedure: Tissue core biopsy

This technique is more useful for evaluation of subcutaneous masses than skin masses.

1. **Action:** Follow steps 1–5 as for a surgical biopsy.
   Rationale: Although there is a smaller wound than in a surgical biopsy, there is still potential for contamination and infection.
2. **Action:** Prime the trigger tissue core biopsy device by drawing back the spring-loaded clip.
   Rationale: This must be done before the needle is inserted into the tissue.
3. **Action:** Make a small cut over the chosen point of entry of the biopsy needle with a no. 11 scalpel blade.
   Rationale: The needle tends to blunt easily, so cutting the skin removes one layer of tissue through which the needle must pass. This also allows more control over placement into a subcutaneous mass.
4. **Action:** Introduce the needle into the mass and depress the plunger to its first point of tension.
   Rationale: This advances the needle into the centre of the mass and exposes the biopsy channel.
5. **Action:** Fully depress the plunger until a click is felt.
   Rationale: The outer sheath is sprung forward, effectively cutting a core of tissue from the mass.
6. **Action:** Remove the needle and pull the plunger out again, reloading the device.
   Rationale: Pressing the plunger to its first tension at this stage exposes the core biopsy within the channel.
7. **Action:** Fill a 5 ml syringe with sterile saline and attach a 23G needle. Use this to rinse the biopsy off the needle and into a biopsy pot containing 10% formol saline (Fig. 12.7).

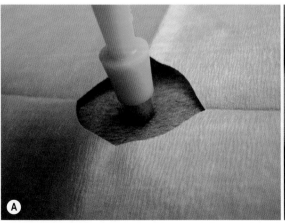
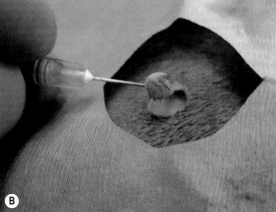

Fig. 12.6 A, Place even pressure on a biopsy punch to cut through the skin. B, Use a needle to lift the biopsy sample without causing any damage to it.

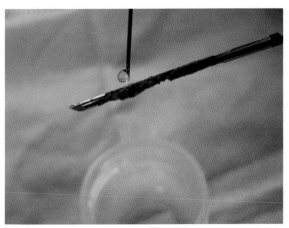

Fig. 12.7 Rinsing biopsy material from a spring-loaded biopsy needle. A small jet of sterile saline is used to wash the sample into a collection pot containing 10% formol saline.

> *Rationale: Using a needle to scrape the tissue off may damage the delicate biopsy.*
8. **Action:** Repeat the process if further biopsies are required.
   Rationale: A new needle must be used if other masses are to be sampled to prevent the risk of spread of other malignant cells.
9. **Action:** Examine the biopsy site for any evidence of bleeding.
   Rationale: If there is bleeding, apply hand pressure over the site for 5 minutes; this should be sufficient to stop the haemorrhage.
10. **Action:** Follow steps 10–12 as above.
    Rationale: The product of this procedure is dealt with in exactly the same way as the surgical biopsy.

Procedure: Fine-needle aspirate (Fig. 12.8)

1. **Action:** Ask an assistant to restrain the patient comfortably and securely.
   Rationale: There is usually no need to sedate or anaesthetize the patient; however, movement may risk placing the needle wrongly.
2. **Action:** Place a 23G needle on a 5 ml syringe and insert the needle into the mass.
   Rationale: To collect cells from the mass.
3. **Action:** Pull back on the plunger to the 3 ml mark and redirect the needle within the mass, pulling it almost out and inserting again.
   Rationale: This tends to suck cells into the hub of the needle. Moving around loosens cells and increases

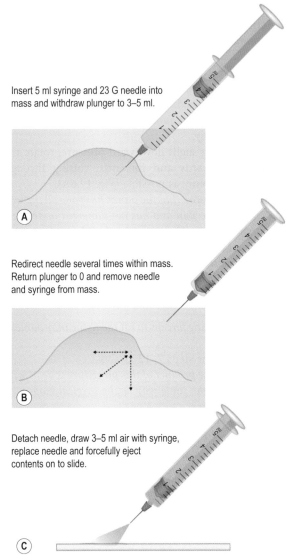

Insert 5 ml syringe and 23 G needle into mass and withdraw plunger to 3–5 ml.

(A)

Redirect needle several times within mass. Return plunger to 0 and remove needle and syringe from mass.

(B)

Detach needle, draw 3–5 ml air with syringe, replace needle and forcefully eject contents on to slide.

(C)

Fig. 12.8 Fine-needle aspiration biopsy method. (Reproduced with permission from Hoad (2006) Elsevier.)

the area that is sampled. An alternative is to place the needle into the mass and redirect without the syringe on.
4. **Action:** Gently release the suction and remove the needle from the mass.
   Rationale: If the suction is not released, the cells will be sucked into the barrel of the syringe and lost.
5. **Action:** Remove the needle from the syringe and fill the syringe with 3–5 ml of air.

Rationale: If the needle is left in place, the cells will be sucked into the barrel of the syringe and lost.

6. **Action:** Replace the needle on to the syringe and sharply press down the plunger over a clean glass slide.
   Rationale: This will squirt the aspirated material on to the slide.

7. **Action:** Gently place another clean glass slide on top of the first slide at a 90° angle and smoothly draw the top slide over the bottom one.
   Rationale: This will spread the cells, reducing clumping. Take care not to press the two slides together as this may crush the cells.

8. **Action:** Wave the slides in the air to dry them, then place them in a slide container.
   Rationale: Air-drying the slides quickly enhances cell preservation.

9. **Action:** Repeat steps 2–7 a further 3–4 times.
   Rationale: Producing several slides increases the chance of the cytologist being able to make a diagnosis.

10. **Action:** Label the slide containers with the patient's details.
    Rationale: To prevent it being mistaken for another patient's sample.

11. **Action:** Send the sample to the pathology laboratory (see Chapter 11) with a completed cytology request form that includes the following information:
    • The patient's details
    • A brief description of the appearance and position of the biopsied tissue
    • How long the mass has been present
    • Any previous or concurrent treatment
    • Whether margins have been included in the biopsy.
    Rationale: The pathologist will be able to take all this information into consideration when considering the prognosis.

12. **Action:** Check the patient for any bleeding.
    Rationale: Any bleeding is likely to be minor and should stop with a little pressure.

WOUND CLOSURE

Wounds may heal in several ways depending on when they happened and how much damage has been done.
• Wounds that are minimally contaminated, that have occurred within the previous 4–6 hours (the 'golden period') and that have suffered little damage to the skin edges may be treated by primary wound closure, i.e. suturing the wound, and then left to heal by first-intention.
• Wounds that are heavily contaminated, involve much skin loss or have been left untreated for more than 4–6 hours must be treated as open wounds prior to either being allowed to granulate (second-intention healing) or being sutured several days later (delayed primary closure).

This section deals with primary wound closure – treatment of contaminated wounds is described in Chapter 8.

Procedure: Primary wound closure

1. **Action:** Administer a premed to the patient as directed by the veterinary surgeon.
   Rationale: A premed should contain an analgesic to reduce pain and a sedative to reduce the total amount of anaesthetic agent required.

2. **Action:** Stabilize the patient under sedation or general anaesthetic.
   Rationale: This will reduce any pain and prevent unwanted movement from the patient.

3. **Action:** Squeeze a layer of water-based lubricant gel into the wound.
   Rationale: To prevent hair getting into the wound whilst clipping.

4. **Action:** Clip the skin surrounding the wound and prep as for aseptic surgery (see Chapter 7).
   Rationale: This reduces infection and wound-healing complications.

5. **Action:** Flush the wound with copious amounts of sterile saline.
   Rationale: The saline will remove any remaining gel and also reduce wound contamination. Using a 19G needle and 20 ml syringe attached to a 500 ml saline bag via a three-way tap helps with the flushing.

6. **Action:** Drape the surgical site with sterile drapes (see Chapter 7).
   Rationale: This reduces contamination of the wound.

7. **Action:** Observe strict aseptic technique: wear gloves, gown and mask.
   Rationale: This reduces contamination of the wound and the risk of infection.

8. **Action:** Using a no. 10 scalpel blade on a holder, scrape the exposed tissue within the wound and the wound edges.

Rationale: This debridement process removes any embedded contaminants such as bacteria, dirt or gravel and also removes a layer of fibrin that may slow down healing. At the end of this process, the deep surface of the wound and the wound edges should ooze a little blood.

9. **Action:** Apply haemostatic forceps to any haemorrhaging blood vessels and ligate using 2 or 1.5 metric (3-0 or 4-0) synthetic absorbable suture material, e.g. Monocryl, Ethicon.

   Rationale: Continuing haemorrhage will interfere with wound healing and increase the risk of infection and wound breakdown and may cause severe blood loss. It will also obscure visualization of the wound.

10. **Action:** Using two pairs of atraumatic forceps, e.g. DeBakey or rat-toothed thumb forceps, attempt to bring the wound edges together.

    Rationale: Wounds should be closed with no tension at the wound edges (Fig. 12.9). It is always a good idea to test in which direction the wound will close most easily before beginning to suture.

11. **Action:** Close any dead space within the wound by suturing with synthetic absorbable suture material in a simple interrupted pattern (Fig. 8.10).

    Rationale: Any dead space will increase the risk of wound breakdown and infection. Dead space also favours the formation of wound seroma. Closing the dead space should reduce the wound size

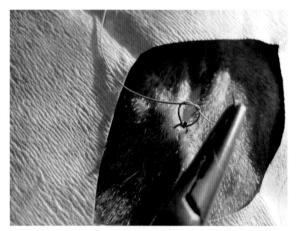

Fig. 12.9 Closing a wound. Note that there is minimal tension at the wound edges.

and bring the wound edges into apposition, thereby reducing tension.

12. **Action:** If the wound is still gaping, then the edges may be brought closer together by placing running or continuous sutures between the subcuticle and the deep tissues of the wound.

    Rationale: Continuous sutures reduce wound tension and decrease dead space.

13. **Action:** Suture the wound, using an appropriate skin suture pattern (see Chapter 8).

    Rationale: The sutures may be placed in the skin or subdermally, depending on surgeon preference.

14. **Action**: Bandage the wound if necessary (see Chapter 8).

    Rationale: Small wounds to the torso or upper limbs usually do not require bandages. Wounds to the distal limb are frequently bandaged to provide some wound support during locomotion.

15. **Action:** Discharge the patient, discussing wound care, care of the bandage if necessary and follow-up appointments with the owner.

    Rationale: A post-operative check should be performed 48–72 hours post-operatively to check the wound for any sign of infection and to make sure the patient has had no adverse reaction to the anaesthetic.

16. **Action:** Remove the sutures at around 10 days post-operatively.

    Rationale: Absorbable sutures will not need removal.

Procedure: Stapling a wound (Fig. 12.10)

Surgical staples provide a very quick means of closing skin wounds, thus reducing operative and anaesthetic time.

1. **Action:** Ensure that the wound to be closed is clean and has a good blood supply.

   Rationale: This reduces the risk of infection and increases the rate of wound healing.

2. **Action:** Ensure that the wound is not under any tension. If necessary, place some subcutaneous sutures.

   Rationale: Skin under tension will not heal well, if at all.

3. **Action:** If the wound is gaping, start at the middle of the wound and use rat-toothed forceps to approximate the wound edges.

   Rationale: Starting at the middle of the wound helps even out skin elastic tension and reduces gathering or puckering of the wound. Forceps will hold the skin in the correct position for the staples.

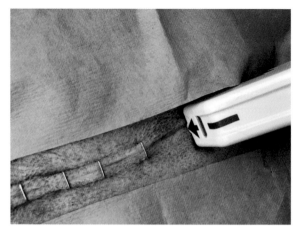

Fig. 12.10 Application of staples to a skin wound.

4. **Action:** Place the stapling device flat on the patient, with the guidance arrow centred on the wound edges and at 90° to the direction of the wound.
   Rationale: If the staples are placed at an angle, they will distort the wound edges and may loosen prematurely.
5. **Action:** Squeeze the stapler trigger firmly to release and set the staple, being careful to maintain even pressure on the wound.
   Rationale: Pressing too hard on the skin will cause puckering of the wound edges. Conversely, too light a pressure may result in the staples not penetrating the skin fully.
6. **Action:** Move the stapler 0.5–1.0 cm along the wound and repeat steps 4 and 5.
   Rationale: The staples should be placed close enough together to allow for good approximation of wound edges. Placing the staples too far apart may allow the wound to gape, whereas placing them too close together is wasteful, can impede the wound's blood supply (thus delaying healing) and will increase the time needed to remove the staples once the wound has healed.

Procedure: Removing surgical staples (Fig. 12.11)

1. **Action:** Always used a sterile staple remover.
   Rationale: A dirty or contaminated staple remover provides a source of infection for the healing wound.
2. **Action:** Ensure the staples are lying flat and are accessible. If necessary, use a pair of forceps to orient any that have spun around in the skin.
   Rationale: It is difficult to remove staples that have spun around, and the patient may find it painful.

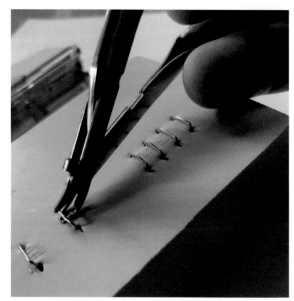

Fig. 12.11 Removal of staples.

3. **Action:** With the removal tool open, slide the lower jaws (double jaws) under the staple.
   Rationale: The staple remover works by bending the staples, allowing them to be lifted from the skin. Bending them the wrong way will make it extremely difficult to remove them.
4. **Action:** Close the jaws of the staple remover.
   Rationale: This folds the staple, lifting it out of the skin.
5. **Action:** Check the wound very carefully for any remaining staples.
   Rationale: Staples may easily be hidden by dried discharge, regrowing hair or folds of skin.

LUMP REMOVAL

As noted in the section on biopsies, there is a wide variety of growths found in or under the skin of dogs and cats. The type of growth will dictate the margin of excision, and the position of the growth will have a huge bearing on the type and pattern of wound closure. For example, a 2 cm diameter benign skin mass on the flank of a dog is amenable to removal by simple excision and primary wound closure as there is plenty of available skin to close the wound with no tension. However, a similar-sized mass on the dorsal carpus of a dog presents a real challenge in wound closure. The excision of the

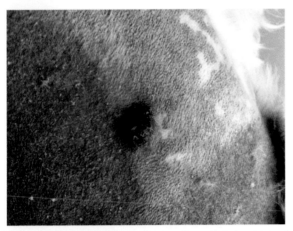

Fig. 12.12 Excision of this small mass allowed it to be removed entirely, and the wound closed with simple sutures.

former mass could be performed by a suitably experienced registered veterinary nurse (RVN), but it is unlikely that the latter one would be.

For the sake of clarity, in this section it will be assumed that the lump to be removed is small enough and in a suitable position to be removed, and the wound closed by simple suturing (Fig. 12.12). It will also be assumed that biopsy, or similar diagnostic test, has shown that the mass is most likely benign.

Procedure: Skin surface lumpectomy

1. **Action:** Admit the patient, taking care to ask the owner to point out the mass (or masses) to be removed.
   Rationale: A clear note of the position should be made on the consent form and, if necessary, a blob of correction fluid may be placed on each lump to aid in location.
2. **Action:** Administer a premed to the patient as directed by the veterinary surgeon.
   Rationale: A premed will contain an analgesic and will also reduce the total amount of anaesthetic agent required.
3. **Action:** Stabilize the patient under sedation or general anaesthetic.
   Rationale: This will reduce any pain and prevent unwanted movement from the patient.
4. **Action:** Clip the skin over and surrounding the lump and prep as for aseptic surgery (see Chapter 7).

Rationale: This reduces infection and wound-healing complications. Shave at least a clipper's width all round the lump to allow for slight movement of the drape or enlargement of the incision if required.

5. **Action:** Drape the surgical site.
   Rationale: This reduces contamination of the wound.
6. **Action:** Observe strict aseptic technique: wear gloves, gown and mask.
   Rationale: This reduces contamination of the wound.
7. **Action:** Open a sterile surgical kit, which should contain a scalpel blade holder, surgical scissors, suture scissors, dressing thumb forceps, rat-toothed or atraumatic thumb forceps, haemostatic forceps and needle holders.
   Rationale: Contents of basic surgical kits will differ but should at least include these instruments.
8. **Action:** Using needle holders, attach a no. 10 or 15 scalpel blade to the holder.
   Rationale: To avoid injuring yourself.
9. **Action:** Apply a little tension to the skin and make an oval or elliptical incision around the lump, allowing at least a 0.5 cm margin.
   Rationale: Even a benign mass can recur if cells are left at the periphery.
10. **Action:** Incise through the skin completely, including the hypodermis.
    Rationale: The subcutaneous fat layer can be removed to extend the deep margin of the excision.
11. **Action:** Apply haemostatic forceps to any haemorrhaging blood vessels and ligate them using 2 or 1.5 metric (3-0 or 4-0) synthetic absorbable suture material, e.g. Monocryl, Ethicon.
    Rationale: Haemorrhage will interfere with wound healing and increase the risk of infection and wound breakdown and may cause severe blood loss. It will also obscure visualization of the wound.
12. **Action:** Use blunt dissection down under the mass and cut it away with scissors.
    Rationale: To separate the skin and subcutaneous tissue from the underlying tissues. Blunt dissection is less likely to cause bleeding or damage to delicate structures such as nerves.

13. **Action**: When the lump has been freed from the tissues, place it in a pot with 10% formol saline ready to be sent to a lab for histopathology.
    Rationale: To identify the type and potential malignancy of the lump.

14. **Action:** Using two pairs of atraumatic forceps, e.g. DeBakey or rat-toothed thumb forceps, attempt to bring the wound edges together.
    Rationale: Wounds should be closed with no tension at the wound edges. It is always a good idea to test in which direction the wound will close more easily before beginning to suture.

15. **Action:** Close any dead space within the wound by suturing with synthetic absorbable suture material in a simple interrupted pattern (see Fig. 8.10).
    Rationale: Any dead space will increase the risk of wound breakdown and infection. Dead space also favours the formation of wound seroma. In addition, closing the dead space should reduce the wound size and bring the wound edges into apposition, thus reducing tension.

16. **Action:** If the wound is still gaping, then the edges may be brought closer together by placing continuous sutures between the subcuticle and the deep tissues of the wound.
    Rationale: Continuous sutures reduce wound tension and decrease dead space.

17. **Action:** Suture the wound, using an appropriate skin suture pattern (see Chapter 8).
    Rationale: The sutures may be placed in the skin or subdermally, depending on surgeon preference.

18. **Action:** Bandage the wound if necessary.
    Rationale: Small wounds to the torso or upper limbs usually do not require dressings. Wounds to the distal limb are frequently dressed to provide some wound support during locomotion.

19. **Action:** Label the pot containing the lump in 10% formol saline with the patient's details.
    Rationale: The mass should be sent for histopathological examination to confirm that it is benign and that it has been completely removed (see Chapter 11).

20. **Action:** Discharge the patient, discussing wound care and follow-up appointments with the owner.
    Rationale: A post-operative check should be made for 48–72 hours post-operatively to check the wound for any sign of infection, to check the bandage if necessary and to make sure the patient has had no adverse reaction to the anaesthetic.

21. **Action:** Remove the sutures at around 10 days post-operatively.
    Rationale: Absorbable sutures will not need removal.

Procedure: Removal of subcutaneous lumps

1. **Action:** Admit the patient, taking care to identify the position of the lumps to be removed (see Skin surface lumpectomy).
   Rationale: It is very important to ensure that all lumps that cause concern to the owner are identified; a common cause for complaint is 'missing a lump'.

2. **Action:** Administer a premed to the patient as directed by the veterinary surgeon.
   Rationale: A premed will contain an analgesic and will also reduce the total amount of anaesthetic agent required.

3. **Action:** Stabilize the patient under sedation or general anaesthetic.
   Rationale: This will reduce any pain and prevent unwanted movement from the patient.

4. **Action:** Clip the skin surrounding the lump and prep as for aseptic surgery (see Chapter 7).
   Rationale: This reduces infection and wound-healing complications. Shave at least a clipper's width all round the lump to allow for slight movement of the drape or enlargement of the incision if required.

5. **Action:** Drape the surgical site.
   Rationale: This reduces contamination of the wound.

6. **Action:** Observe strict aseptic technique: wear gloves, gown and mask.
   Rationale: This reduces contamination of the wound.

7. **Action:** Open a sterile surgical kit, which should contain a scalpel blade holder, surgical scissors, suture scissors, dressing thumb forceps, rat-tooth or atraumatic thumb forceps, haemostatic forceps and needle holders. A pair of surgical retractors, e.g. Gelpi retractors, may be useful.
   Rationale: Contents of basic surgical kits will differ but should at least include the above. Gelpi retractors improve visualization within a deep wound.

8. **Action:** Using needle holders, attach a no. 10 or 15 scalpel blade to the holder.
   Rationale: *To avoid injuring yourself.*

9. **Action:** Apply a little tension to the skin with your finger and thumb and make a straight incision over the lump, extending to just a little beyond the margins.
   Rationale: *Some subcutaneous lumps, such as small lipomata, can be removed through a small wound; however, the wound should be large enough to allow visualization of the lump's margins and to be able to remove the lump intact. In any case, the incision should follow tension lines to facilitate closure.*

10. **Action:** Use blunt dissection to separate the mass from surrounding tissues. If the lump has a capsule, try to avoid tearing or cutting the capsule.
    Rationale: *Blunt dissection is less likely to cause bleeding or damage to delicate structures such as nerves. Tearing the capsule may result in dissemination of the mass, increasing the risk of recurrence or spread.*

11. **Action:** Apply haemostatic forceps to any haemorrhaging blood vessels and ligate those using 2 or 1.5 metric (3-0 or 4-0) synthetic absorbable suture materials, e.g. Monocryl, Ethicon.
    Rationale: *Haemorrhage will interfere with wound healing and increase the risk of infection and wound breakdown and may cause severe blood loss. It will also obscure visualization of the wound.*

12. **Action:** Close the wound and bandage as necessary (steps 14–17 as for Skin surface lumpectomy).

13. **Action:** Place the excised lump in a histopathology pot containing 10% formol saline and label the pot with the patient's details (see Chapter 11).
    Rationale: *The mass should be sent for histopathological examination to confirm that it is benign and has been completely removed.*

14. **Action:** Discharge the patient, discussing wound care and follow-up appointments with the owner.
    Rationale: *A post-operative check should be made for 48–72 hours post-operatively to check the wound for any sign of infection and to make sure the patient has had no adverse reaction to the anaesthetic.*

15. **Action:** Remove the sutures at around 10 days post-operatively.
    Rationale: *Absorbable sutures will not need removal.*

CATHETER PLACEMENT FOR THE DELIVERY OF FLUID THERAPY

Whilst peripheral catheters, e.g. in the cephalic vein or saphenous vein, are generally sufficient for most instances of fluid therapy, it is occasionally necessary to consider alternative circulatory system access. In severely debilitated and dehydrated patients, for example, the peripheral pressure veins may be difficult to cannulate. Additionally, jugular catheters provide a means of measuring central venous pressure and may be left in place for a week or longer. Placement of a regular 'over-the-needle' intravenous cannula into the jugular vein is described in Chapter 4, whilst the technique described here refers to placement of a dedicated jugular catheter.

Procedure: Placing a jugular catheter using the Seldinger technique

1. **Action:** Prepare the equipment and warm the fluids to body temperature.
   Rationale: *Administering cold fluids will lower the body temperature and is uncomfortable to the patient.*

2. **Action:** Ask an assistant to restrain the patient in lateral recumbency on a treatment table.
   Rationale: *Sedation is often not necessary and may be contraindicated as these patients may be quite debilitated. However, a frightened animal may try to escape, and movement makes placement difficult. Two assistants may be required to restrain the patient to prevent movement.*

3. **Action:** Clip an area of skin overlying the jugular vein and prep as for surgery, including the use of sterile drapes.
   Rationale: *Contamination of the catheter could result in local infection, or even septicaemia.*

4. **Action:** Observe strict aseptic technique: wear gloves, gown and mask.
   Rationale: *This reduces the risk of introducing infection.*

5. **Action:** Using a fine-gauge needle, e.g. 25G or 23G, inject a bleb (0.2–0.4 ml) of local anaesthetic, e.g. lidocaine or mepivacaine, subcutaneously at the catheterization site.
   Rationale: *To desensitize the skin as placing a jugular catheter can be painful.*

6. **Action:** Make a small incision through the skin over the jugular vein using a no. 15 scalpel blade.

Rationale: The incision reduces drag of the cannula sheath and makes it easier to insert it into the jugular vein.

7. **Action:** Take the introducer needle (a thin-walled intravenous cannula) from the jugular catheter pack and insert it into the jugular vein, directing it towards the patient's torso.

   Rationale: The presence of blood in the hub of the needle will confirm placement.

8. **Action:** Insert the wire guide into the hub of the introducer needle and thread the J-wire through the needle (Fig. 12.13A).

   Rationale: The curved end of the J-wire will catch in the jugular vein and act as a guide for the catheter.

9. **Action:** Remove the introducer needle, leaving the J-wire in place (Fig. 12.13B). Apply pressure with two fingers over the puncture site.

   Rationale: The finger pressure will reduce leakage of blood around the punctured vein and prevent haematoma formation.

10. **Action:** Thread the widener down the J-wire into the vein (Fig. 12.13C), turn it slowly and then remove it, keeping the wire in place and maintaining finger pressure on the vein.

    Rationale: The widener makes it easier to pass the soft, flexible jugular catheter.

11. **Action:** Thread the soft flexible catheter over the J-wire and into the jugular vein, suturing it in place with non-absorbable suture material (Fig. 12.13D).

    Rationale: Suturing the catheter prevents it slipping out.

12. **Action**: Remove the J-wire and flush the catheter with 2–5 ml of heparinized saline.

    Rationale: This reduces clot formation and blockage of the catheter.

13. **Action:** Connect the catheter to a pre-filled giving set or place a sterile injection bung on the Luer end of the catheter.

    Rationale: Care must be taken to avoid air bubbles entering the catheter at this stage.

14. **Action:** Place a sterile adherent dressing over the catheterization site and bandage the neck.

    Rationale: The catheterization site must be checked daily to inspect placement and check for signs of infection. Bandaging reduces the risk of removal or damage by the patient.

15. **Action:** Return the patient to the cage. The catheter should be flushed at least four times daily.

Rationale: To prevent the catheter becoming blocked.

Procedure: Placing an intraosseous catheter

Placing a catheter into the medullary cavity allows a fluid delivery rate that equals that of intravenous catheterization. The technique is useful in small animals, where the veins are often fragile and easily damaged. If the catheter becomes dislodged, haemorrhage from the site is less likely.

The most common sites for intraosseous placement are the greater tubercle of the humerus, the dorsal iliac wing of the bird, the tibial tuberosity or the trochanteric fossa of the femur. Also refer to placement of an intraosseous catheter in the rabbit in Chapter 13.

The following description details placement into the trochanteric fossa of the femur.

1. **Action:** Prepare the equipment and warm the fluids to body temperature.

   Rationale: Administering cold fluids will lower the body temperature and is uncomfortable to the patient.

2. **Action:** Stabilize the patient under sedation or general anaesthetic.

   Rationale: Placement of an intraosseous needle is painful. An alternative to sedation is to administer local anaesthetic, e.g. lidocaine, mepivacaine, to the area.

3. **Action:** Place the patient in lateral recumbency.

4. **Action:** Clip an area of skin overlying the hip joint and prep as for aseptic surgery, including the use of sterile drapes.

   Rationale: Contamination of the catheter may result in local infection, or even septicaemia.

5. **Action:** Observe strict aseptic technique: wear gloves, gown and mask.

   Rationale: This reduces the risk of introducing infection.

6. **Action:** Palpate the greater trochanter of the femur. The palpation is helped by rotation of the hind limb.

   Rationale: The trochanteric fossa lies between the greater trochanter and the acetabulum, i.e. the hip socket. Rotating the limb will help to identify the hip joint.

7. **Action:** Using a no. 15 scalpel blade, make a small stab incision through the skin overlying the greater trochanter.

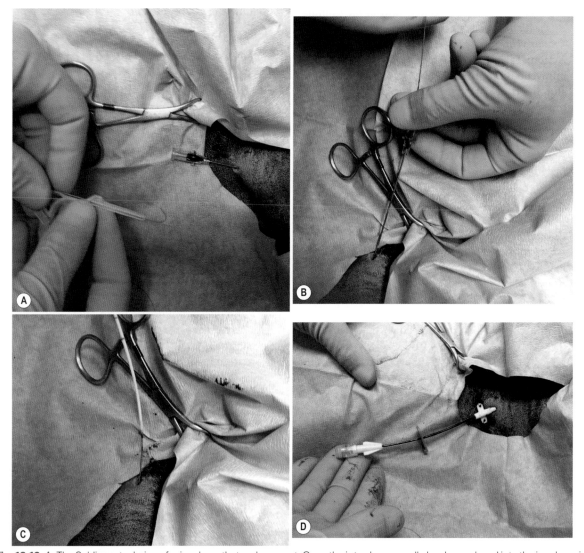

Fig. 12.13 A, The Seldinger technique for jugular catheter placement. Once the introducer needle has been placed into the jugular vein, the J-wire is fed down into the vein. B, The introducer needle is then withdrawn, leaving the J-wire in place. C, The cannula is then threaded down the J-wire (a widener may or may not be used prior to this step – see text). D, The J-wire is removed, and the cannula is sutured in place.

>   ***Rationale:*** *Making the incision over the bone, rather than over soft tissue, reduces the risk of damage to the ischial nerve.*

8. **Action:** Glide the intraosseous needle and stylet down the medial side of the greater trochanter until the bottom of the fossa is felt.

>   ***Rationale:*** *The stylet must be kept in place until the needle is placed in the medullary cavity to prevent the needle getting blocked with soft tissue or bone.*

9. **Action:** Rotate the needle back and forth, applying firm pressure.

>   ***Rationale:*** *The needle must penetrate the bone cortex. When this happens, a slight loss of resistance is felt.*

10. **Action:** Check for placement of the needle by moving the pelvic limb.

>   ***Rationale:*** *If the placement is correct, the needle should be rigidly held and move as the limb moves.*

11. **Action:** Remove the stylet and immediately flush the catheter with 1–2 ml of heparinized saline.
    Rationale: It is important not to allow clots to form as they could block the catheter.
12. **Action:** Place an adherent dressing over the catheter and bandage the limb and pelvis.
    Rationale: It is important not to let the patient self-traumatize or dislodge the catheter.
13. **Action:** Attach a giving set or injection bung to the catheter.
    Rationale: Intraosseous fluids may be administered in the same manner as intravenous fluids (see Chapter 4).
14. **Action:** Flush the catheter at least four times daily with heparinized saline.
    Rationale: It is important not to allow clots to form as they could block the catheter.

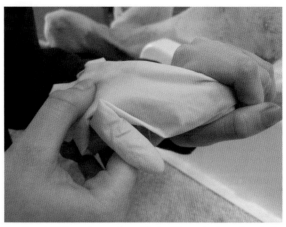

Fig. 12.14 Using a latex glove filled with surgical scrub solution to prep a paw prior to nail removal.

OTHER TECHNIQUES

Procedure: Onychectomy (nail removal)

Indications for onychectomy include trauma, chronic nail bed infections or biopsy for suspected neoplasia. Removal of nails for reasons of behaviour or management is considered mutilation and unethical.

1. **Action:** Administer a premed to the patient as directed by the veterinary surgeon.
   Rationale: A premed will contain an analgesic and will also reduce the total amount of anaesthetic agent required.
2. **Action:** Stabilize the patient under sedation or general anaesthetic.
   Rationale: This will reduce any pain and prevent unwanted movement from the patient. If only one nail is to be removed, sedation may be sufficient.
3. **Action:** Ask the veterinary surgeon to administer local anaesthesia.
   Rationale: Administering 0.5–1.0 ml 0.5% mepivacaine into the distal interphalangeal joint will provide powerful analgesia and reduce pain 'wind-up', which is a major cause of post-operative pain.
4. **Action:** Clip the skin of the digit and paw and prep for aseptic surgery. Scrubbing the paw may be difficult but a useful tip is to half-fill a latex glove with scrub solution. Place this over the patient's paw and thoroughly massage the scrub solution around the foot (Fig. 12.14).
   Rationale: Thorough scrubbing reduces infection and wound-healing complications.
5. **Action:** Drape the surgical site.
   Rationale: This reduces contamination of the wound.
6. **Action:** Observe strict aseptic technique: wear gloves, gown and mask.
   Rationale: This reduces contamination of the wound.
7. **Action:** Open a sterile surgical kit, which should contain a scalpel blade holder, surgical scissors, suture scissors, dressing thumb forceps, rat-toothed or atraumatic thumb forceps, haemostatic forceps and needle holders. Alternatively, a pair of sterile 'guillotine'-type nail clippers may be used.

There are two methods for removal of the nail:
    Method 1
1. **Action:** Using a no. 10 or 15 scalpel blade on a holder, make an incision through the thin skin surrounding the base of the claw (Fig. 12.15A).
   Rationale: Any haemorrhage may be controlled by pressure or application of fine mosquito forceps and ligation of the vessels.
2. **Action:** Transect the common digital extensor tendon, then the deep digital flexor tendon, the medial collateral ligaments and the joint capsule. In cats, the dorsal elastic ligament must also be cut.
   Rationale: This method removes the entire distal phalanx.

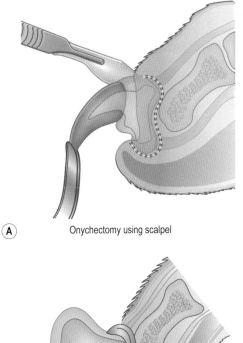

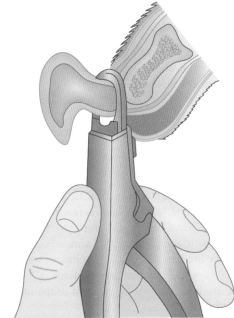

(A) Onychectomy using scalpel

(B) Onychectomy using guillotine nail clippers

Fig. 12.15 A, Onychectomy using a scalpel. B, Onychectomy using guillotine nail clippers.

Method 2

1. **Action:** Place a sterile pair of guillotine nail clippers at the level of the distal interphalangeal joint and close them to amputate the nail (Fig. 12.15B).

   Rationale: *Although much quicker, this method will not remove the entire distal phalanx. It is also*

difficult to identify any bleeding vessels and ligate them.

2. **Action:** Once the nail has been removed by either method, if the nail is to be sent off to the laboratory for examination, it should be placed into 10% formol saline (for histology), or else into a transport pot (for bacteriology/microbiology). The sample should be clearly labelled with the patient's name, and a laboratory request form should be filled out.

   Rationale: *If the sample is to be sent for culture, it should not be placed into formol saline – this will kill the microorganisms.*

3. **Action:** Close the wound using 1.5 or 2 metric synthetic non-absorbable suture material in a simple interrupted skin pattern.

   Rationale: *If preferred, subcutaneous sutures of 1.5 or 2 metric synthetic absorbable suture material may be placed instead. This obviates the need for suture removal.*

4. **Action:** Place a non-adherent dressing and foot bandage (see Chapter 8).

   Rationale: *This helps prevent self-mutilation.*

5. **Action:** Discharge the patient with a 5-day course of non-steroidal anti-inflammatory drugs (NSAIDs). Antibiotics should be given as required.

   Rationale: *If the sample is sent for culture, it may be best to await the results and then opt for a more appropriate antibiotic based on sensitivity studies. Alternatively, a broad-spectrum antibiotic may be administered until results are back.*

6. **Action:** Change the dressing 2–3 days post-operatively.

   Rationale: *It is usually necessary to keep the wound dressed for 5–7 days.*

7. **Action:** Remove the sutures at 7–10 days post-operatively.

   Rationale: *If subcutaneous sutures have been placed, this is not necessary.*

Procedure: Flushing the nasolacrimal duct

A common cause of epiphora, i.e. excessive tears and a build-up of secretions around the eyes, is blockage of the nasolacrimal or tear duct. The lacrimal puncta or duct openings are situated towards the medial canthus on the upper and lower eyelids of dogs and cats. Ocular secretions drain into these puncta and are carried down the nasolacrimal ducts to the ventral surface of the nasal cavity in dogs and cats (Fig. 12.16). Ducts are especially

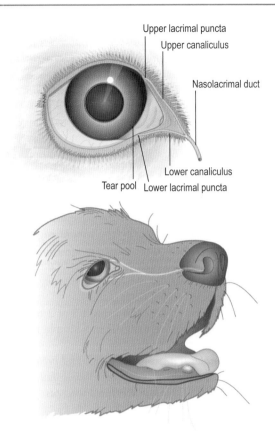

Upper lacrimal puncta
Upper canaliculus
Nasolacrimal duct
Lower canaliculus
Tear pool   Lower lacrimal puncta

Fig. 12.16 Anatomy of the nasolacrimal duct in the dog and cat. (Reproduced with permission from Hoad (2006), Elsevier.)

prone to blockage in toy breeds, due to the combination of small puncta and tortuous nasolacrimal ducts.

1. **Action:** Prepare an instrument trolley with warmed sterile saline, a sterile irrigating cannula, Minims 1% fluorescein drops (Chauvin Pharmaceuticals), 5 ml syringes and 21G needles. Prepare a syringe by filling it with sterile saline and then drawing up a drop of fluorescein dye.

   Rationale: *Irrigating cannulae (Portex) come in two sizes – 0.91 mm outside diameter (OD) and 0.76 mm OD – and are colour-coded pink and blue, respectively. The fluorescein dye helps to identify correct placement of the irrigating cannula as it can be seen exiting the nostril.*

2. **Action:** Stabilize the patient under sedation.

   Rationale: *The procedure can be carried out in a conscious patient using good restraint and topical local analgesia if it is calm and well behaved; however,*

the majority of patients are easier to manage when sedated, and this reduces the risk of damage to the eye caused by unexpected movement.

3. **Action:** Apply 1–2 drops of local anaesthetic, e.g. amethocaine 0.5% drops (Minims, Chauvin Pharmaceuticals), to each eye.

   Rationale: *This will desensitize the eyelid and make it easier to place a cannula. Always remember that local anaesthetics take a little time (2–3 minutes) to take effect. An injection of NSAIDs may also help to reduce post-operative pain in the case of inflammatory blockage.*

4. **Action:** Perform a surgical hand wash and wear sterile surgical gloves.

   Rationale: *Although it is not possible to perform this technique in a sterile manner, it is good practice to reduce the risk of nosocomial infection.*

5. **Action:** Identify the upper and lower lacrimal puncta.

   Rationale: *The puncta are 0.5–1 mm in diameter and may appear as little slits or depressions about 2 mm from the inner margin of the eyelids. Magnification, e.g. by means of loupes, is very helpful.*

6. **Action:** Insert the tip of the cannula into one of the puncta.

   Rationale: *It can be difficult to place the cannula, especially when chronic inflammation has caused scarring of the duct opening. Stiff, monofilament suture material may be used to insert into the opening, and the cannula slid over the top.*

7. **Action:** Attach the 5 ml syringe containing saline and dye to the Luer end of the irrigating cannula.

   Rationale: *Be careful at this stage not to dislodge the cannula. Holding the eyelids gently closed helps to keep the tip in position.*

8. **Action:** Depress the syringe plunger gently but firmly to flush the duct.

   Rationale: *Fluorescein dye should be seen to exit the nostril. Excessive force should be avoided as this may damage the duct and, if it is blocked, dye will squirt out all over you.*

9. **Action:** Steps 5–8 should be repeated on the upper and lower puncta of both pairs of eyelids. At least 10 ml of saline should be used to flush each side. If directed to do so by a veterinary surgeon, a small amount of antibiotic, e.g. gentamicin, may be added to the flush solution.

   Rationale: *To counteract any infection in the ducts.*

Procedure: Suturing wounds to the pinna

Although the fundamental principles of suturing wounds to the ear are similar to those of other wounds, there are a few differences that require further explanation. The pinna is essentially a sandwich of two layers of skin separated by cartilage. The cartilage is very poorly vascularized, which means that the skin of the ear derives its blood supply from vessels that run longitudinally from the base to the tip. Any injury to the blood supply results in poor healing of tissues distal to the injured vessel. In some cases, this can result in necrosis of the ear tip. Thus, any lacerations to the pinna should be examined well to ensure that the blood supply has not been interrupted. If so, amputation of the distal portion may be a better option. To examine for the presence of a blood supply, the colour of the pinna skin should be noted. A healthy pink colour that blanches when pressed is indicative of a good blood supply, whereas a dull greyish or pale colour often results from lack of perfusion. A narrow-gauge needle, e.g. 23G, can be used to prick the skin – the presence of fresh blood ooze is a good indication of blood supply.

1. **Action:** Examine the patient thoroughly prior to general anaesthesia.
   Rationale: There may be other wounds present.
2. **Action:** Assess the clotting ability of the patient by taking a small sample in a plain blood tube and observing the clotting time.
   Rationale: To make sure that there is no underlying coagulopathy.
3. **Action:** Perform a packed cell volume test on the patient (see Chapter 11).
   Rationale: To ensure that any blood loss has not caused anaemia.
4. **Action:** Prepare an instrument trolley with a surgical kit suitable for suturing wounds.
   Rationale: No specialist instruments are required for this procedure.
5. **Action:** Stabilize the patient under sedation or general anaesthetic.
   Rationale: This will reduce any pain and prevent unwanted movement from the patient.
6. **Action:** Clip the pinna and surrounding skin and prep for aseptic surgery.
   Rationale: This reduces infection and wound-healing complications. The ear can be difficult to prepare aseptically, especially in patients with long pendulous ears. It may be helpful to have a scrubbed assistant or trolley nurse to hold the pinna or use atraumatic forceps such as Babcock's to hold the pinna whilst the final skin prep is carried out.
7. **Action:** Drape the surgical site.
   Rationale: This reduces contamination of the wound.
8. **Action:** Observe strict aseptic technique: wear gloves, gown and mask.
   Rationale: This reduces contamination of the wound.
9. **Action:** Carefully debride the wound edges to remove any devitalized tissue.
   Rationale: Avoid removing too much skin, as this will cause tension on the wound edges and will lead to distortion of the pinna. This is not only unsightly but can cause changes in the microenvironment of the ear canal, increasing the risk of otitis.
10. **Action:** Repair the skin using 1.5 or 2 metric non-absorbable suture material in a simple interrupted pattern.
    Rationale: If any part of the wound breaks down, a continuous suture pattern will fail along the length of the suture line, whereas interrupted sutures will not.
11. **Action:** Tack down any loose flap of skin to the underlying cartilage, using a full-thickness mattress suture (see Chapter 8).
    Rationale: Tacking the skin down reduces the risk of haematoma. The vertical mattress pattern, placed parallel to the base tip orientation of the ear, resists pull-out and has little effect on blood supply to the ear. If the sutures are placed perpendicular to the line of the ear, they may cross over blood vessels.
12. **Action:** Place an ear bandage, or other suitable dressing and an Elizabethan collar (see Chapter 8).
    Rationale: If the patient self-mutilates, this could cause wound breakdown and bleeding.

Procedure: Treating aural haematoma

An aural haematoma (pl. haematomata) is most commonly seen in dogs, although it can also occur in cats, particularly unneutered tomcats who are more likely to fight. Although it can occur idiopathically, it more often results from self-trauma due to otitis, so otoscopy should always be performed on these patients. If left to resolve without any intervention, a misshapen 'cauliflower' ear often results. Medical management –

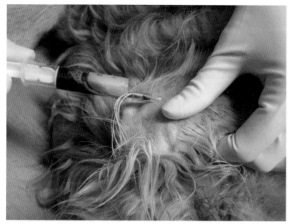

Fig. 12.17 Aspirating serosanguineous fluid from an aural haematoma prior to instilling a depot-acting corticosteroid.

involving draining the pinna and instilling a depot-acting corticosteroid (Fig. 12.17) – is usually an effective treatment, but surgery may benefit those cases that fail to respond.

1. **Action:** Prepare an instrument trolley with a surgical kit suitable for suturing wounds.

    Rationale: No specialist instruments are required for this procedure.

2. **Action:** Stabilize the patient under sedation or general anaesthetic.

    Rationale: This will reduce any pain and prevent unwanted movement from the patient. Ear surgery is very painful – ensure attention is paid to the most suitable selection of analgesia. Patients with aural haematoma may have had corticosteroids, so exercise caution if considering the use of NSAIDs.

3. **Action:** Clip the pinna and surrounding skin and prep for aseptic surgery.

    Rationale: This reduces infection and wound-healing complications. The ear can be difficult to prepare aseptically, especially in patients with long pendulous ears. It may be helpful to have a scrubbed assistant or trolley nurse to hold the pinna or use atraumatic forceps such as Babcock's to hold the pinna whilst the final skin prep is carried out.

4. **Action:** Drape the surgical site.

    Rationale: This reduces contamination of the wound.

5. **Action:** Observe strict aseptic technique: wear gloves, gown and mask.

    Rationale: This reduces contamination of the wound.

6. **Action:** Using a no. 10 blade on a scalpel holder, make a curving, S-shaped incision over the length of the haematoma on the inner surface of the pinna (Fig. 12.18).

    Rationale: The curved wound results in less distortion of the ear during healing.

7. **Action:** Drain the haematoma and, using the scalpel blade or a sterile curette, scrape the cavity of the haematoma.

    Rationale: The lining of the haematoma contains fibrin, which may retard the healing process.

8. **Action:** Suture the ear using 2–3 rows of 1.5 metric non-absorbable suture material in a full-thickness vertical mattress pattern (see Chapter 8).

    Rationale: It is vital not to place too much tension on the sutures as this will be painful and lead to wound breakdown. The tips of the needle holders should be able to be inserted under the sutures when placed. Stenting material, such as buttons, radiographic film or stiff bandage material, may be used to distribute the suture pressure more evenly, but this should not be necessary if attention is paid to suture placement.

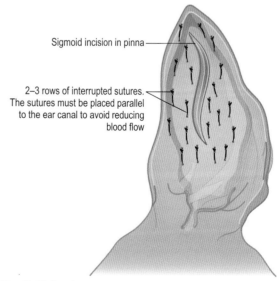

Sigmoid incision in pinna

2–3 rows of interrupted sutures. The sutures must be placed parallel to the ear canal to avoid reducing blood flow

Fig. 12.18 Surgical treatment of aural haematoma. (Reproduced with permission from Hoad (2006), Elsevier.)

9. **Action:** Place a non-adherent dressing and ear bandage (see Chapter 8). An Elizabethan collar should be fitted.

    Rationale: If the patient self-mutilates, this could cause wound breakdown and bleeding.

10. **Action:** Change the bandage after 2–3 days.

    Rationale: Leaving the bandage on longer increases the risk of wound infection. The ear should be checked to ensure healing is proceeding well.

11. **Action:** Remove the sutures at 10–14 days postoperatively.

    Rationale: Removing the sutures too soon can lead to recurrence.

Procedure: Tail tip removal

In 2006, the docking of tails was made illegal in the UK, with very few exceptions. Indications for tail tip removal (partial caudectomy) include neoplasia, intractable infection and trauma.

1. **Action:** Administer a premed to the patient as directed by the veterinary surgeon.

    Rationale: A premed will contain an analgesic and will also reduce the total amount of anaesthetic agent required.

2. **Action:** Stabilize the patient under sedation or general anaesthetic.

    Rationale: This will reduce any pain and prevent unwanted movement from the patient. It is worth considering the use of a local anaesthetic to reduce post-operative pain and reduce the risk of chronic pain, which could lead to tail tip self-injury.

3. **Action:** Clip the tail and prep for aseptic surgery. The tail can be difficult to prepare aseptically. It may be helpful to have a scrubbed assistant or trolley nurse hold the tail or use atraumatic forceps such as Babcock's to hold the tail tip while the final skin prep is carried out.

    Rationale: This reduces infection and wound-healing complications.

4. **Action:** Drape the surgical site.

    Rationale: This reduces contamination of the wound. A fenestrated drape is quite useful for this purpose.

5. **Action:** Observe strict aseptic technique: wear gloves, gown and mask.

    Rationale: This reduces contamination of the wound.

6. **Action:** Open a sterile surgical kit, which should contain a scalpel blade holder, surgical scissors, suture scissors, dressing thumb forceps, rat-toothed or atraumatic thumb forceps, haemostatic forceps and needle holders.

    Rationale: Contents of basic surgical kits will differ but should at least include the above.

7. **Action:** Using needle holders, affix a no. 10 or 15 scalpel blade to the holder.

    Rationale: Avoid injuring yourself.

8. **Action:** Make a V-shaped full-thickness skin incision on the dorsal and ventral aspects of the tail, starting laterally just proximal to the intervertebral space at the level of amputation and extending to the mid-vertebral body (Fig. 12.19).

    Rationale: As little of the tail should be removed as possible – usually one vertebral body clear of the diseased portion is sufficient. The incision should

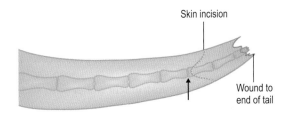
Skin incision
Wound to end of tail

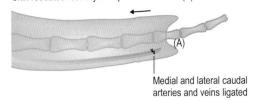
Skin retracted rostrally to expose articulation (A)
(A)
Medial and lateral caudal arteries and veins ligated

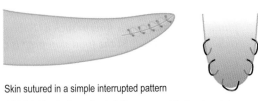
Skin sutured in a simple interrupted pattern

Fig. 12.19 Technique for tail tip removal following injury.

leave enough skin to close over the amputation site with no tension.

9. **Action:** Double ligate any blood vessels immediately proximal to the transaction site with 1.5 or 2 metric synthetic absorbable suture material.

   Rationale: *Caudal arteries run ventrally to the tail. Smaller vessels may be present laterally. Any haemorrhage may delay healing and lead to self-mutilation.*

10. **Action:** Transect the tail through the intervertebral joint using a scalpel blade.

    Rationale: *Although the tail can be removed by cutting through the vertebral body with bone cutters, this can cause splintering of the bone and lead to chronic pain.*

11. **Action:** Ligate any further sources of bleeding.

    Rationale: *As in step 9.*

12. **Action:** Oppose the subcutaneous tissue and muscle with simple interrupted or horizontal mattress sutures of 1.5 or 2 metric synthetic absorbable suture material.

    Rationale: *All dead space should be closed to avoid seroma formation.*

13. **Action:** Oppose the skin edges using 1.5 or 2 metric suture material.

    Rationale: *Either subcutaneous or skin sutures may be used, depending on preference.*

14. **Action:** Place a non-adherent wound dressing and tail bandage. Patients should be fitted with an Elizabethan collar.

    Rationale: *Self-mutilation is to be avoided as it may lead to wound breakdown or persistent tail tip pain.*

15. **Action:** Continue pain relief for at least 5 days post-surgery.

    Rationale: *Pain will increase the risk of self-trauma.*

16. **Action:** Remove sutures at 7–10 days post-surgery.

    Rationale: *By this time the wound should have healed.*

REFERENCES AND FURTHER READING

Ackerman, N., 2016. Aspinall's Complete Textbook of Veterinary Nursing, third ed. Elsevier, Oxford.

Aspinall, V., 2011. The Complete Textbook of Veterinary Nursing, second ed. Elsevier, Oxford.

Fowler, D., Williams, J.M. (Eds.), 1999. BSAVA Manual of Canine and Feline Wound Management and Reconstruction. BSAVA, Gloucester.

Hoad, J., 2006. Minor Veterinary Surgery – A Handbook for Veterinary Nurses. Elsevier, Oxford.

Hotston-Moore, A. (Ed.), 1999. Manual of Advanced Veterinary Nursing. BSAVA, Gloucester.

Lane, D.R., Cooper, B. (Eds.), 2003. Veterinary Nursing. third ed. Butterworth-Heinemann, Oxford.

Seymour, C., Duke-Novakovski, T. (Eds.), 2007. BSAVA Manual of Canine and Feline Anaesthesia and Analgesia. BSAVA, Gloucester.

Tobias, K.M., Johnston, S.A. (Eds.), 2012. Veterinary Surgery: Small Animal. Elsevier Saunders, Missouri.

13

Treatment of exotic species

Rachel Mowbray

CHAPTER OUTLINE

INTRODUCTION

The presentation of various exotic species of animal to the veterinary surgeon for treatment is now an everyday occurrence. The care and handling needed by these animals differs from that required by dogs and cats in the following ways:

- **Response to human contact** – most exotic species have an innate fear of humans and any form of human contact is likely to induce a degree of distress. Certain individual animals, e.g. some rabbits, guinea pigs and ferrets, may tolerate or actively seek human company but for most the instinct is to run, or in some cases, to attack. This must be taken into consideration when providing nursing care – observe the patient unobtrusively, avoid unnecessary physical contact and be aware that most 'exotics' do not appreciate the sound of the human voice.

- **Methods of restraint** – some species are small and agile and can be easily injured by inept handling, whilst others have wings, providing a different means of escape. Reptiles are ectothermic, depending on their environment for heat and energy – they may suddenly become very active in the warmth of your hands. All are capable of causing injury to the ill-prepared handler.

- **Reaction to anaesthesia** – the term 'exotics' covers a wide range of species showing an equally wide range of differing responses to anaesthetic agents. It is not the brief of this chapter to describe the action of each anaesthetic agent, but veterinary nurses must ensure that they are familiar with the clinical parameters and the reflexes that can be used to monitor the level of anaesthesia.

By understanding that the nursing care required by exotic species is different from that normally given to dogs and cats, the veterinary nurse can significantly increase the chances of recovery and survival of the exotic patient.

THE RABBIT – *ORYCTOLAGUS CUNICULUS*

For biological data, see Table 13.1.

HANDLING AND RESTRAINT

Procedure: To restrain a rabbit

1. **Action:** Observe the rabbit before handling.
   Rationale: To assess the nature and condition of the rabbit – if it is aggressive, you may need to ask for assistance. Restraint may cause respiratory arrest in dyspnoeic animals. Severe stress and fear may lead to cardiac arrest.
2. **Action:** Rabbits should be handled gently but firmly.
   Rationale: Rabbits have an innate fear of humans, whom they perceive as predators.
3. **Action:** Talk quietly to the rabbit and approach from behind the head.
   Rationale: The eyes of the rabbit are placed on each side of the head, providing good lateral vision, but very poor backwards vision. There is no need to offer a hand for the rabbit to sniff – it may be mistaken for food.
4. **Action:** If the animal is fractious, grasp by the scruff and support the weight with one hand under the hindquarters (Fig. 13.1).
   Rationale: Never pick a rabbit up by the ears! The hind legs must be supported at all times. Rabbits have a fragile skeleton and large lumbar muscles. By struggling or kicking, rabbits can easily break their hind legs or dislocate or fracture their spines, resulting in paralysis. They also have large claws, which may injure you.
5. **Action:** More docile rabbits may be restrained by placing one hand under the thorax and gripping the forelegs between the thumb and forefingers of that hand. Support the hind end with your other hand.
   Rationale: Some rabbits may resent being scruffed. The back should be kept in a normal curved position to avoid spinal fracture.
6. **Action:** To carry the rabbit, tuck the head and front feet under your upper arm and support the body along your forearm (Fig. 13.2).
   Rationale: Keeping the rabbit close to your body avoids the risk of it kicking and scratching you. Keeping its head in the dark makes the rabbit relax.
7. **Action:** A large towel can be used as an additional means of restraint. Place the rabbit on the opened towel with its head projecting from one side. Wrap the towel around the body, covering the feet and leaving the head exposed (Fig. 13.3).
   Rationale: Covering the feet protects the handler from injury, whilst the head is available for examination and administration of medicines.
8. **Action:** An excessively aggressive rabbit may be removed from a cage by throwing a towel over the animal and covering it completely. The rabbit can be unwrapped when it is safely on the examination table.
   Rationale: Care must be taken to avoid injuring the rabbit or being injured yourself.

Procedure: To sex a rabbit

1. **Action:** Hold the scruff of the rabbit and support its weight by placing one hand under its hindquarters.
   Rationale: The rabbit must be held firmly to avoid possible injury to itself or to you.
2. **Action:** Gently lower the rabbit onto an examination table so that it lies in dorsal recumbency. Maintain your hold on the scruff and tilt the animal so that it is almost upside down.
   Rationale: In this position the rabbit is almost 'hypnotized' and is easier to examine.
3. **Action:** Using your forefinger and middle finger, apply pressure to the vent area just in front of the anus. It may be easier for the examination to be carried out by an assistant while you maintain a firm hold on the rabbit (Fig. 13.4).
   Rationale: In both sexes, the area will protrude. Bucks (males) under 5 weeks old will show a blunt white tube without a central line, whilst older bucks will show a pink tube with a pointed end that resembles a bullet; the doe (female) has a central slit-like opening to the vulva with a band of pink tissue on either side.

N.B.: Young rabbits are difficult to sex up to the age of about 3 weeks. Adult bucks have large scrotal sacs, which are visible lateral and cranial to the penis. The testes can be retracted. Adult does often have a prominent fur-covered dewlap under the chin.

TABLE 13.1 Biological data relating to rabbits and small rodents

	Chinchilla	Gerbil	Guinea pig	Golden hamster	Mouse	Rat	Rabbit
Lifespan (years)	10–12	3–4	4–8	2–3	2–3	3–4	5–12
Adult weight	400–600 g	50–60 g	750–1000 g	80–120 g	20–40 g	400–800 g	1–8 kg
Body temperature (°C)	38–39	37.4–39	38.6	36.2–37.5	37.5	38.0	38.3–39.4
Respiratory rate (breaths/min)	40–80	90–140	90–150	70–80	100–250	70–150	35–60
Pulse rate (beats/min)	100–150	250–500	130–190	280–412	500–600	260–450	130–325
Oestrus cycle (days)	41 Seasonally polyoestrous	4–6	15–17	4	4–5	4–5	No regular cycle. Induced ovulator
Age at puberty	8 months	10 weeks	M 8–10 weeks F 4–5 weeks	6–10 weeks	6–7 weeks	8–10 weeks	4–6 months
Gestation period (days)	111	24–26	63	16	19–21	20–22	28–32
Development of young at birth	Precocial	Altricial	Precocial	Altricial	Altricial	Altricial	Altricial
Weaning age	6–8 weeks	24–27 days	2–3 weeks	3–4 weeks	3–4 weeks	3–4 weeks	4–6 weeks
Type of diet	Herbivorous Coprophagic	Omnivorous Coprophagic	Herbivorous Need vitamin C	Omnivorous Coprophagic	Omnivorous Coprophagic	Omnivorous Coprophagic	Herbivorous Coprophagic
Natural behaviour	Nocturnal Social	Nocturnal Monogamous	Diurnal Social	Nocturnal Solitary	Nocturnal Social	Nocturnal Social	Crepuscular Social

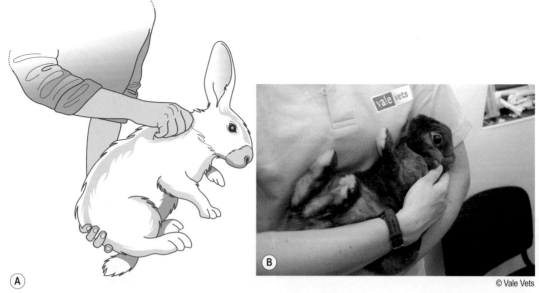

Fig. 13.1 Restraining a rabbit.

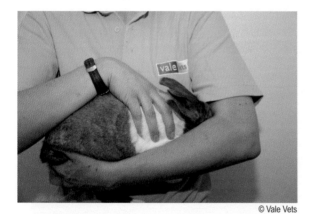

Fig. 13.2 Carrying a rabbit with the head tucked under the arm.

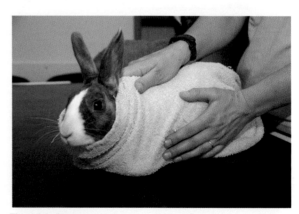

Fig. 13.3 A large towel wrapped securely around the rabbit can be very helpful for restraint.

ADMINISTRATION OF MEDICINES

Procedure: To administer oral fluids or liquid medication

1. **Action:** Place the rabbit in sternal recumbency on an examination table and wrap it in a towel, as previously described (Fig. 13.3).
   Rationale: Using this method, the legs are restrained but the head is exposed, providing access to the mouth.

2. **Action:** Take the head in one hand and tilt slightly to one side.

Rationale: In this position, one corner of the mouth is uppermost.

3. **Action:** Using a syringe of an appropriate size containing the liquid medication, place the nozzle into the uppermost corner of the mouth.
   Rationale: Avoid using large syringes as they are difficult to control.

4. **Action:** Apply gentle pressure to the syringe and give the medication. Allow time for the rabbit to swallow.
   Rationale: Give fluid in boluses of 0.25–0.5 ml. If the fluid is given too fast, the rabbit will choke, or the liquid may escape out of the mouth.

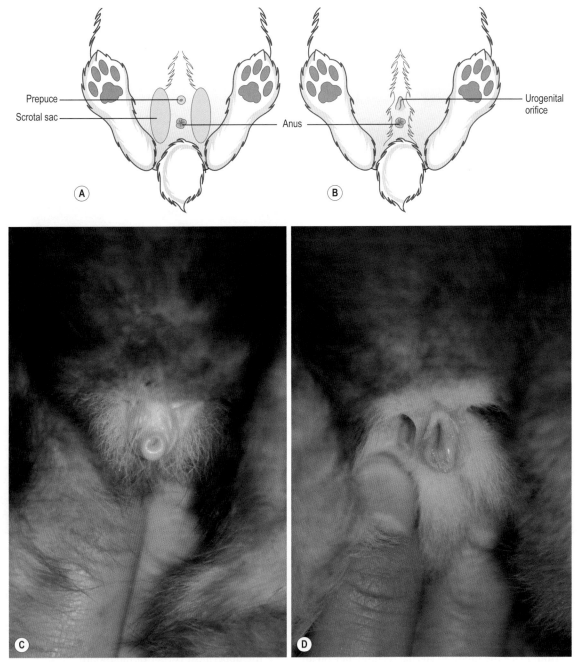

Fig. 13.4 Sexing a rabbit. A, C, Male rabbit; B, D, female rabbit.

Procedure: To place a naso-oesophageal feeding tube

Rabbits always breathe through their noses, so this procedure is not recommended for rabbits showing signs of respiratory distress.

1. **Action:** Select a 5–8F (French gauge) feeding tube.
   Rationale: *The size depends on the size of the rabbit.*
2. **Action:** Lay the tube along the outside of the rabbit's body, from the external nares to the caudal end of the

sternum. Mark the point of the external nares with a tape or ballpoint pen.

Rationale: As the tube is passed through the nasal cavity and down the oesophagus, the pen or tape mark will reach the opening to the nasal cavity, indicating that the end of the tube has reached the distal oesophagus, close to the entrance to the stomach.

3. **Action:** Restrain the rabbit in sternal recumbency and wrap in a towel as previously described.
   Rationale: In this position the body is restrained but there is access to the head.

4. **Action:** Apply local anaesthetic spray to one of the rabbit's nostrils. Wait for 3–5 minutes.
   Rationale: This desensitizes the opening to the nasal cavity and facilitates tube placement.

5. **Action:** Apply lidocaine gel to the end of the tube.
   Rationale: This lubricates the passage of the tube so that it can be inserted without resistance.

6. **Action:** Raise the rabbit's head and place the tip of the tube into the selected nostril at the ventral meatus. Gently advance the tube medially and ventrally. Return the head to a normal position as the pharynx is approached. Continue until the mark on the tube lies at the entrance to the nasal cavity.
   Rationale: This ensures that the tube passes down into the distal oesophagus.

7. **Action:** Take a radiograph of the lateral thorax and abdomen.
   Rationale: It is important to check that the tube is in the oesophagus and not in the trachea. Introducing a small volume of saline down the tube is a simple means of monitoring, but rabbits do not always cough when this is done. The use of a lateral radiograph is a more reliable method. The rabbit will be conscious and must be restrained – make sure that correct radiological protection measures are carried out.

8. **Action:** Pass the external part of the tube over the bridge of the nose and between the ears. Fix in place using superglue, tape or sutures at the external nares and at the base of one ear.
   Rationale: It is important that the tube is not dislodged by patient interference.

9. **Action:** If necessary, use an Elizabethan collar.

N.B.: This technique can be used to administer liquid oral medication or to feed hospitalized rabbits.

Procedure: Subcutaneous injection

1. **Action:** Place the rabbit in sternal recumbency on a suitable examination table with a non-slip surface.
   Rationale: If the rabbit feels secure, it will be less likely to struggle and injure itself. Minimal restraint is needed, but the rabbit must be prevented from leaping off the table.

2. **Action:** Select a sterile 21G or 23G needle and a syringe of an appropriate size. Draw up the drug to be administered.
   Rationale: Large volumes can be given by subcutaneous injection.

3. **Action:** Grasp the loose skin of the scruff and inject the drug into the subcuticular space.
   Rationale: You may draw back on the syringe prior to injection of the drug to check that a vein has not been penetrated, but this is not usually necessary with a subcutaneous injection.

4. **Action:** Withdraw the needle and gently massage the site.
   Rationale: To aid dispersion of the drug. Absorption of a drug from this area takes about 30–40 minutes.

Procedure: Intramuscular injection

1. **Action:** Place the rabbit in sternal recumbency on a suitable examination table with a non-slip surface.
   Rationale: If the rabbit feels secure, it will be less likely to struggle and injure itself.

2. **Action:** Select a 23G needle and a syringe of appropriate size. Draw up the drug to be administered.
   Rationale: A volume of 0.5–1.00 ml can be given by this route. Large volumes will cause pain and damage to muscle tissue.

3. **Action:** Grasp the scruff of the rabbit with one hand.
   Rationale: This prevents the rabbit from moving or leaping off the table.

4. **Action:** Inject into the lumbar muscles.
   Rationale: This is a large muscle mass that is easily accessible. The procedure can be performed single-handedly in docile rabbits. Assistance may be required if the patient is more active.

5. **Action:** Alternatively, the quadriceps group of muscles on the cranial aspect of the thigh may be used. Restrain the rabbit in sternal recumbency and extend a hind leg towards the veterinary surgeon.
   Rationale: This position provides easy access to the muscle group.

6. **Action:** The veterinary surgeon will hold the muscle between the finger and thumb of the left hand and introduce the needle into the muscle with the right hand.
   Rationale: Assuming that the veterinary surgeon is right-handed.
7. **Action:** Draw back on the syringe to check that a vein has not been penetrated.
   Rationale: Muscle tissue is well supplied with blood vessels and there is a danger of accidental venepuncture. Care must also be taken to avoid the sciatic nerve, which runs behind the femur.
8. **Action:** If no blood appears in the hub of the needle, inject the drug into the muscle.
9. **Action:** Withdraw the needle, applying gentle pressure over the site.
   Rationale: To aid dispersion of the drug. Absorption from this area takes approximately 15–20 minutes.

Procedure: Intravenous injection (venepuncture)

1. **Action:** Place the rabbit in sternal recumbency on an examination table with a non-slip surface.
   Rationale: If the rabbit feels secure, it will be less likely to struggle and injure itself.
2. **Action:** Wrap the rabbit in a towel with the head uncovered, as previously described.
   Rationale: This restrains the body while providing access to the head.
3. **Action:** Clip the fur lying over the marginal ear vein of one ear. Clean the site but avoid the use of spirit.
   Rationale: The marginal ear vein runs down the side of each ear. The use of spirit can collapse the vein, making sampling and injection more difficult (Fig 13.5).
4. **Action:** Apply local anaesthetic cream to the site. Wait for 10 minutes.
   Rationale: This desensitizes the area so that the rabbit is less likely to shake its head when the needle is introduced.
5. **Action:** Place a ball of cotton wool soaked in hot water under the ear.
   Rationale: This causes the vein to dilate, making it easier to visualize.
6. **Action:** Apply pressure to the base of the selected ear.
   Rationale: This pressure acts as a tourniquet, preventing blood returning from the ear pinna to the heart, thereby dilating or 'raising the vein' and making it more visible.

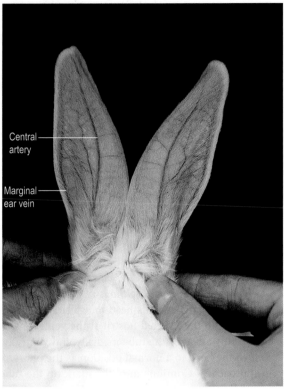

Fig. 13.5 The blood vessels within the pinna of the rabbit – the central artery is clearly visible. The marginal ear veins can be used for venepuncture. (Taken from Aspinall and Aspinall (2013) Clinical Procedures in Small Animal Veterinary Practice, Elsevier.)

7. **Action:** Maintain the pressure while the veterinary surgeon inserts a 23G needle through the overlying skin into the marginal ear vein.
   Rationale: The vein should be clearly visible (Fig 13.5).
8. **Action:** The veterinary surgeon will draw back on the syringe.
   Rationale: If blood appears in the hub of the needle, the vein has been penetrated.
9. **Action:** If blood appears in the hub of the needle, release the pressure on the vein a little while the veterinary surgeon injects the drug to be given.
   Rationale: Do not inject more than 1.5 ml, as larger volumes may cause damage to the vein.
10. **Action:** When the procedure is complete, the veterinary surgeon will slowly withdraw the needle while you apply pressure over the injection site for a few seconds.

Rationale: *This prevents haemorrhage into the surrounding tissues.*

N.B.: If repeated injections are to be given, use an intravenous or a butterfly catheter held firmly in place with superglue or tape. If collecting a blood sample, use the saphenous, the cephalic or the jugular veins. The maximum volume that can be collected at one time is 2.5 ml.

Procedure: Intraperitoneal injection

1. **Action:** Place the rabbit in sternal recumbency on an examination table with a non-slip surface.
   Rationale: *If the rabbit feels secure, it will be less likely to struggle and injure itself.*
2. **Action:** Grasp the scruff with one hand and the hind legs with the other hand.
   Rationale: *The rabbit must be held firmly to prevent it struggling during the procedure.*
3. **Action:** Pick the rabbit up and hold it in dorsal recumbency with its spine against your chest (Fig. 13.6).
   Rationale: *This position exposes the abdomen for injection, but care must be taken with dyspnoeic patients.*

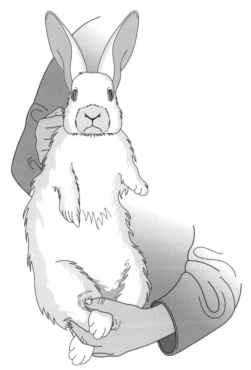

Fig. 13.6 Restraining a rabbit for an intraperitoneal injection.

4. **Action:** The veterinary surgeon will introduce a short needle at a point midway between the xiphisternum and the pubis.
   Rationale: *This position should avoid accidental penetration of the bladder or stomach. Rabbit skin is thin, and a short needle easily penetrates the abdominal wall.*
5. **Action:** Draw back on the syringe and examine the contents.
   Rationale: *If blood, urine or gut contents appear, reposition the needle. If nothing appears in the hub of the needle, it is safe to proceed with the injection.*
6. **Action:** If there is nothing in the syringe, gently inject the contents of the syringe.
   Rationale: *Up to 50 ml of fluid can be given by this route.*
7. **Action:** When the procedure is complete, withdraw the needle.

N.B.: This technique can be used to collect samples of fluid from the peritoneal cavity and samples of urine from the bladder.

Procedure: To place an intraosseous catheter

1. **Action:** Select an appropriate site.
   Rationale: *In the rabbit, the proximal femur and the proximal tibia provide ease of access and a medullary cavity from which fluid can be rapidly absorbed.*
2. **Action:** Prepare the site aseptically.
   Rationale: *To prevent the introduction of infection.*
3. **Action:** Infiltrate the area with local anaesthetic.
   Rationale: *To desensitize the tissues. The rabbit may be under a general anaesthetic but this depends on the nature and condition of the individual patient.*
4. **Action:** Select a spinal needle or plain needle of an appropriate size and insert it into the bone.
   Rationale: *The needle must be of a size that will enter the medullary cavity – use a radiograph of the leg or previous experience to assess the size.*
5. **Action:** Flush the needle with heparinized saline.
   Rationale: *The needle may become blocked with tissue fragments. Heparinized saline will ensure that it is patent.*
6. **Action:** Fix the needle in place with tissue glue or by suturing.
   Rationale: *It is important that the needle does not become dislodged.*

7. **Action:** Attach a short length of tubing and a syringe or attach a fluid giving set to the needle.
   Rationale: *This procedure may be used to give a bolus of fluid or a slow infusion. Absorption from this site is as rapid as it is by the intravenous route.*
8. **Action:** If the needle is to be left in situ, bandage the area. You may need to use an Elizabethan collar.
   Rationale: *To prevent the risk of infection, to reduce limb mobility and to prevent patient interference. An Elizabethan collar will also prevent interference, but intraosseous catheters are usually well tolerated.*
9. **Action:** When giving further fluid or drugs through the needle, maintain an aseptic technique.
   Rationale: *To prevent the introduction of infection.*
10. **Action:** Flush with heparinized saline before each use.
    Rationale: *To flush out any blood clots.*
11. **Action:** Keep the needle patent by flushing with heparinized saline at least three times daily, even if it is not being used.
    Rationale: *To maintain patency.*

N.B.: This route is useful for small animals whose veins are often fragile and easily damaged by needles and catheters. If the needle is dislodged, haemorrhage from the site is unlikely to occur.

GENERAL ANAESTHESIA

For general considerations, see Table 13.2.

Procedure: Induction of anaesthesia

1. **Action:** Weigh the rabbit.
   Rationale: *To calculate the correct dose of anaesthetic. It is important not to overdose the patient.*
2. **Action:** During the induction process, the rabbit must be handled gently and calmly.
   Rationale: *This process easily distresses a rabbit, and it may contribute to cardiac or respiratory arrest or gut stasis which may occur post-surgery.*
3. **Action:** If using an injectable agent, e.g. fentanyl/fluanisone or ketamine/medetomidine, give by the appropriate route; restrain the patient as described previously (Table 13.3).
   Rationale: *Injectable agents provide a rapid and stress-free induction. Use small syringes for more accurate dosing.*
4. **Action:** Supplement with oxygen by mask or by intubating the patient.
   Rationale: *This should be done even when using injectable agents.*
5. **Action:** If using inhalation anaesthesia, e.g. isoflurane, induce using a mask or an induction chamber.

TABLE 13.2 **Points to be considered during anaesthesia of the rabbit**	
Action	**Rationale**
1. There is no need for pre-operative starvation of rabbits	1. Rabbits are unable to vomit. Starvation may cause a fatal hypoglycaemia, especially in smaller individuals. The stomach is never completely empty as rabbits exhibit coprophagia
2. Avoid dehydration by giving fluids intravenously, subcutaneously, intraperitoneally or intraosseously	2. Rabbits undergoing a routine procedure can be given a bolus of fluid
3. Keep the patient warm at all times using a heat pad or by wrapping in 'bubble wrap', but check regularly for signs of hyperthermia	3. Hypothermia may be a problem in small animals, particularly during anaesthesia and post-operatively, as they have a large surface area in relation to their body weight. Anaesthetics depress temperature regulation and may cause vasodilation. If viscera are exposed during surgery, heat loss will be increased
4. Apply an ophthalmic lubricant to protect the eyes	4. Rabbits have bulging eyes, which are prone to drying out during anaesthesia. If ketamine is used in any anaesthetic combination, the eyes will remain central and fixed
5. Make sure that the tongue is pulled forward if the patient is not intubated	5. A rabbit's tongue is large and may obstruct the airway

TABLE 13.3 Anaesthetic agents used in small rodents and rabbits

Drug	Species, dose rate and route of administration				Duration of anaesthesia
	Mouse	Rat	Guinea pig	Rabbit	
Fentanyl/fluanisone (Hypnorm)	0.2–0.5 ml IM 0.3–0.6 mg/ml IP	As mouse	–	0.2–0.4 ml	Sedation only 30–45 min
Fentanyl/fluanisone (Hypnorm)/diazepam	0.4 ml/kg 5 mg/kg	0.3 ml/kg 2.5 mg/kg	1 ml/kg IM 2.5 ml/kg	0.3 ml/kg IM 2 mg/kg IP	45–60 min
Fentanyl/fluanisone (Hypnorm)/midazolam*	10 ml/kg*	2.7 ml/kg*	8 ml/kg*	0.3 ml/kg IM 0.5–1 ml/kg IV	45–60 min
Ketamine/medetomidine	200 mg/kg 0.5 mg/kg	90 mg/kg 0.5 mg/kg	40 mg/kg 0.5 mg/kg	35 mg/kg 0.5 mg/kg	20–30 min
Propofol	26 mg/kg IV	10 mg/kg IV	–	10 mg/kg IV	5 min
Atipamezole	1 mg/kg IM, IP, SC, IV to reverse any combination using medetomidine				

IM, intramuscular; IP, intraperitoneal; IV, intravenous; SC, subcutaneous.
*One part fentanyl/fluanisone (Hypnorm) to one part midazolam (5 mg/ml) to two parts water.
Hotston-Moore (1999), Gloucester.

Rationale: Using a mask is easier if the rabbit has been given a premed. An induction chamber of a suitable size for the patient may take several minutes to fill. Induction by either of these methods is not recommended as the rabbit may hold its breath or may struggle violently, injuring its back. The most commonly used anaesthetic, isoflurane, is irritant to mucous membranes.

6. **Action:** Give 100% oxygen for 1–2 minutes before attempting to intubate the rabbit.

   Rationale: To increase the oxygen concentration in the anaesthetic mixture. Intubation is more difficult than in the dog and the cat and may take longer as the glottis and larynx are not visible.

7. **Action:** Intubate the rabbit by placing it in sternal or dorsal recumbency with the head and neck extended. Use a laryngoscope to illuminate the area and use an introducer, such as that found inside a cat urinary catheter, to stiffen the endotracheal tube. Slide the tube over the introducer into the trachea and remove the introducer.

   Rationale: The glottis of the rabbit is small and obscured by the tongue. A fatal laryngospasm may occur if care is not taken.

8. **Action:** Alternatively, intubation may be performed 'blind'. Estimate the position of the larynx externally and advance the endotracheal tube until it lies in the correct position. Check for correct positioning.

   Rationale: The larynx may be palpated externally. Listen for respiratory sounds through the tube to check positioning. A transparent tube may show evidence of condensation from the moisture in the exhaled breath.

9. **Action:** Attach the endotracheal tube to the anaesthetic circuit.

   Rationale: Circuit must be appropriate to the species, e.g. Ayre's or Jackson Rees modified T-piece.

10. **Action:** Take appropriate steps to keep the rabbit warm at all times.

    Rationale: Heat loss can be reduced by wrapping in 'bubble wrap' or a 'space blanket' and by use of a heat pad.

11. **Action:** If possible, raise the chest above the abdominal cavity.

    Rationale: The thoracic cavity is small and can be compressed by the abdominal contents.

Procedure: Maintenance and monitoring of anaesthesia

1. **Action:** Make sure that you are familiar with the reactions of the rabbit under general anaesthesia.

   Rationale: Rabbits are not as relaxed as dogs and cats.

2. **Action:** Pay particular attention to the rate and depth of respiration.

   Rationale: This is the most reliable method of monitoring the depth of anaesthesia. Laboured breathing and pauses between breaths indicate deep anaesthesia.

3. **Action:** Monitor the tension of the jaw.
4. **Action:** Pinch the ear.
   Rationale: Absence of a head shake indicates an acceptable level of surgical anaesthesia.
5. **Action:** Assess the pedal reflex.
   Rationale: This reflex remains for longer than in the dog and cat and is only lost under deep anaesthesia.
6. **Action:** The corneal and palpebral reflexes can also be used to assess depth of anaesthesia.
   Rationale: These are similar to those in the dog and cat.

Procedure: Post-operative care

1. **Action:** The rabbit must be monitored until it is completely conscious and behaving normally.
   Rationale: Avoid too much direct attention, e.g. talking to the rabbit, as this will increase the levels of stress. Observe from a discreet distance.
2. **Action:** Place the rabbit in a cage in a room that is warm, quiet and dimly lit.
   Rationale: Bright lights and noise will distress the rabbit during recovery.
3. **Action:** Ensure that the rabbit is kept warm using a heat pad or Vetbed, or blankets or towels placed under and over the body. Avoid the use of shavings or hay.
   Rationale: Hypothermia can be fatal or will prolong the recovery period. Loose bedding such as shavings may clog the mouth and nose.
4. **Action:** Monitor the core temperature until the animal is completely conscious.
   Rationale: Use a rectal thermometer but try to avoid excessive manipulation of the recovering rabbit.
5. **Action:** Be prepared to give oxygen if necessary.
   Rationale: This will increase the rate of recovery.
6. **Action:** If the rabbit shows signs of pain, e.g. tooth grinding, grunting, lack of appetite, or if the condition warrants it, provide analgesia.
   Rationale: Any procedure that would cause pain in any other species should be considered to cause pain in the rabbit and would warrant the use of analgesics. Correct use of analgesics, e.g. carprofen or buprenorphine, will do no harm.
7. **Action:** If the rabbit does not eat or drink soon after recovery, consider providing fluid therapy – either intravenously or intraperitoneally; this should include glucose.
   Rationale: Lack of fluid may rapidly cause serious dehydration. Lack of food may lead to a fatal hypoglycaemia. Both will compromise recovery.

8. **Action:** Monitor urine and faeces output.
   Rationale: General anaesthesia and surgery may impair both kidney and intestinal function. Overhandling of the intestine may cause paralytic ileus, which is indicated by a lack of faeces.

SMALL RODENTS

For biological data, see Table 13.1.

HANDLING AND RESTRAINT

It is the natural response of a frightened rodent to bite. This can be avoided by knowing how to handle each species correctly, but if you are bitten:

- Replace the rodent in its cage with your finger still in its mouth. As soon as the rodent feels its feet on a firm surface, it should let go!
- Do not attempt to pull your finger from the rodent's mouth, as the injury will be made worse by the backward-pointing curved teeth.
- Do not shake the rodent off your finger, as this will cause serious injury to the rodent.
- Wash the bite thoroughly under running water, apply antiseptic ointment and cover for as long as you are working with the animals.
- Consult your doctor if it becomes excessively painful or swollen.
- Keep your tetanus vaccination up to date.

THE CHINCHILLA – *CHINCHILLA LANIGERA*

Procedure: To restrain a chinchilla

1. **Action:** If the chinchilla is tame, pick it up by placing one hand around its shoulders.
   Rationale: Chinchillas are relatively easy to handle; most are not aggressive and rarely bite. Be aware of the pressure you are putting on the chest as this can restrict normal breathing.
2. **Action:** Avoid grasping hold of the fur.
   Rationale: Rough handling can cause patches of fur to come away in your hand – a condition known as 'fur slip'. In the wild, this mechanism enables the chinchilla to escape from predators. New fur may take several months to grow back and may be of a different shade.

3. **Action:** Once removed from the cage, most chinchillas will sit quietly on your forearm, gently restrained by the base of the tail.
   Rationale: If the animal feels supported and secure, it will be unlikely to try to escape.
4. **Action:** More nervous or active animals can be lifted by the base of the tail, with your other hand supporting the body.
   Rationale: Only lift by the base of the tail as further down may injure the tail. Do not leave the animal unsupported for any longer than is necessary.
5. **Action:** To restrain for any clinical procedure, hold the base of the tail with one hand and place the other around the shoulder and chest.
   Rationale: This can be used to hold the animal firmly for procedures such as injection and examination.

Procedure: To sex a chinchilla

1. **Action:** Grasp the base of the tail with one hand and support the body around the shoulders.
   Rationale: If the animal feels supported and secure, it will be unlikely to try to escape.
2. **Action:** Hold the chinchilla in dorsal recumbency, moving the tail to expose the genital area.
   Rationale: This can be done single-handedly unless the chinchilla struggles.
3. **Action:** Examine the genital area and measure the anogenital distance.
   Rationale: This is the distance between the anus and the opening of the vulva (female) or the penis (male) and is longer in the male than in the female (Fig. 13.7).
   The female chinchilla has a relatively large cone-shaped clitoris, which may be mistaken for the penis of the male. Adult male chinchillas have a pair of large testes which are very obvious during the breeding season of November–March.

THE GERBIL – *MERIONES UNGUICULATUS*

For biological data, see Table 13.1.

Procedure: To restrain a gerbil

1. **Action:** If the gerbil is tame and used to being handled, scoop it into your cupped hands.
   Rationale: Gerbils are extremely active creatures and can jump horizontally and vertically.
2. **Action:** If the gerbil is less tame, immobilize it by placing your hand over it.

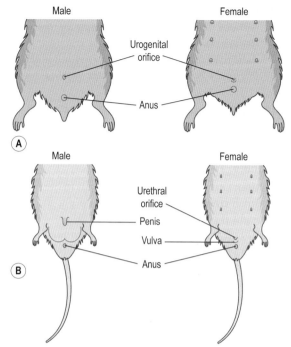

Fig. 13.7 General method of sexing rodents. A, Hamsters; B, mice.

   Rationale: This will prevent it escaping. The darkness will temporarily calm it.
3. **Action:** Move your hand to grasp the scruff and lift the animal clear of the cage.
   Rationale: Most gerbils are not aggressive, but some will try to bite – make sure that you grasp enough scruff to prevent it turning around to bite.
4. **Action:** Further restraint can be achieved by using your other hand to hold the base of the tail.
   Rationale: Do not hold the tip of the tail as the skin may be shed, leaving a raw and painful tail.

Procedure: To sex a gerbil

1. **Action:** Restrain the gerbil by grasping the scruff as described previously.
   Rationale: If the gerbil feels secure and comfortable, it will be less likely to struggle or to attempt to bite you.
2. **Action:** Examine the ventral surface of the gerbil.
   Rationale: Male gerbils have no teats; females have four pairs of teats arranged along the ventral body wall of the thorax and the abdomen.
3. **Action:** Examine the genital area and measure the anogenital distance (Fig. 13.7).

Rationale: The anogenital distance is the distance between the anus and the opening of the vulva (female) or the penis (male) and is longer in the male than in the female (Fig. 13.7). Adult male gerbils have a pair of testes lying in the inguinal region.

THE GUINEA PIG – *CAVIA PORCELLUS*

For biological data, see Table 13.1.

Procedure: To restrain a guinea pig

1. **Action:** Guinea pigs should be brought to the surgery in small covered boxes. A companion pig should be brought if possible.
   Rationale: Guinea pigs are nervous animals, and a box provides security and darkness, which will calm them. They like to be in close contact with their own species (Fig. 13.8).

2. **Action:** Open the box in a dim light if possible.
   Rationale: This will reduce stress, but you must be able to examine the patient.

3. **Action:** Pick up the animal by placing one hand around its shoulders and chest (Fig. 13.9).
   Rationale: Guinea pigs are generally non-aggressive and can be handled gently but firmly.

4. **Action:** Lift the guinea pig clear of the cage or box, supporting its weight with your other hand.
   Rationale: This is important if the animal is pregnant or heavy.

5. **Action:** Move your thumb from around the shoulders and place it under the mandible (Fig. 13.9).
   Rationale: This prevents the animal from lowering its head to bite.

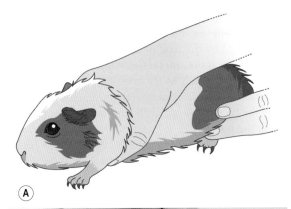

A

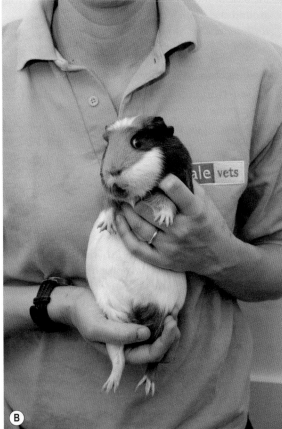

B

© Vale Vets

Fig. 13.9 Restraining a guinea pig for examination. A, Initial restraint is achieved by grasping the animal around the shoulders. B, The hindquarters should be supported if the animal weighs more than 200–300 g.

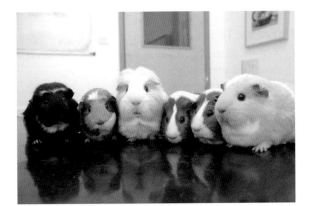

Fig. 13.8 The guinea pig – a popular children's pet.

6. **Action:** If further restraint is needed, place the guinea pig in dorsal recumbency and extend the hind legs.
   Rationale: The animal will be unable to move.

Procedure: To sex a guinea pig

1. **Action:** Restrain the guinea pig in dorsal recumbency as previously described.
   Rationale: This provides good exposure of the genital area.
2. **Action:** Examine the inguinal region.
   Rationale: Both male (boar) and female (sow) have a single pair of nipples in the inguinal region. Adult males have a pair of large testes.
3. **Action:** Examine the genital opening.
   Rationale: Females have a Y-shaped opening; males have a slit-shaped opening (Fig. 13.10).
4. **Action:** Apply gentle pressure on either side of the genital opening.
   Rationale: In the male, the penis will extend and protrude. Female guinea pigs have a pale-coloured clitoris that may protrude, but is much less obvious than the male penis.

N.B.: Guinea pigs can be sexed as early as 1–2 days old.

HAMSTER – *MESOCRICETUS AURATUS* (SYRIAN OR GOLDEN HAMSTER)

Procedure: To restrain a hamster

For biological data, see Table 13.1.

1. **Action:** Allow the hamster time to wake up before attempting to pick it up.
   Rationale: Waking a sleeping hamster can provoke an aggressive response.
2. **Action:** As the hamster runs around on the floor of the cage or box, grasp a large section of the scruff (Fig. 13.11).
   Rationale: Hamsters are unpredictable and often aggressive. It is important to take a large area of scruff to prevent the animal turning around to bite you.
3. **Action:** Lift the hamster upwards.
   Rationale: Hamsters are not very heavy and can be lifted with one hand.

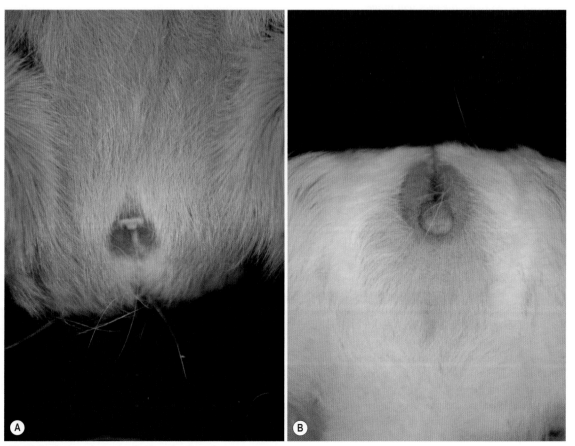

Fig. 13.10 Sexing a guinea pig. A, Female; B, male.

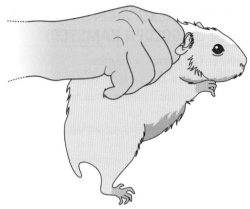

Fig. 13.11 Picking up a hamster by the scruff of the neck.

4. **Action:** Draw the scruff tight to prevent the hamster from moving around.
   Rationale: In this position you can inject the animal and examine the teeth and the oral pouches. If the scruff is too tight, the eyes will bulge.
5. **Action:** If the hamster does not need to be examined or injected, you can pick it up in your cupped hands or allow it to run into a small cup or jug.
   Rationale: The hamster can be moved from cage or box to an induction chamber but is not sufficiently restrained for any clinical procedure.

Procedure: To sex a hamster

1. **Action:** Restrain the hamster in one hand using the scruff as previously described.
   Rationale: Make sure you are holding enough of the scruff to prevent the hamster turning around and biting you.
2. **Action:** Examine the genital area and measure the anogenital distance (Fig. 13.7).
   Rationale: Adult males have a pair of large testes. These are visible from the dorsal surface as the hamster runs around. The anogenital distance is the distance between the anus and the opening of the vulva (female) or the penis (male) and is longer in the male than in the female (Fig. 13.7).
3. **Action:** Examine the ventral surface of the hamster.
   Rationale: The male hamster has no teats; the female has six pairs arranged along the ventral body wall of the thorax and abdomen.
4. **Action:** If the hamster is mature, examine the region of the hips.

Rationale: Male hamsters have a scent gland over each hip. This becomes pigmented as the animal ages. The gland is not present in the female.

N.B.: The much smaller Chinese and Russian hamsters are also popular children's pets. The techniques for handling and sexing these species are exactly the same as described for the Syrian hamster.

THE MOUSE – *MUS MUSCULUS*

For biological data, see Table 13.1.

Procedure: To restrain a mouse

1. **Action:** If the mouse is tame and used to being handled, scoop it into your cupped hands.
   Rationale: This works well for tame mice, but many mice are very nervous and may attempt to bite – a careful approach is essential.
2. **Action:** If the mouse is not used to being handled, pick it up by the base of the tail (Fig. 13.12).
   Rationale: Do not pick it up by the tip of the tail as the outer skin may be shed, leaving the tail raw and painful.
3. **Action:** Lift the mouse clear of the cage and place it on a rough surface such as a towel, your sleeve or the top of the wire cage.
   Rationale: Mice are light enough to be lifted by the tail without the need to support the body.
4. **Action:** Pull the mouse gently backwards (Fig. 13.12).
   Rationale: The mouse will grip the surface and is sufficiently restrained for an initial examination.
5. **Action:** With your other hand, grasp a large amount of scruff between your finger and the base of your thumb, while keeping control of the tail.
   Rationale: If you do not take enough of the scruff, the mouse will be able to turn round and bite you.
6. **Action:** Lift the mouse up and transfer your hold on the tail to between the third and fourth fingers of that hand (Fig. 13.12).
   Rationale: The mouse is restrained securely and, as it is held in one hand only, your other hand is free to examine or inject it.

Procedure: To sex a mouse

1. **Action:** Restrain the mouse by the scruff and tail as previously described.
   Rationale: Mice can easily struggle and escape if not held securely.

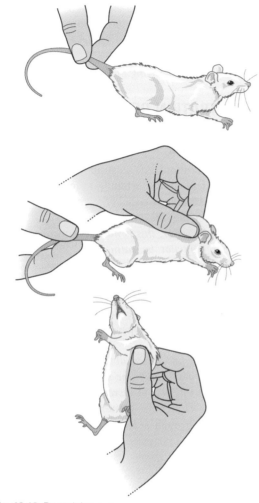

Fig. 13.12 Restraining a mouse.

2. **Action:** Examine the ventral surface of the body.

    Rationale: *Male mice do not have teats; females have seven pairs arranged along the ventral body wall of the thorax and abdomen.*

3. **Action:** Examine the genital region and measure the anogenital distance (Fig. 13.7).

    Rationale: *The anogenital distance is the distance between the anus and the opening of the vulva (female) or the penis (male) and is longer in the male than in the female (Fig. 13.7). Adult males have a pair of large testes lying in the inguinal region.*

THE RAT – *RATTUS NORVEGICUS*

For biological data, see Table 13.1.

Procedure: To restrain a rat

1. **Action:** With one hand, grasp the body around the shoulders and lift clear of the cage.

    Rationale: *Rats are intelligent, docile animals that rarely bite unless they are frightened or in pain. Be aware of how much pressure you are applying to the chest – too little will allow the animal to escape; too much will compress the chest and may make the animal bite you.*

2. **Action:** Position your thumb so that it lies under the lower jaw (Fig. 13.13).

    Rationale: *Use your thumb to apply pressure and to push the jaw up. This will prevent the animal from biting.*

3. **Action:** Alternatively, if the rat is aggressive or unused to being handled, pick it up by the base of the tail.

    Rationale: *Do not pick up by the tip of the tail as the outer skin may be shed, leaving a raw and painful tail.*

4. **Action:** Place the rat on the cage lid or on a rough surface, maintaining your grip on the tail.

    Rationale: *This provides something for the rat to grip.*

5. **Action:** As the rat moves forward, place your other hand over the shoulders and chest.

    Rationale: *Do not hold too tightly as this will affect the rat's respiration and may cause distress.*

6. **Action:** Move your thumb and forefinger to lie behind the rat's elbows so that the forelegs are pushed forward to cross under the chin.

    Rationale: *The rat is held securely, and it can be examined without the risk of being bitten.*

7. **Action:** If the rat struggles when first restrained, allow it to rest on your sleeve with a minimum of restraint.

    Rationale: *After a short time, the rat will relax.*

N.B.: Rats do not like being picked up by the scruff and doing this may cause the animal to bite.

Procedure: To sex a rat

1. **Action:** Restrain the rat by picking it up around the shoulders.

    Rationale: *If the rat feels secure, it will be less likely to struggle or to bite.*

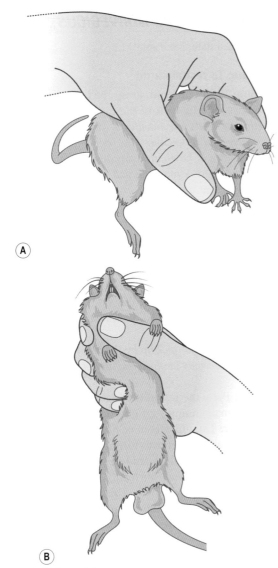

(A)

(B)

Fig. 13.13 Restraining a rat.

2. **Action:** Lift it clear of the cage and hold it in dorsal recumbency.
   Rationale: In this position you have access to the relevant parts of the animal.
3. **Action:** Examine the ventral surface of the body.
   Rationale: Male rats do not have teats; females have five pairs arranged along the ventral body wall of the thorax and abdomen.
4. **Action:** Examine the genital area and measure the anogenital distance (Fig. 13.7).

Rationale: The anogenital distance is the distance between the anus and the opening of the vulva (female) or the penis (male) and is longer in the male than in the female (Fig. 13.7). Adult males have a pair of large testes lying in the inguinal region.

ADMINISTRATION OF MEDICINES

Procedure: To administer oral fluids or liquid medication

1. **Action:** Medication such as antibiotics can be given to small rodents in the drinking water or in food.
   Rationale: All other sources of water or food can be withheld so that the animal has to take in the medication. However, this is not recommended as the animal may not be eating or drinking normal amounts – the precise dose is unknown.
2. **Action:** If the animal is not drinking, liquid medication or replacement fluids can be given by inserting a syringe or pipette into the side of the mouth at the level of the diastema (space between the incisors and molar teeth).
   Rationale: Use an unbreakable syringe to prevent the animal biting through the nozzle. Sweeten the liquid with fruit juice to increase acceptability.
3. **Action:** The chinchilla, guinea pig and rat can be given liquid through a 3–4F catheter inserted into the pharynx, oesophagus or stomach. Make a mouth gag by drilling a hole crossways through a 1 ml syringe case. Place the 'gag' across the mouth of the patient and pass the catheter through the hole and down the pharynx. Ensure that the catheter is correctly placed before injecting any fluids by listening for respiratory sounds in the tube or by taking a lateral radiograph of the animal.
   Rationale: This technique enables you to give volumes of up to 5 ml. The use of the gag prevents the patient biting through the catheter. It is vital to check that the catheter is not in the trachea as the administration of fluid into the lungs may 'drown' the animal or cause aspiration pneumonia.

Procedure: To administer medication by parenteral routes

For details of injection sites, see Table 13.4.
   General points to be considered:
1. **Action:** For most procedures, use a 23G or 25G needle.

TABLE 13.4	**Parenteral routes for the administration of medicines in small rodents**			
Species of rodent	**Subcutaneous**	**Intramuscular**	**Intraperitoneal**	**Intravenous**
Chinchilla	Scruff or the flank Avoid rough handling as this causes 'fur slip' 5–10 ml	Quadriceps group on cranial thigh or semimembranosus/ semitendinosus on caudal thigh No more than 0.3 ml	Restrain with head lower than hindquarters. Insert needle in posterior quadrant to the right of the midline 2.5 cm in front of pubis	Use the cephalic, saphenous or jugular veins
Gerbil	Scruff Up to 2 ml	Quadriceps group No more than 0.3 ml Not recommended	Restrain with head downwards Insert needle into lower left quadrant Give 3–4 ml	Not recommended
Guinea pig	Lift the skin between the scapulae Up to 10 ml	Quadriceps group No more than 0.3 ml	Restrain with head lower than hindquarters. Insert needle in posterior quadrant to the right of the midline 2.5 cm in front of pubis at 45° angle	Cephalic or lateral saphenous veins
Hamster	Scruff Up to 3–4 ml	Quadriceps group No more than 0.1 ml Not recommended	Restrain with head downwards. Insert needle either side of midline in inguinal region, caudal to umbilicus which avoids the caecum, at 45° angle. Aspirate before injecting	Not recommended
Mouse	Scruff Up to 2 ml	Quadriceps group No more than 0.05 ml Not recommended	Insert needle into lower right quadrant to avoid caecum on the left at 20° angle. Aspirate before injecting – should be a vacuum. Give 2–3 ml	Lateral tail veins Warm complete mouse or tail to dilate the veins; 0.2 ml can be injected
Rat	Scruff or flank Up to 5–10 ml	Quadriceps group No more than 0.3 ml	Insert needle into lower right quadrant (to avoid caecum on the left) at 20° angle. Aspirate before injecting – should be a vacuum. Give 10–15 ml	Lateral tail veins. Warm complete rat or the tail to dilate the veins; 0.5 ml can be injected

    Rationale: *Small needles cause less damage to the tissues.*

2. **Action:** If giving small volumes of drugs, use small syringes.
   Rationale: *Larger sizes are more difficult to handle when restraining small, struggling rodents.*

3. **Action:** When using the intramuscular route, give small volumes.
   Rationale: *Large volumes may cause tissue damage, pain, irritation and possible self-mutilation at the*

site. This route is not recommended in very small rodents, e.g. mice.

4. **Action:** When restraining an animal for an intraperitoneal injection, hold the animal with its head downwards.
   Rationale: *This allows the intestines to fall cranially, making them less likely to be punctured by the needle. This is not recommended for debilitated or dyspnoeic animals as downward movement of the abdominal contents may restrict respiratory movements – restrain them vertically.*

Procedure: To collect a blood sample

1. **Action:** The sample required may be as small as a drop of blood or may be a larger volume.
   Rationale: *A drop of blood can be used to make a smear to examine the red or white cells. Larger volumes may be used for biochemical analysis.*

2. **Action:** In any species, no more than 10% of the total blood volume may be taken at any one time.
   Rationale: *For details of blood volumes, see Table 13.5.*

3. **Action:** Select the appropriate site for the species (Table 13.5).
   Rationale: *In all the small rodents, clipping a nail may yield a small volume of blood, but this is not recommended unless really necessary as it causes pain and distress.*

4. **Action:** Prepare the site aseptically.
   Rationale: *To prevent the introduction of infection.*

5. **Action:** Select a suitably sized needle and a 1 ml syringe.
   Rationale: *Choose a size that is as large as is practicable for the species. The needle must be able to enter the vein and must not be so small that it impedes the flow of blood and damages the red cells, leading to haemolysis of the sample.*

6. **Action:** Ask an assistant to restrain the animal appropriately and to apply pressure to the selected vein – known as 'raising the vein'.
   Rationale: *When collecting blood, it will be necessary for an assistant to restrain the animal to avoid injuring the animal and causing it distress. Pressure should be applied to the vein to dilate it, making it more obvious for venepuncture.*

7. **Action:** Introduce the needle into the vein at an angle to the skin with the bevel uppermost. Once the needle is in the vein, advance it parallel to the skin.

TABLE 13.5 Blood sampling in small rodents

Species	Adult blood volume (ml/kg)	Total adult blood volume (ml)	Maximum sample volume (ml)	Site for venepuncture	Comments
Rabbit	57–65	58.5–585	5–50	Cephalic, jugular, lateral saphenous, ear vein	Large variation in size, care with ear vein as trauma can lead to ear necrosis
Chinchilla	100	40–60	5	Cephalic, jugular, lateral saphenous, femoral vein; cranial vena cava	For femoral vein: dorsal recumbency, palpate femoral artery and direct needle parallel to this
Gerbil	66–78	8	0.5	Cephalic, lateral saphenous	Blood can be collected from needle into heparinized haematocrit tubes
Guinea pig	69–75	50–60	5	Cephalic, lateral saphenous, femoral vein; cranial vena cava. For vena cava: puncture with a 25- or 27G needle inserted cranial to last rib at 45° angle directed towards the opposite hip	
Hamster	78	8	0.5	Cephalic, lateral saphenous vein. Blood can be collected from needle into heparinized haematocrit tubes	
Mouse	58.5	2	0.25	Lateral tail, cephalic, lateral saphenous vein	Dilate the vein by warming the tail
Rat	54–70	30	3	Lateral tail, jugular, cephalic, lateral saphenous vein	Dilate the vein by warming the tail

Rationale: The body of the needle now lies within the lumen of the vein.

8. **Action:** Either allow blood to drip from the hub of the needle into a collecting pot or attach the syringe and gently pull back the plunger.

   Rationale: Larger volumes can be collected by using a syringe. The vein will collapse around the needle if you try to withdraw the blood too quickly. The blood sample may also be haemolysed as a result of red cell damage.

9. **Action:** Empty the syringe into an appropriate collecting pot and rotate gently.

   Rationale: If the sample is to be analysed, the pot must contain an appropriate anticoagulant, e.g. ethylenediamine tetraacetic acid (EDTA) or lithium heparin. Gentle rotation will mix the blood with the anticoagulant; over-enthusiastic mixing will damage the blood cells.

10. **Action:** Ask your assistant to apply pressure over the site of venepuncture while you slowly withdraw the needle from the vein.

    Rationale: To prevent haemorrhage into the surrounding tissues and to encourage clotting.

11. **Action:** Dress the site appropriately.

    Rationale: To prevent infection and to prevent self-mutilation at the site.

GENERAL ANAESTHESIA

Procedure: Induction of anaesthesia

1. **Action:** Many patients to be anaesthetized are geriatric.

   Rationale: Small rodents have a short lifespan, which must be considered when undertaking anaesthesia.

2. **Action:** The patient may already be debilitated, in poor condition or obese before it is presented to the veterinary surgeon.

   Rationale: These all increase the risks of anaesthesia.

3. **Action:** The patient may be affected by a pre-existing illness.

   Rationale: Make a careful clinical examination to identify any risk factors, e.g. chronic respiratory disease.

4. **Action:** The patient may be anorexic and dehydrated. Always assess the level of dehydration and delay anaesthesia until it has been corrected.

   Rationale: Provide replacement fluid therapy by the appropriate route.

5. **Action:** There is no need for pre-operative fasting in small rodents.

Rationale: Fasting may lead to a fatal hypoglycaemia. Many species exhibit coprophagia, so the stomach and intestines are rarely completely empty.

6. **Action:** Weigh the patient.

   Rationale: This enables accurate anaesthetic doses to be calculated and provides a baseline for clinical assessment during recovery, e.g. whether the animal is eating or drinking.

7. **Action:** Anaesthetic induction may be performed in an induction chamber or by mask using an inhalation anaesthetic agent such as isoflurane or sevoflurane.

   Rationale: Induction chambers are preferred as masks are often too big for small rodents. Induction by inhalation is stressful to the patient, and there is a risk of injury as the patient may struggle during the procedure. The advantage is rapid recovery, which reduces the risk of hypothermia.

8. **Action:** Induction can be performed using injectable agents (see Table 13.3).

   Rationale: These provide a smooth, stress-free induction but recovery rates may be longer, depending on the choice of drug.

Procedure: Maintenance and monitoring of anaesthesia

1. **Action:** Once the patient is anaesthetized, maintain using an inhalation anaesthetic agent, e.g. isoflurane or sevoflurane delivered by mask, or supplement injectable drugs with oxygen by mask.

   Rationale: Small rodents are difficult to intubate. Inhalation anaesthesia delivered by mask may lead to fluctuations in depth.

2. **Action:** Monitor body temperature and keep the patient warm at all times by using a heat pad and wrapping in 'bubble wrap' or a 'space blanket'.

   Rationale: Small rodents have a large surface area to bodyweight ratio, which means that they lose heat rapidly. Under anaesthesia, the body's ability to regulate the core temperature is impaired, adding to the risk of hypothermia.

3. **Action:** Prepare the surgical site carefully.

   Rationale: Rodent skin is thin and can be easily nicked by clippers. Avoid the use of spirit to sterilize the site as this will further cool the patient.

4. **Action:** Apply ophthalmic ointment to the eyes.

   Rationale: Rodents have prominent eyes, which can be dried by the heat of the operating light and the lack of a blink reflex under anaesthesia, leading to keratitis and corneal ulceration.

5. **Action:** Monitor the depth of anaesthesia using reflexes and monitoring equipment.
   Rationale: *Each species varies in its response to anaesthesia, and it is important to become familiar with these variations. The use of electronic monitoring equipment may be difficult as it is designed and calibrated for use in larger animals, such as the cat and the dog.*
6. **Action:** Monitor respiration.
   Rationale: *Respiratory depression or arrest can be overcome by delivering oxygen by mask or using respiratory stimulants such as doxapram.*

Procedure: Post-operative care

1. **Action:** After the surgical procedure is complete, place the patient in a secure, warm cage in a quiet, warm, darkened room and cover with a towel, blanket, 'bubble wrap' or a 'space blanket,' as appropriate.
   Rationale: *Hypothermia during recovery can be fatal. Initially, the temperature of the cage should be kept at 35°C, falling to 26–28°C as the animal regains consciousness. Any noise or bright light will overstimulate a recovering animal.*
2. **Action:** Observe the patient quietly and unobtrusively.
   Rationale: *Rodents do not appreciate being touched or talked to as a dog would. Look at the animal from a distance and only interfere if it is really necessary.*
3. **Action:** Monitor the core temperature.
   Rationale: *To be aware of hypothermia before it becomes critical.*
4. **Action:** Monitor respiration.
   Rationale: *Respiratory depression or arrest may also occur during the recovery period.*
5. **Action:** If the patient shows signs of pain, e.g. tooth grinding, vocalization, aggression or a hunched position, provide analgesia.
   Rationale: *Any procedure that would cause pain in any other species should be considered to cause pain in the rodent and would warrant the use of analgesics. Correct use of analgesics, e.g. carprofen or buprenorphine, will do no harm.*
6. **Action:** Continue to monitor the patient after it has regained consciousness.
   Rationale: *Observe whether the animal is eating or drinking. Note the production of faeces and urine.*

7. **Action:** Instruct the owner of the warning signs to watch out for when the patient is taken home.
   Rationale: *The owner should monitor the patient for at least 24 hours after the surgical procedure.*

THE FERRET – *MUSTELA PUTORIUS FURO*

For biological data, see Table 13.6.

HANDLING AND RESTRAINT

Procedure: To restrain a ferret

1. **Action:** Allow the ferret to come out of its box first.
   Rationale: *Reaching into the box may startle the ferret, causing it to bite.*
2. **Action:** Place one hand around the shoulders and the neck.
   Rationale: *Ferrets vary in temperament – some are quite tame and relax when handled, whilst others may be aggressive. The ferret has a well-muscled neck that must be held firmly.*
3. **Action:** Lift the ferret clear of the cage and support the hind end with your other hand (Fig. 13.14).
   Rationale: *Ferrets can be quite heavy and need to be supported. The body should not be stretched as this causes them to struggle. Some ferrets like to be dangled by the front end while their knuckles are rubbed! Heavy or pregnant animals should always be supported under the hind end.*
4. **Action:** Move your thumb so that it lies under the lower jaw. Place your forefinger around the neck, leaving the other fingers under the forelegs (Fig. 13.14).
   Rationale: *This prevents the ferret from moving its head to bite you.*
5. **Action:** Hold the ferret gently but firmly.
   Rationale: *Ferrets are very agile creatures designed for going down holes, and they can wriggle free if not held firmly.*
6. **Action:** Tame ferrets may rest along the handler's forearm.
   Rationale: *Gentle restraint is usually adequate for a physical examination. Handle ferrets that may be in pain with caution as they may bite.*
7. **Action:** If a more secure hold is required, grasp a large portion of scruff and suspend the body.
   Rationale: *The ferret has a large area of scruff. Suspending the animal induces relaxation.*

TABLE 13.6 Ferrets – biological data

Parameter	Measurement	Comment
Lifespan	5–11 years	
Adult weight	Jill: 600–900 g	Weight fluctuates with the time of year – heavier in the winter
	Hob: 1–2 kg	
Body temperature	38.8°C (37.8–40°C)	Rises to 40°C when the ferret is excited
Respiratory rate	33–36 breaths/min	
Pulse rate	200–400 beats/min	
Oestrous cycle	Seasonally monoestrous Induced ovulator	Season starts in March and continues until September. Female remains in oestrus until she is mated. Ovulation occurs 30–40 hours after mating
Age at puberty	Jill: 7–10 months	Puberty occurs in the spring after birth, so age varies
	Hob: 5–14 months	
Gestation period	38–44 days	Young are altricial. May be eaten by the jill if disturbed
Litter size	2–6	
Weaning age	6–8 weeks	
Diet	Carnivorous	Require 35–40% animal protein, >20% fat, <2.5% fibre, <25% carbohydrate

Procedure: To sex a ferret

1. **Action:** Restrain the ferret by the scruff or by holding around the shoulders as previously described.
   Rationale: *This position leaves one hand free to examine the ferret.*
2. **Action:** Examine the genital area.
   Rationale: *In the male (hob), the opening to the penis is situated on the ventral abdomen just caudal to the umbilicus, giving a long anogenital distance (Fig. 13.15A). Male ferrets have a pair of testes that enlarge during the breeding season. In the female (jill), the vulva lies close to the anus and becomes swollen when the female is in oestrus (Fig. 13.15B).*

ADMINISTRATION OF MEDICINES

Procedure: To administer oral fluids or liquid medication

1. **Action:** Restrain the ferret by the neck and shoulders and support the hind end on a table or allow it to dangle.
   Rationale: *In this position you have control of the head. Supporting the hind end on a table may encourage the ferret to struggle. This will depend on the weight, temperament and condition of the ferret.*
2. **Action:** Using a small syringe filled with the liquid, place the nozzle into the side of the mouth.
   Rationale: *Avoid using large syringes as they are difficult to manipulate while holding the patient. This procedure may be used to give liquid medication or replacement fluid.*
3. **Action:** Slowly deposit the liquid towards the back of the tongue.
   Rationale: *Do not give the medication too fast as the ferret lacks a cough reflex and may aspirate the liquid.*

Procedure: Subcutaneous injection

1. **Action:** Grasp a large section of the scruff of the ferret.
   Rationale: *Ferrets have a large scruff, and this position both restrains the ferret and provides a suitable site for the injection.*
2. **Action:** Select a sterile 23G needle and a syringe of an appropriate size, fill with the medication and introduce the needle into the scruff.
   Rationale: *A maximum of 5–10 ml can be given at this site.*
3. **Action:** Apply pressure to the plunger and inject the drug.
   Rationale: *There is no need to draw back on the syringe for a subcutaneous injection as the risk of penetrating a blood capillary is low.*
4. **Action:** Remove the needle from the scruff.
   Rationale: *Absorption of the drug from this site takes about 30 minutes.*

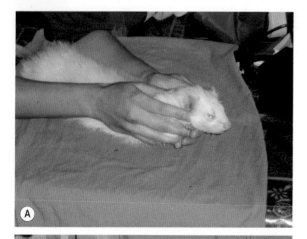

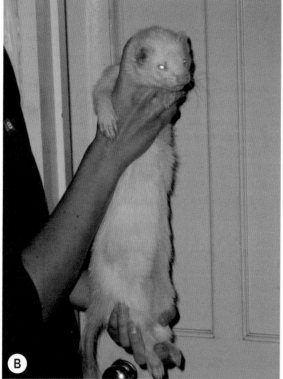

Fig. 13.14 A, Restraining a ferret by placing it on a towel on a table. B, Lifting a ferret and supporting the hind end with the other hand.

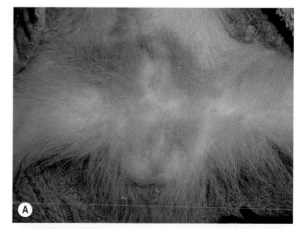

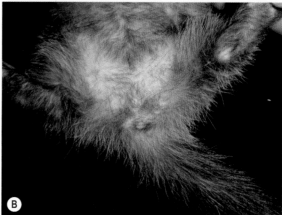

Fig. 13.15 Sexing a ferret. A, Male ferret; B, female ferret.

Procedure: Intramuscular injection

1. **Action:** Ask an assistant to restrain the ferret in sternal recumbency on the examination table, placing one hand behind the head and using the other to pin the lumbar region to the table.

Rationale: This restrains the body firmly, preventing struggling and possible injury to the ferret and to the handler.

2. **Action:** Locate the quadriceps group on the cranial aspect of the thigh or the epaxial muscles in the cervical region or, for amounts of less than 0.25 ml, the lumbar region.

Rationale: These muscles are relatively large and can be easily located between the finger and thumb. Take care with the lumbar muscles as these are thin and penetration of a kidney is a risk if the ferret struggles. The cervical muscles are a good choice in hobs, less so in smaller jills.

3. **Action:** Select a sterile 23G needle and a syringe of an appropriate size, fill with the drug and introduce the needle into the muscle.

Rationale: The muscle mass is small, so only small volumes can be given by this route – maximum of 0.5 ml.

4. **Action:** Draw back on the syringe.
   Rationale: Muscle tissue has a good blood supply, and there is a risk of penetrating a blood vessel.

5. **Action:** If no blood appears in the hub of the needle, gently inject the drug.
   Rationale: Do not inject too rapidly as the pressure may cause the drug to spurt out of the hub.

6. **Action:** Apply gentle pressure over the injection site and withdraw the needle.
   Rationale: This aids dispersion of the drug. The rate of absorption from this site is 15–20 minutes.

Procedure: Intraperitoneal injection

1. **Action:** Ask an assistant to restrain the ferret by holding it around the shoulders and chest with the thumb under the chin and the fingers under the forelegs as previously described (Fig. 13.14).
   Rationale: This restrains the body firmly, preventing struggling and possible injury to the ferret and to the handler.

2. **Action:** Use the other hand to support the hind end.
   Rationale: The hind end must be held firmly to prevent the ferret moving around and injuring itself during the procedure.

3. **Action:** In this position the assistant should rest the body against his or her chest, presenting the ventral abdomen towards you.
   Rationale: The ventral abdomen is the site of the injection.

4. **Action:** Select a 21–23G needle and a small syringe and fill it with the drug to be administered.
   Rationale: This procedure may also be used to administer fluid therapy. A maximum of 8 ml can be given at any one time.

5. **Action:** Introduce the needle to one side of the midline and into one of the lower quadrants of the abdomen. The needle should be pointing cranially.
   Rationale: This will decrease the risk of entering one of the abdominal organs.

6. **Action:** Draw back on the syringe.
   Rationale: To check that you have not penetrated an organ. If urine, intestinal contents or blood appear in the syringe, reposition the needle.

7. **Action:** If the hub of the needle is empty, inject the drug into the peritoneal cavity and withdraw slowly.

Procedure: Intravenous injection

1. **Action:** Restrain the ferret in sternal recumbency by grasping a large section of the scruff and placing the legs firmly on a table.
   Rationale: If the ferret feels secure, it will be less likely to try to escape.

2. **Action:** Extend one of the forelegs towards the veterinary surgeon with the elbow in the palm of your hand.
   Rationale: This is the same position as is used in the dog or the cat.

3. **Action:** Place the thumb of this hand across the crook of the ferret's elbow and apply gentle pressure.
   Rationale: This pressure will cause the cephalic vein to dilate and become more obvious.

4. **Action:** Gently rotate your thumb outwards.
   Rationale: This completes the dilation of the vein.

5. **Action:** The veterinary surgeon will clip a small area over the cephalic vein and prepare it aseptically.
   Rationale: To prevent the introduction of infection into the vein.

6. **Action:** The veterinary surgeon will select a 23G needle and a small syringe filled with the drug to be administered and insert the needle through the skin and into the vein.
   Rationale: Use a small-gauge needle as the vein has a narrow diameter.

7. **Action:** The veterinary surgeon will draw back on the syringe.
   Rationale: To check that the needle is in the lumen of the vein.

8. **Action:** If blood appears at the hub of the needle, the veterinary surgeon will inject the drug slowly into the vein.
   Rationale: Drugs given by the intravenous route are instantly absorbed.

9. **Action:** When the procedure is complete, you should apply gentle pressure over the injection site while the veterinary surgeon slowly withdraws the needle.
   Rationale: This pressure prevents haemorrhage into the surrounding tissues.

10. **Action:** Dress the site appropriately.
    Rationale: To prevent infection and self-mutilation of the wound.

N.B.: The lateral saphenous vein running over the lateral aspect of the hock may also be used. If intravenous fluid therapy is to be given, place a catheter into the cephalic, saphenous or jugular vein. Blood samples can also be collected from these veins.

GENERAL ANAESTHESIA

Procedure: Induction of anaesthesia

1. **Action:** Starve the ferret for 4–6 hours before anaesthesia but allow free access to water.

   Rationale: Ferrets are able to vomit, so it is important to ensure that the stomach is empty. Older ferrets should not be starved for longer than 2 hours, as there is a risk of an insulinoma precipitating a hypoglycaemic attack. Access to water should minimize dehydration.

2. **Action:** Weigh and examine the animal before giving the anaesthetic.

   Rationale: This provides an accurate weight from which to calculate your dose and guarantees that there are no underlying problems that may affect the anaesthetic.

3. **Action:** Atropine given subcutaneously or intramuscularly and famotidine given orally can be used as a premed.

   Rationale: Atropine reduces salivation and gastrointestinal secretions and minimizes cardiac arrhythmias. Famotidine reduces the risk of stress-induced gastric ulceration.

4. **Action:** If inducing anaesthesia by using an inhalation agent such as isoflurane or sevoflurane given by mask, premedicate with a sedative such as midazolam first.

   Rationale: This reduces the stress of inhalation induction, which can cause anaesthetic problems and gastric ulceration.

5. **Action:** Induction can also be achieved by using an appropriate injectable agent, e.g. ketamine and medetomidine given by the correct route.

   Rationale: Do not use injectable agents in sick or debilitated patients.

6. **Action:** Once the ferret is anaesthetized, intubate with a 1.5–3.0 mm uncuffed endotracheal tube.

   Rationale: This is an easy procedure as the ferret is able to open its mouth wide for visualization of the larynx. Ferrets do not seem to suffer from laryngospasm.

Procedure: Maintenance and monitoring of anaesthesia

1. **Action:** To maintain the anaesthetic, use a non-rebreathing circuit delivering isoflurane or sevoflurane.

   Rationale: The type of circuit must be appropriate to the size of the animal.

2. **Action:** During anaesthesia, make sure that the ferret is kept warm by placing on a heat pad or wrapping in 'bubble wrap' or a 'space blanket'.

   Rationale: Hypothermia may be a problem as the ferret has a large surface area in relation to its bodyweight and thus loses heat very rapidly.

3. **Action:** Monitor the hydration status of the patient.

   Rationale: Give intravenous fluids to sick or debilitated animals during surgery.

4. **Action:** Monitor the depth of anaesthesia by assessing respiratory rate and depth, heart rate, jaw tone, withdrawal and palpebral reflexes.

   Rationale: Response to anaesthesia is similar to that of the cat.

5. **Action:** If the procedure is painful or likely to be painful, provide analgesia such as buprenorphine and a non-steroidal anti-inflammatory drug.

   Rationale: Pre-emptive analgesia, i.e. that given before the onset of pain, is the most effective. The use of analgesics reduces the dose of anaesthetic required and increases the rate of recovery post-operatively.

Procedure: Post-operative care

1. **Action:** After the surgical procedure is complete, place the patient in a secure, warm cage in a quiet, warm, darkened room and cover with a towel, blanket, 'bubble wrap' or a 'space blanket,' as appropriate.

   Rationale: Hypothermia during recovery can be fatal. Any noise or bright light will overstimulate a recovering animal.

2. **Action:** Observe the patient quietly and unobtrusively.

   Rationale: Ferrets do not appreciate being touched or talked to. Look at the animal from a distance and only interfere if it is really necessary.

3. **Action:** Monitor the core temperature.

   Rationale: To be aware of hypothermia before it becomes critical.

4. **Action:** Monitor respiration.

   Rationale: Respiratory depression or arrest may also occur during the recovery period.

5. **Action:** If the patient shows signs of pain, e.g. vocalization, aggression or hunched position, provide additional analgesia.

   Rationale: Any procedure that would cause pain in any other species should be considered to cause pain in the ferret and would warrant the use of analgesics. Correct use of analgesics, e.g. flunixin or buprenorphine, will do no harm.

6. **Action:** Continue to monitor the patient after it has regained consciousness.
   Rationale: Observe whether the animal is eating or drinking. Note the production of faeces and urine.
7. **Action:** Instruct the owner of the warning signs to watch out for when the patient is taken home.
   Rationale: The owner should monitor the patient for at least 24 hours after the surgical procedure.

CAGE AND AVIARY BIRDS

HANDLING AND RESTRAINT

Procedure: To capture and restrain a bird

1. **Action:** Make sure that all doors and windows are closed and that the extractor fans are turned off.
   Rationale: If the bird escapes from its cage, it will not be able to get out of the room or be injured in the extractor fan.
2. **Action:** Remove all movable objects, e.g. perches, feeding bowls, toys, from the cage.
   Rationale: This makes capture quicker and easier, and therefore less stressful for the bird.
3. **Action:** Turn the lights off or, if possible, dim them. Use a small hand torch covered in a red or blue filter for illumination.
   Rationale: Most common species of cage and aviary birds are active in daylight. A dim light will simulate night and induce quiet behaviour. Birds do not see well in red or blue light.
4. **Action:** Tip the cage on its side.
   Rationale: This enables you to approach the bird from the bottom of the cage and provides more room for manoeuvre.
5. **Action:** Approach the bird slowly.
   Rationale: This avoids causing air movement, which will startle the bird.
6. **Action:** Quickly grab the bird around its neck or close your hands around the wings and body, creating a 'net' (Fig. 13.16).
   Rationale: It is important to catch the bird quickly, firmly and gently to avoid causing distress. Closing your hands around the body holds the wings closed and prevents them flapping and possibly breaking. This method can be used to catch small psittacine birds, e.g. budgerigars and lovebirds, and others such as canaries and finches.

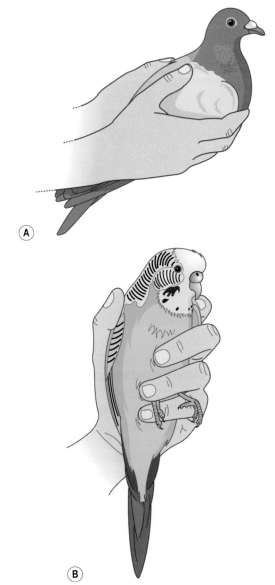

Fig. 13.16 Handling small birds. A, A pigeon held in the hands. Note how the two hands encompass the wings and prevent the bird from flapping. B, A budgerigar in the hand. Note how the fingers form a 'net' around the bird: undue pressure must not be applied.

7. **Action:** Wear clean, strong gloves if catching larger birds such as cockatoos and macaws (Fig. 13.17).
   Rationale: These birds have vicious beaks. The use of gloves when handling small birds is not recommended as it reduces your sense of touch.

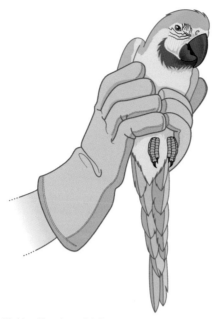

Fig. 13.17 Handling large birds.

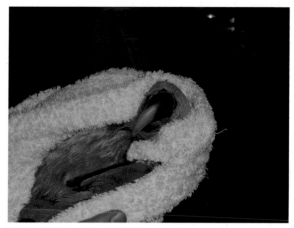

Fig. 13.18 Restraining a bird in a towel.

Procedure: To capture a bird using the towel method

1. **Action:** Select a suitable towel.
   Rationale: A hand towel is about the right size.
2. **Action:** Drape the towel over one hand.
   Rationale: This disguises your hand.
3. **Action:** Advance your towelled hand towards the bird and trap it in a corner of the cage.
   a. *Rationale: Trap the bird as quickly as possible. Making several attempts to catch the bird causes fear and distress and may damage the wings and plumage (Fig. 13.18).*
4. **Action:** Catch hold of the bird by the neck.
   Rationale: The bird cannot bite you if the head and neck are controlled. There is very little chance of you strangling the bird because your hand is covered in the towel, which reduces the pressure you are able to apply.
5. **Action:** Taking your hand out of the towel, place your thumb and forefinger over the temporomandibular joint on either side of the head.
   Rationale: This prevents the bird from biting you.
6. **Action:** Take care with larger psittacines, e.g. macaws and cockatoos.
   Rationale: These species can deliver a nasty bite.
N.B.: If you are bitten you can try:

- Blowing on the bird's face
- Squeezing the top of the bird's head
- As a last resort, open the beak with whelping forceps – take care, as you may damage the beak
- Avoid pulling your finger out of the beak as it is curved, and you may lose a chunk of flesh!

It is often better if owners are not present during capture and treatment, as the more intelligent species will associate their experience with the owner.

Procedure: To clip the wings

This procedure is controversial, particularly in cage birds such as parrots. Clipping does not prevent flying completely and should be viewed as a short-term measure to allow training of the bird. Birds such as parrots can climb.

1. **Action:** Ask an assistant to restrain the bird and extend one wing in turn.
   Rationale: Both wings are clipped.
2. **Action:** Primary feathers 5–10 are clipped using a small pair of sharp scissors. Blood feathers should not be cut.
   Rationale: This reduces the chance of damage – splintered feather ends can induce feather plucking. Blood feathers will bleed, and if one or more are found in the area to be clipped, the clip should be deferred.
3. **Action:** The bird should be flight-tested.
   Rationale: If the bird can fly more than 7.5 metres, another primary is cut.

Procedure: To clip the claws

1. **Action:** Use bird nail clippers or small cat nail clippers to cut the nail from side to side.
   Rationale: This squeezes the nail over the artery and reduces haemorrhage.
2. **Action:** Clip small amounts off each nail until they are the right length or until bleeding starts.
   Rationale: The artery is often near the end of the nail.
3. **Action:** Control any bleeding with silver nitrate sticks or potassium permanganate.

ADMINISTRATION OF MEDICINES

Procedure: To administer oral fluid via a crop tube

1. **Action:** Select some form of metal catheter or crop tube and attach to the end of a syringe filled with warmed fluid.
   Rationale: Metal crop tubing catheters are available, but a Spreull needle can be used. Plastic and rubber tubing may be bitten through.
2. **Action:** Place the crop tube against the bird and mark the approximate area of the crop with a felt or ball-point pen.
   Rationale: This measures the length of crop tube that must be inserted down the oesophagus to reach the crop. Ingesta travel from the mouth down the oesophagus into the crop, which is a diverticulum of the oesophagus, lying outside the body cavity in the ventral part of the neck (Fig. 13.19).
3. **Action:** Lubricate the crop tube.
   Rationale: To facilitate the passage of the crop tube down the oesophagus. K-Y jelly is a suitable lubricant.
4. **Action:** Restrain the bird by the neck.
   Rationale: You may need an assistant to hold the wings close to the body.
5. **Action:** Insert the crop tube on the left side at the junction of the upper and lower beak (Fig. 13.19). Extend the neck as you advance the tube.
   Rationale: Extending the neck stretches the oesophagus, making placement easier.
6. **Action:** Direct the tube upwards towards the roof of the oropharynx and then down towards the oesophagus.
   Rationale: This ensures that the tube does not enter the glottis and trachea of the bird. Birds have a poor cough reflex and may asphyxiate or develop pneumonia if fluid enters the lungs or air sacs. Using a tube that is wider than the glottis may help to prevent incorrect positioning.

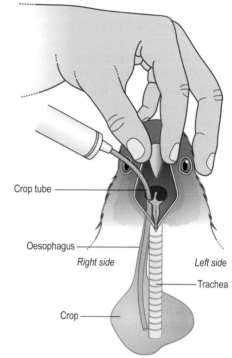

Fig. 13.19 Crop tubing a parrot.

7. **Action:** Advance the crop tube down the right dorsal side of the oesophagus until it enters the crop.
   Rationale: The crop lies on the right side of the neck. The end of the tube can be palpated when it enters the crop. In fledglings, the tube can be seen passing down the oesophagus.
8. **Action:** Slowly administer an appropriate volume of fluid.
   Rationale: Slow infusion prevents the fluid refluxing up the oesophagus.
9. **Action:** Slowly withdraw the crop tube and observe the patient.
   Rationale: Slow withdrawal prevents damage to the tissues. It is important to observe the patient for adverse reactions.

Procedure: Intramuscular injection

1. **Action:** Restrain the bird so that it cannot struggle, holding its wings close to the body.
   Rationale: Small birds such as finches can be restrained and injected single-handedly but be aware of the pressure that you are applying around the chest as this may restrict respiration. You may need an assistant to restrain larger species while you inject.

2. **Action:** Identify the pectoral muscles forming the breast of the bird. Select an area in the caudal part of the muscle group.
   Rationale: The pectoral muscles form the largest area of muscle in the bird.

3. **Action:** Using a sterile 23–25G needle and a syringe of an appropriate size, part the feathers and introduce the needle into the muscle.
   Rationale: Feathers should never be plucked unless it is essential. They will only grow back at the next moult, and this may take months. Lack of feathers may affect insulation, flight and appearance, depending on the site and the species.

4. **Action:** Draw back on the syringe.
   Rationale: To check that you have not penetrated a blood vessel.

5. **Action:** If no blood appears in the hub of the needle, inject the drug.
   Rationale: Drugs are rapidly absorbed from this site. Absorption from subcutaneous injections is slow, so intramuscular injections are more commonly performed.

6. **Action:** Withdraw the needle and apply pressure over the site.
   Rationale: To prevent haemorrhage into the surrounding tissues. Birds bleed readily from injection sites.

Procedure: Intravenous injection

1. **Action:** Restrain the bird in the appropriate position to expose the vein. Ask an assistant to hold the head or hold the mask if the patient is anaesthetized. The following veins may be used for venepuncture:
   - Brachial (or basilic) vein – on the medial side of the elbow within the wing (Fig. 13.20)
   - Jugular vein – on either side of the neck. The right jugular vein is larger than the left (Fig. 13.21)
   - Medial metatarsal – on the caudal aspect of the leg. Easily visualized in larger species.

2. **Action:** Wet the feathers to enable the vein to be more easily visualized.
   Rationale: Avoid plucking the feathers to expose the vein. New feathers will not grow back until the next moult. Loss of feathers may affect the bird's ability to fly or to keep warm. In show birds, it may affect their appearance.

3. **Action:** Prepare the site aseptically.
   Rationale: To prevent the introduction of infection.

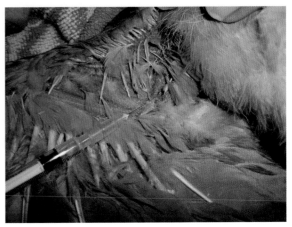

Fig. 13.20 Using the brachial vein in the wing to give an intravenous injection.

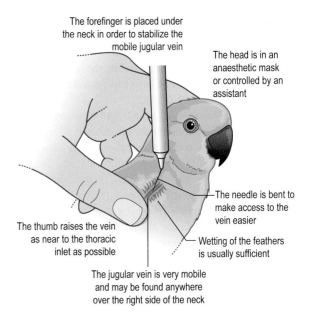

The forefinger is placed under the neck in order to stabilize the mobile jugular vein

The head is in an anaesthetic mask or controlled by an assistant

The needle is bent to make access to the vein easier

Wetting of the feathers is usually sufficient

The thumb raises the vein as near to the thoracic inlet as possible

The jugular vein is very mobile and may be found anywhere over the right side of the neck

Fig. 13.21 Using the right jugular vein to give an intravenous injection. (Redrawn from Beynon and Forbes (1996), BSAVA.)

4. **Action:** Raise the vein by applying pressure at the base of the right side of the neck (jugular), proximal to the injection site on the upper wing (brachial) or around the lower leg (median metatarsal).
   Rationale: Veins carry blood towards the heart. Pressure applied between the chosen site and the heart will prevent venous return and cause the vein to dilate or be 'raised'.

5. **Action:** Insert a small needle at an angle into the vein and draw back on the syringe. If using the jugular vein, you may need to bend the needle (Figs 13.20 and 13.21).
   Rationale: To check that the needle has penetrated the vein. Bending the needle facilitates access to the jugular vein.
6. **Action:** If blood appears in the hub of the needle, inject the drug slowly.
   Rationale: If the drug is injected too quickly, the pressure may cause it to spurt out of the hub of the needle.
7. **Action:** If the injection is to be repeated or if fluid is to be given intravenously, an indwelling 20G catheter can be inserted into the jugular vein.
   Rationale: This prevents damage to the vein by repeated injection.
8. **Action:** Suture or glue the catheter in place and cover with a light dressing.
   Rationale: It is important that the catheter does not become dislodged by the bird's movement or by self-mutilation.

Procedure: Intraosseous injection

1. **Action:** This should be performed under anaesthesia.
   Rationale: This is a painful procedure.
2. **Action:** The optimum site for an intraosseous injection is the ulna or the proximal tibiotarsus.
   Rationale: These bones have a medullary cavity from which fluid can be rapidly absorbed.
3. **Action:** Prepare the site aseptically.
   Rationale: To prevent the introduction of infection. Avoid plucking the feathers to expose the site. New feathers will not grow back until the next moult. Loss of feathers may affect the bird's ability to fly or to keep warm. In show birds, it may affect their appearance.
4. **Action:** Select a 20–22G needle.
   Rationale: This size will be able to enter the medullary cavity.
5. **Action:** Introduce the needle into the bone and flush with heparinized saline.
   Rationale: The saline will flush out any blood or bony tissue that accumulates as the needle is pushed through the cortex of the bone.
6. **Action:** Connect to a syringe or to a giving set and bag of fluid.
   Rationale: This procedure can be used to administer a bolus of fluid or for continuous infusion.

7. **Action:** Calculate the fluid requirement:

   Maintenance volume $= 75$ ml/kg bodyweight
   Fluid deficit of $4 - 10\% = 40 - 10$ml/Kg bodyweight replaced over 48 hours

   Rationale: The majority of ill birds are dehydrated. Birds that are dehydrated and anorexic may suffer from a metabolic acidosis – correct this with lactated Ringer's (Hartmann's) solution.
8. **Action:** Set the fluid running at the required drip rate.
   Rationale: Volumes required are usually small.
9. **Action:** Cover the site with a bandage.
   Rationale: It is important that the needle or catheter is not dislodged by the bird's movement or by self-mutilation.

Procedure: To collect a blood sample

1. **Action:** Restrain the bird on its back on a soft surface with one wing extended – if you are right-handed, use the right wing.
   Rationale: The site for collecting a reasonable sample of blood is the brachial vein, which lies on the ventral aspect of the wing, distal to the elbow (Fig. 13.20). A small sample can be collected by clipping a toenail. Small samples can be used for sexing the bird, but the cells are often distorted, which may affect haematological studies.
2. **Action:** Wet the feathers over the site.
   Rationale: This enables you to see the vein more clearly. Avoid plucking the feathers to expose the vein. New feathers will not grow back until the next moult. Loss of feathers may affect the bird's ability to fly or to keep warm. In show birds, it may affect their appearance.
3. **Action:** Prepare the site aseptically.
   Rationale: To prevent the introduction of infection.
4. **Action:** Place the first and second finger of the left hand on the mid-distal humerus with the palm on the carpus of the wing.
   Rationale: This keeps the wing extended and restrained.
5. **Action:** Raise the vein with the thumb of your left hand.
   Rationale: Your right hand is free for sample collection.
6. **Action:** Select a 23–27G needle and a 1 ml syringe.

Rationale: The needle must be able to enter the vein but must not be so small that it impedes the flow of blood and damages the red cells, leading to haemolysis of the sample.

7. **Action:** Flush the needle and syringe with dilute heparin (1:100) before use.
   Rationale: This prevents the blood from clotting if the sample collection is slow.

8. **Action:** Introduce the needle into the vein and draw back on the syringe.
   Rationale: If blood appears at the hub of the needle, the needle is correctly positioned in the vein.

9. **Action:** Collect the blood sample.

10. **Action:** Withdraw the needle, applying gentle pressure over the site for 2–3 minutes as you do so.
    Rationale: This prevents haematoma formation.

N.B.: The jugular vein can also be used for blood sampling.

GENERAL ANAESTHESIA

Procedure: Induction of anaesthesia

1. **Action:** Do not starve birds that are less than 120 g in weight. Large psittacines may be starved for 1–2 hours. Fruit-eaters and waterfowl should be starved for 4–10 hours.
   Rationale: Starvation in small birds may cause a fatal hypoglycaemia and increase the anaesthetic risk. Grain-eaters, e.g. psittacines, seldom regurgitate.

2. **Action:** Make sure that all equipment is ready before you start the procedure.
   Rationale: The procedure should run as smoothly and as quickly as possible to reduce stress to the patient and thus reduce anaesthetic risk.

3. **Action:** Handle the bird as little as possible.
   Rationale: To reduce stress.

4. **Action:** Induce anaesthesia by using a mask and an inhalation agent, e.g. isoflurane or sevoflurane, or by using an injectable agent.
   Rationale: For dose rates, see Table 13.7.

5. **Action:** Intubate the bird. This should be done for all but very short procedures.
   Rationale: Use an uncuffed tube as birds have complete tracheal rings that may be ruptured by inflation of the cuff. Intubation protects the airway and allows intermittent positive pressure ventilation to be performed if necessary. Psittacines have large fleshy tongues that obscure the view of the glottis, making intubation difficult – use a tongue depressor.

6. **Action:** Attach to an appropriate type of anaesthetic circuit.
   Rationale: The circuit should provide low resistance, particularly for small birds.

Procedure: Maintenance and monitoring of anaesthesia

1. **Action:** Maintain anaesthesia using an inhalation agent, e.g. isoflurane or sevoflurane (Table 13.7).

TABLE 13.7 **Anaesthetic agents for use in birds**	
Anaesthetic agent	**Comments**
Mask induction is usually performed. It is quick and effective due to the bird's respiratory system; most birds can then be intubated	
Halothane	This is no longer considered a safe anaesthetic for birds
Isoflurane	Induction 3–5%; maintenance 1.5–2%; rapid induction and recovery
Sevoflurane	Induction 5–8%; maintenance 2–4%; more rapid recovery than isoflorane but considerably more expensive
Diazepam	Can be used as a premedication to reduce stress on induction: 0.2–0.5 mg/kg IM; 0.05–0.15 mg/kg IV
Midazolam	Can be used as a premedication to reduce stress on induction: 0.1–0.5 mg/kg IM; 0.05–0.15 mg/kg IV
Ketamine/diazepam	Can be given to large birds IV to induce anaesthesia: Ketamine: 30–40 mg/kg Diazepam: 1–1.5 mg/kg; inject slowly

IM, intramuscularly; IV, intravenously.

Rationale: If an injectable agent has been used, supplement with oxygen via a mask or endotracheal tube.

2. **Action:** Flow rate through the circuit should be three times the minute volume.
   Rationale: Flow rate is approximately 3 ml/g bodyweight and should not be less than 0.75 l/min. A high flow rate prevents hypercapnia.

3. **Action:** At all times, ensure that the patient is warm. Use a heat pad or wrap in 'bubble wrap' or a 'space blanket'.
   Rationale: Birds have a high core temperature of 40–44°C due to a high metabolic rate.

4. **Action:** Assess the need for fluid therapy. If necessary, give intravenously or by intraosseous injection, as previously described.
   Rationale: Ill birds are often dehydrated, and provision of fluid will increase the chances of recovery.

5. **Action:** Monitor the depth of anaesthesia using appropriate reflexes.
   Rationale: Toe, cere and wing reflexes are lost on a medium plane, palpebral reflex is lost on a deeper plane and the corneal reflex is lost when the bird is very deeply anaesthetized.

6. **Action:** Monitor respiration.
   Rationale: The rate and depth of respiration decrease as anaesthesia deepens. The rate should not fall below half the normal resting rate. The respiratory pattern should remain stable.

7. **Action:** Monitor the heart rate.
   Rationale: Use a cardiac monitor or an oesophageal stethoscope. Heart rate is a good indicator of pain – it increases when the bird feels pain.

8. **Action:** Place electrocardiography leads over the distal tarsometatarsus and carpal joints of each wing.
   Rationale: To monitor the rate and pattern of the heartbeat.

Procedure: Post-operative care

1. **Action:** After the surgical procedure is complete, remove the endotracheal tube and wrap the bird in a towel.
   Rationale: This keeps the bird warm and prevents the wings from flapping during recovery, causing possible damage. If isoflurane is used, the bird can be allowed to recover slowly in your hands before being placed in its cage.

2. **Action:** Place the bird into its own cage to recover in a warm, quiet, darkened room.
   Rationale: Remove all portable object such as toys, feeding bowls and perches to facilitate handling of the bird if necessary. If the bird is placed in a normal recovery cage, it will have to be caught to place it back into its own cage – this increases the stress to the bird.

3. **Action:** Keep the bird under discreet observation.
   Rationale: Many problems can develop during the recovery period. Birds do not need to be talked to or touched.

4. **Action:** Continue to monitor the bird's progress for a few days after the operation.
   Rationale: It is important that the bird begins to eat and drink. Small birds cannot survive for long without a source of energy.

5. **Action:** If necessary, feed the bird using a crop tube as previously described.
   Rationale: To prevent the onset of dehydration and hypoglycaemia.

REPTILES

ZOONOSES

All species should be handled with care as many reptiles are known to carry zoonotic diseases. Infection by *Salmonella* spp. is the most common. It is difficult to determine whether or not an individual is infected as the bacteria may be shed intermittently in the faeces, and bacterial culture may not detect all species. *Salmonella* is spread by ingestion of the faeces, so although careful handling is not a risk, you must wash your hands after touching any reptile species.

As a general rule, the species of reptile most commonly kept as pets can be handled safely. However, precautions should be taken when handling venomous species. Large constrictors such as pythons should not be handled on your own as you might need assistance if they wind themselves around your arm or your neck.

SNAKES

Procedure: To restrain a snake

1. **Action:** Ask the owner if the snake is used to being handled.
   Rationale: This gives an indication of the response the snake may have to being handled and examined.

2. **Action:** A snake should be transported in a soft bag that is closed securely by doubling over the top and then tying it.
   Rationale: Bumping against the hard surfaces of a cage or box can easily damage a snake. Snakes are very good at pushing through loosely tied knots. A pillowcase makes a good snake bag.
3. **Action:** Avoid wearing gloves when handling snakes.
   Rationale: Wearing gloves makes it difficult to appreciate the pressure you are putting on the snake and may result in damage to the animal.
4. **Action:** Open the bag or vivarium and look inside.
   Rationale: This helps you to locate the position of the snake's head.
5. **Action:** If the snake is tame, pick it up gently around the body and lift it from the bag or the vivarium. Snakes over 2 metres in length must be lifted by two people.
   Rationale: Handle gently but positively. Snakes bruise easily but, as they have a slow metabolism, the injury may not show for several weeks. A snake may die from severe bruising.
6. **Action:** Avoid making sudden movements or waving your hand in front of the snake.
   Rationale: This may cause the snake to strike.
7. **Action:** As soon as possible, support the body and allow the snake to move around.
   Rationale: Never suspend the body by the head – snakes have a single occipital condyle, and the neck is easily broken. Use minimal restraint. Snakes do not like being held tightly or being stretched out.
8. **Action:** If further restraint is needed, place a finger and thumb on either side of the head and one finger on the top of the head (Fig. 13.22). Support the body with your other hand.
   Rationale: In this position, the snake is prevented from biting.
9. **Action:** To handle more aggressive or vicious snakes, use a towel. Move the towel towards the snake and catch the snake behind the head with your towel-covered hand.
   Rationale: If the snake strikes, it will hit the towel. Snake hooks can be used.

Procedure: To administer fluids or liquid medication

1. **Action:** Select and lubricate a 5–8F catheter.
   Rationale: The type used for dogs and cats is appropriate. Lubrication aids the introduction of the catheter.

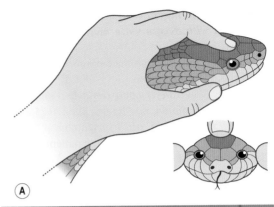

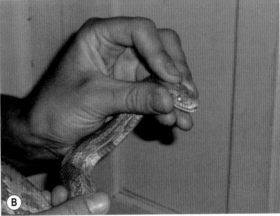

Fig. 13.22 Restraining the head of a snake.

2. **Action:** Lay the catheter along the outside of the snake. Mark the approximate position of the stomach on the catheter using a ballpoint pen.
   Rationale: The stomach lies approximately halfway down the length of the snake.
3. **Action:** Select an appropriate size of syringe and fill with fluid.
   Rationale: It is good practice to have all equipment ready before you begin to handle the snake as this reduces the stress caused by the procedure.
4. **Action:** With the snake on a table, restrain the head and open the mouth using a blunt metal spatula.
   Rationale: Snakes' teeth are very sharp and may point backwards in some species. They are also very dirty, and any bite may become infected. Take steps to avoid being bitten.
5. **Action:** Use a mouth gag if necessary.
   Rationale: Most snakes will open their mouths quite easily when gentle pressure is applied. Make a gag by folding a small piece of radiographic film and

cutting a hole in the centre. The catheter is passed through the hole.

6. **Action:** Support the weight of the body on the table or ask an assistant to help you.

    Rationale: Never suspend the body by the head – snakes have a single occipital condyle, and the neck is easily broken.

7. **Action:** Slowly insert the catheter into the back of the mouth and down the oesophagus.

    Rationale: The glottis, which leads to the trachea and lungs, sits forward in the oral cavity to avoid asphyxiation when the snake is swallowing prey. It is easy to see, and there is little risk of the catheter entering it.

8. **Action:** Insert the catheter to the level of the stomach.

    Rationale: The ballpoint pen mark will lie at the level of the mouth.

9. **Action:** Introduce the fluid in the syringe slowly.

    Rationale: If you introduce the fluid too quickly, the pressure applied may cause the fluid to spurt out of the junction with the syringe.

10. **Action:** Gently withdraw the catheter and observe the snake.

    Rationale: To check that there are no adverse effects.

Procedure: Intravenous injection or blood sampling

1. **Action:** Restrain the snake appropriately.

    Rationale: The site for intravenous injection is the ventral venous sinus in the midline of the ventral tail (Fig. 13.23). The jugular vein can be used but may require a surgical cut-down. The palatine veins can be seen when the mouth is open, but the snake must be anaesthetized or sedated if these are used.

2. **Action:** Prepare the site aseptically using povidone-iodine or 70% ethanol.

    Rationale: To prevent the introduction of infection.

3. **Action:** Select a small needle and syringe.

    Rationale: The needle must be small enough to enter the vein.

4. **Action:** Insert the needle between the paired caudal scales distal to the cloaca. Angle the needle at a 45° angle to the tail. Draw back on the syringe.

    Rationale: In the male, care must be taken to avoid damaging the hemipenes, which lie here. If blood appears in the hub of the needle, the needle is correctly positioned in the vein.

5. **Action:** Collect the sample into a lithium heparin tube.

    Rationale: EDTA lyses the cells.

6. **Action:** A drop of blood can be used to make a blood smear.

    Rationale: This is useful for haematology.

7. **Action:** If injecting intravenously, slowly inject the drug into the vein.

8. **Action:** Withdraw the needle.

N.B.: The total volume of blood is approximately 5–8% of bodyweight. This is about 70 ml/kg, and 10% of this can be collected in one withdrawal.

Sites for the Administration of Parenteral Drugs

- Subcutaneous – under the loose skin over the ribs
- Intramuscular – into the longissimus muscles parallel to spine.

Injections may be given into the tail, but snakes have a renal portal venous system in which blood flows from the hind end of the body to the kidneys before returning to the heart. Any drug injected into the hind end may be eliminated by the kidneys without being absorbed. Nephrotoxic drugs must not be injected into the hind end.

CHELONIANS

These are the shelled reptiles, e.g. tortoises and terrapins.

Procedure: To restrain a tortoise or terrapin

1. **Action:** Consider the species you are to handle.

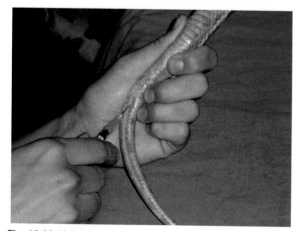

Fig. 13.23 Using the ventral venous sinus in the tail to give an intravenous injection.

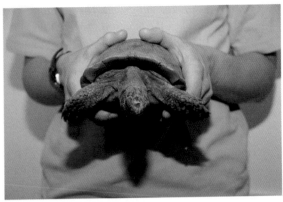

Fig. 13.24 How to pick up a tortoise.

Rationale: Most tortoises are non-aggressive and used to being handled. They may withdraw into their shells. Some species of terrapin, particularly the snapping turtle, are aggressive and may bite rather than withdraw into their shells.

2. **Action:** Pick a tortoise up by placing both hands around the middle of the shell or carapace and supporting the whole body (Fig. 13.24).

   Rationale: Some individuals can be heavy. Watch out for the hind legs, which may push against your hands and push the body out of your grip.

3. **Action:** If handling a terrapin, wear plastic gloves.

   Rationale: Terrapins are known to carry Salmonella, and you should take precautions to protect yourself from this zoonosis. This is important if you have to remove the animal from water.

4. **Action:** Pick a terrapin up by placing your hands at the rear of the carapace just cranial to the hind legs. To achieve a better grip, place your fingers into the inguinal area.

   Rationale: This will prevent the terrapin from biting your fingers. If the terrapin has been in water, it will be slippery. Some terrapins also have long claws, which can scratch.

5. **Action:** More aggressive individuals, e.g. snapping turtles, can be restrained in a towel while you move your hands towards the back of the carapace.

   Rationale: The towel will cover the head, preventing the animal from biting.

6. **Action:** Soft-shelled terrapins should be handled wearing leather gloves.

   Rationale: To prevent damage to the carapace and to prevent you being bitten.

7. **Action:** In any species of chelonian, extend the head by placing your finger and thumb behind the occipital condyle and pulling slowly against the action of the retractor muscles of the neck.

   Rationale: Gentle but firm and constant pressure must be applied. The muscles will become tired and relax. Holding a tortoise with its forelegs against the shell and its body downwards may induce the head to come out far enough for you to grasp it.

8. **Action:** Forcing the hind legs into the inguinal region may bring the head and forelegs out.

   Rationale: The use of padded forceps may help extraction of the head but be careful not to cause any damage.

Procedure: To administer fluids or liquid medication

1. **Action:** Select an appropriate type of stomach tube and lubricate it.

   Rationale: Tubes designed for use in chelonians can be obtained, but small dog catheters may also be used.

2. **Action:** Calculate the required dose of fluid or medication and fill a syringe of an appropriate size.

   Rationale: It is good practice to have all equipment ready before you begin to handle the tortoise as this reduces the stress caused by the procedure.

3. **Action:** Holding the tortoise on its back for a short time, place the tube along the length of the plastron and mark the approximate position of the stomach on the tube using a ballpoint pen (Fig. 13.25).

   Rationale: The stomach lies under the abdominal scute of the plastron. Lay the tube from the gular notch to the caudal border of the abdominal scute (Fig. 13.25).

4. **Action:** Restrain the tortoise so that it is resting on its caudal scutes and extend the head and neck.

   Rationale: If the patient withdraws into its shell, you may need to ask for assistance.

5. **Action:** Pull the mandible down with one finger and insert your index finger into the commissure of the lips (Fig. 13.26).

   Rationale: Your index finger acts as a gag. Tortoises have a beak but no teeth and placing your finger at the angle of the lips is unlikely to be painful for you.

6. **Action:** Slide the lubricated tube towards the back of the mouth, down the oesophagus and into the stomach (Fig. 13.27).

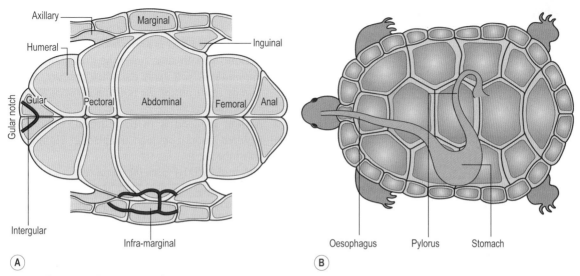

Fig. 13.25 The position of the stomach in relation to the scutes of A, the plastron and B, the carapace of a tortoise.

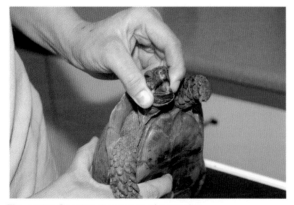

Fig. 13.26 Opening the mouth of a tortoise.

> *Rationale: The glottis is easy to see and to avoid. You will feel the tube pass through the cardiac sphincter into the stomach. The ballpoint pen mark will lie at the mouth.*

7. **Action:** Introduce the fluid in the syringe slowly.
   > *Rationale: If you introduce the fluid too quickly, the pressure applied may cause the fluid to spurt out of the junction with the syringe.*

8. **Action:** Gently withdraw the catheter and observe the patient.
   > *Rationale: To check that there are no adverse effects.*

N.B.: This method is suitable for all types of chelonian.

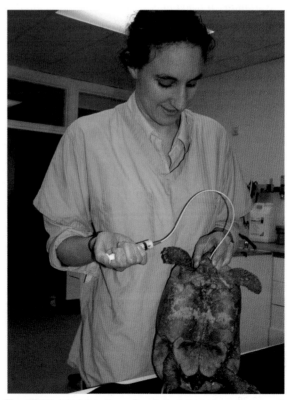

Fig. 13.27 Administration of anthelminthics to a tortoise via stomach tube.

Procedure: Intravenous injection or blood sampling

1. **Action:** Restrain the tortoise appropriately. You may need an assistant to hold the body.
   Rationale: The sites most commonly used in chelonians are the jugular vein and the dorsal venous sinus. If an assistant is not available, you can hold the shell between your knees.
2. **Action:** To use the jugular vein, extend the head and extend the neck fully by placing your finger and thumb behind the occipital condyle and pulling slowly against the action of the retractor muscles of the neck.
   Rationale: The jugular vein runs from the level of the eardrum to the base of the neck and may be visible (Fig. 13.28).
3. **Action:** Ask your assistant to raise the vein by applying pressure at the base of the neck.
   Rationale: The jugular vein carries blood from the head and neck towards the heart.
4. **Action:** Insert a small needle parallel to the neck, pointing towards the body (Fig. 13.28), and draw back on the syringe.
   Rationale: If blood appears in the hub of the needle, the needle is correctly placed.
5. **Action:** To use the dorsal venous sinus, extend the tail fully.
   Rationale: The vein is located in the dorsal midline of the tail.
6. **Action:** Insert a small needle in the exact midline at an angle of 45° and advance the needle until it touches the bone. Aspirate the syringe and withdraw the needle slightly until blood appears in the hub of the needle.

Rationale: At first the needle goes through the sinus, but as you withdraw the needle, it re-enters the sinus and blood is aspirated.

7. **Action:** At both sites, inject the drug slowly.
   Rationale: If you apply too much pressure, the drug may spurt out of the junction between the needle and syringe.
8. **Action:** If blood is to be collected, withdraw the required amount of blood and place in a lithium heparin tube.
   Rationale: EDTA lyses the blood cells.
9. **Action:** After the procedure is complete, withdraw the needle and apply gentle pressure over the site.
   Rationale: To prevent the formation of a haematoma.

N.B.: The total volume of blood is approx. 5–8% of body-weight. This is about 70 ml/kg, and 10% of this can be collected in one withdrawal.

Sites for the Administration of Parenteral Drugs

- Subcutaneous – use the loose skin around the neck
- Intramuscular – triceps muscle in the forelimb; pectoral muscles at the angle of the forelimb and neck; muscles of the hindlimb.

Injections may be given into the hindlimb, but chelonians have a renal portal venous system in which blood flows from the hindlimbs to the kidneys before returning to the heart. Any drug injected into the hindlimbs and tail may be eliminated by the kidneys without being absorbed. Nephrotoxic drugs must not be injected into the hindlimb.

LIZARDS

Procedure: To restrain a lizard

1. **Action:** Identify the species of lizard and ask the owner whether it is used to being handled.
   Rationale: There are many species of lizard commonly kept as pets. They vary in size and in nature. Most are amenable to handling but some, notably the Tokay gecko, are aggressive. There are only two venomous lizards – Heloderma suspectum (the Gila monster) and Heloderma horridum (the beaded lizard) – but neither is particularly aggressive.
2. **Action:** Place your hand around the shoulders and lift the animal clear of the cage.

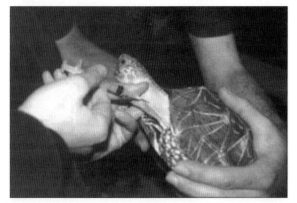
Fig. 13.28 Intravenous injection in a tortoise using the jugular vein.

Rationale: Never lift a lizard by the tail. Many species are able to shed their tails as a means of defence – a process known as autotomy. The tail will regrow, but it never looks the same again.

3. **Action:** Restrain the lizard by placing one hand around the pectoral girdle and the other around the pelvic girdle and hind legs. Hold the hind legs against the tail.

   Rationale: In this position the lizard is unable to struggle or to thrash its tail around.

4. **Action:** You may need to wear gloves when handling larger lizards.

   Rationale: Some species may bite or scratch, lash out with their tails or graze you with their scales.

5. **Action:** More aggressive specimens can be induced to lie still by placing a towel over the head.

   Rationale: If the head is in the dark, the lizard will remain motionless, and the body can be examined.

Procedure: To administer fluids or liquid medication

1. **Action:** Select a 5–8F catheter and lubricate it.

   Rationale: The type used for dogs and cats is appropriate. Lubrication aids the introduction of the catheter.

2. **Action:** Lay the catheter along the outside of the lizard. Mark the approximate position of the stomach on the catheter using a ballpoint pen.

   Rationale: The stomach lies at a point just caudal to the caudal border of the ribs.

3. **Action:** Select an appropriate size of syringe and fill with fluid.

   Rationale: It is good practice to have all equipment ready before you begin to handle the lizard as this reduces the stress caused by the procedure.

4. **Action:** With the lizard on a table, restrain the body and open the mouth using a blunt metal spatula.

   Rationale: Take steps to avoid being bitten.

5. **Action:** Use a mouth gag if necessary.

   Rationale: Most lizards will open their mouths quite easily when gentle pressure is applied. Make a gag by folding a small piece of radiographic film and cutting a hole in the centre. The catheter is passed through the hole.

6. **Action:** Slowly insert the catheter into the back of the mouth and down the oesophagus.

   Rationale: The glottis, which leads to the trachea and lungs, sits forward in the oral cavity. It is easy to see, and there is little risk of the catheter entering it.

7. **Action:** Insert the catheter to the level of the stomach.

   Rationale: The ballpoint pen mark will lie at the level of the mouth.

8. **Action:** Introduce the fluid in the syringe slowly.

   Rationale: If you introduce the fluid too quickly, the pressure applied may cause the fluid to spurt out of the junction with the syringe.

9. **Action:** Gently withdraw the catheter and observe the lizard.

   Rationale: To check that there are no adverse effects.

Procedure: Intravenous injection or blood sampling

1. **Action:** Restrain the lizard appropriately.

   Rationale: The site most commonly used in large lizards is the ventral venous sinus lying in the midline of the ventral surface of the tail. In smaller species a toe nail can be clipped to provide enough blood to fill a capillary tube.

2. **Action:** Prepare the site aseptically using povidone-iodine or 70% ethanol.

   Rationale: To prevent the introduction of infection.

3. **Action:** Select a small needle and syringe.

   Rationale: The needle must be small enough to enter the vein.

4. **Action:** Introduce the needle in the exact midline of the ventral surface of the tail distal to the vent, at an angle of 45°. Advance the needle until you touch bone.

   Rationale: The needle will go through the sinus and touch the underlying vertebra.

5. **Action:** Slowly withdraw the needle and aspirate the syringe at the same time until blood appears in the hub of the needle.

   Rationale: As you pull the needle back, it will re-enter the sinus, and blood will be aspirated into the syringe.

6. **Action:** Collect the sample into a lithium heparin tube.

   Rationale: EDTA lyses the cells.

7. **Action:** A drop of blood can be used to make a blood smear.

   Rationale: This is useful for haematology.

8. **Action:** If giving medication, slowly introduce the drug into the vein.

9. **Action:** Withdraw the needle.

N.B.: The total volume of blood is approx. 5–8% of bodyweight. This is about 70 ml/kg, and 10% of this can be collected in one withdrawal.

Sites for the Administration of Parenteral Drugs

- Subcutaneous – under the loose skin of the ribs
- Intramuscular – into the caudal muscles of the fore-limb, the hindlimb (Fig. 13.29) or into the tail, but care must be taken in those species that show autotomy as they may slough their tails.

Injections may be given into the hindlimb, but lizards have a renal portal venous system in which blood flows from the hindlimbs and tail to the kidneys before returning to the heart. Any drug injected into the hindlimbs may be eliminated by the kidneys without being absorbed. Nephrotoxic drugs must not be injected into the hindlimb.

GENERAL ANAESTHESIA

(General points to be considered for all species of reptile.)

Procedure: Induction of anaesthesia

1. **Action:** Have all anaesthetic equipment ready, organize assistance if required and be familiar with all the procedures involved before you get the patient from the cage.
   Rationale: This will minimize the stress caused to the patient. Reptiles are not as used to being handled as dogs and cats, and this increase in stress will increase the anaesthesia risk.

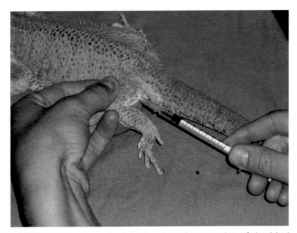

Fig. 13.29 Intramuscular injection into the muscles of the hindlimb of a lizard.

2. **Action:** Small species of reptile do not need to be starved before an anaesthetic. Starve larger lizards and chelonians for 18 hours and large snakes for 72–96 hours. Avoid feeding reptiles with live insects just before an anaesthetic.
   Rationale: The presence of live insects in the stomach may cause a problem. Vomiting does not occur in reptiles.

3. **Action:** Weigh the animal accurately.
   Rationale: This enables you to calculate an accurate dose of anaesthetic and the replacement fluid requirement.

4. **Action:** Sedatives may be used as premedication, but the use of atropine to reduce the production of saliva is unnecessary.
   Rationale: The use of sedatives will facilitate handling and reduce the stress caused to the patient. Salivary secretions are not a problem in reptiles.

5. **Action:** Induce anaesthesia using injectable agents administered by the appropriate method.
   Rationale: For drugs and dose rates, see Table 13.8.

TABLE 13.8 Anaesthetic agents for use in reptiles

Anaesthetic agent	Dose rate (mg/kg)	Site
Ketamine	20–50 (larger dose to smaller animals)	SC, IM, IP for sedation/ premedication
Medetomidine/ ketamine	<2 kg: 0.2 mg/kg medetomidine, 10 mg/kg ketamine >2 kg: 0.1 mg/kg medetomidine, 10 mg/kg ketamine	IM
Propofol	Tortoises 14 mg/kg Lizards 10 mg/kg Snakes 10 mg/kg	IV (agent of choice for induction)
Sevoflurane	5–8% induction 3–5% maintenance	
Isoflurane	3–5% induction 2–3% maintenance	

IM, intramuscular; IP, intraperitoneal; IV, intravenous; SC, subcutaneous.

6. **Action:** Induce anaesthesia by inhalational agents using a mask for large lizards and for snakes, but not for chelonians.
   Rationale: *The use of a mask may be difficult in chelonians. For drugs and dose rates, see Table 13.8.*
7. **Action:** Induction chambers can be used to deliver inhalational agents for most reptiles except terrapins.
   Rationale: *Terrapins are aquatic chelonians and are able to hold their breath and revert to anaerobic metabolism for up to 27 hours. This delays the uptake and activity of the anaesthetic agent.*
8. **Action:** Reptiles can be intubated relatively easily using an uncuffed tube. The glottis is easily visualized in snakes, but the large fleshy tongue of some lizards and chelonians may obscure the view.
   Rationale: *Reptiles have complete tracheal rings, which may be ruptured by inflation of a cuff. Use a gag to keep the mouth open. Dog and cat intravenous catheters can be used to intubate small reptiles.*
9. **Action:** Dehydration may increase the risks of anaesthesia.
   Rationale: *Correct fluid imbalance before anaesthesia.*
10. **Action:** Reptiles should be kept at their preferred body temperature (PBT) throughout the anaesthetic and during the recovery period.
    Rationale: *All reptiles have their own PBT at which the metabolic rate is at its most efficient. If the PBT is too low, the rate of recovery and healing will be reduced.*

Procedure: Maintenance and monitoring of anaesthesia

1. **Action:** Closed anaesthetic circuits are commonly used in reptile anaesthesia.
   Rationale: *The respiratory rate required to maintain an adequate level of anaesthesia is often greater than the rate shown by a conscious animal. A closed circuit will keep the gas concentration higher than a semi-closed circuit will.*
2. **Action:** Intermittent positive pressure ventilation (IPPV) may be used as a continuous means of ventilation during the anaesthetic.
   Rationale: *Reptiles have a low respiratory rate, and apnoea is common. Administer at the rate of 2 breaths/min.*

3. **Action:** Monitor the respiratory rate by observation.
   Rationale: *Observation of the respiratory rate may be difficult as the rate is often slow.*
4. **Action:** The corneal and palpebral reflexes may be used to monitor the depth of anaesthesia, except in the snake.
   Rationale: *Snakes have no eyelids, and the cornea is covered in a transparent skin scale known as a spectacle. The palpebral reflex is lost when the surgical plane of anaesthesia is reached.*
5. **Action:** The tongue withdrawal reflex is a useful means of monitoring the depth of anaesthesia in snakes and in some lizards.
   Rationale: *Pull out the tongue gently and note whether it flicks or is withdrawn. This is lost when the surgical plane of anaesthesia is reached.*
6. **Action:** Monitor jaw tone and pedal and tail reflexes.
   Rationale: *The pedal and tail reflexes are lost when the surgical plane of anaesthesia is reached.*
7. **Action:** Monitor the heart rate by oesophageal stethoscope, Doppler ultrasound or electrocardiography.
   Rationale: *During deep anaesthesia the heart rate slows and the pupils become fixed and dilated.*

Procedure: Post-operative care

1. **Action:** If a reptile has been induced with an injectable anaesthetic agent, it may take hours to regain complete consciousness.
   Rationale: *Reptiles have a slow metabolic rate, so anaesthetic drugs are broken down slowly, and recovery will be slow.*
2. **Action:** Continue to give oxygen by IPPV until the reptile has begun to breathe spontaneously.
   Rationale: *To maintain adequate levels of oxygen to the tissues.*
3. **Action:** Keep the patient warm at all times. Once the surgical procedure is complete, transfer it to its vivarium maintained at its PBT. Monitor the environmental temperature to avoid overheating.
   Rationale: *Reptiles are cold-blooded, and the environmental temperature influences their metabolic rate. If the reptile is kept at its PBT, the recovery will occur more quickly than if the reptile is cold.*
4. **Action:** Monitor the respiratory rate until the patient is fully conscious and moving around.
   Rationale: *Respiratory stimulants, e.g. doxapram, can be used.*

5. **Action:** Give replacement fluid therapy orally, intravenously or intraperitoneally – up to 4% of bodyweight.
   Rationale: *Dehydration can lead to visceral gout – the build-up of urates in the visceral organs.*

6. **Action:** Monitor the patient until it is fully conscious.
   Rationale: *Problems may occur during the post-operative period. Appetite is often difficult to measure, as many reptiles eat infrequently.*

REFERENCES AND FURTHER READING

Ackerman, N., 2016. Aspinall's Complete Textbook of Veterinary Nursing, third ed. Elsevier, Oxford.

Aspinall, V., 2011. The Complete Textbook of Veterinary Nursing, second ed. Elsevier, Oxford.

Aspinall, R., Aspinall, V., 2013. Clinical Procedures in Small Animal Veterinary Practice. Saunders, Oxford.

Aspinall, V., O'Reilly, M., 2009. Introduction to Veterinary Anatomy and Physiology, second ed. Butterworth-Heinemann, Oxford.

Beynon, P., Forbes, N. (Eds.), 1996. Manual of Psittacine Birds. BSAVA, Gloucester.

Debmark Rabbit Education Resource, 13 May 2006. Online. Available, http://www.debmark.com/rabbits/sexing.htm.

Girling, S.J., Raiti, P., 2004. Manual of Reptiles. BSAVA, Gloucester.

Harcourt-Brown, N., Chitty, J., 2005. Manual of Psittacine Birds, second ed. BSAVA, Gloucester.

Hillyer, E.V., Quesenberry, K.E., 1997. Ferrets, Rabbits and Rodents, Clinical Medicine and Surgery. W B Saunders, Philadelphia.

Hotston-Moore, A. (Ed.), 1999. Manual of Advanced Veterinary Nursing. BSAVA, Gloucester.

Keeble, E., Meredith, A., 2009. Manual of Rodents and Ferrets. BSAVA, Gloucester.

Laber-Laird, K., Swindle, M., Flecknell, P., 1991. Handbook of Rodent and Rabbit Medicine. Pergamon, Oxford.

O'Malley, B., 2005. Clinical Anatomy and Physiology of Exotic Species. Elsevier Saunders, Oxford.

14

Basic clinical procedures in the horse

Lucy Middlecote

CHAPTER OUTLINE

INTRODUCTION

Working with horses in veterinary practice involves assisting the veterinary surgeon with a wide range of clinical procedures. It is highly important that all of these procedures are carried out in a professional manner to ensure the safety and wellbeing of patients, staff and clients. The aim of this chapter is to provide a useful overview of some of the more basic and commonly carried out procedures that the veterinary nurse may encounter when working in equine veterinary practice.

HANDLING AND RESTRAINT

With training, horses are generally very amenable to handling, but by nature they are unpredictable, flight animals, and even the quietest horse can become excitable or distressed. Horses are large, strong animals that may become anxious when placed in an unfamiliar environment and will often attempt to escape if they suspect that a situation is dangerous. Some horses may show aggressive behaviour as a result of anxiety or fear, whilst others may use aggression as a method of protection or dominance. It is important to be aware of the nature of the individual patient and the type of behaviour that is being displayed.

When carrying out any task with a horse, it is important that health and safety is adhered to at all times. Long hair should be tied back, jewellery should not be worn, and personal protective equipment (PPE) should be utilized. PPE should include a skull cap, gloves and suitable clothing, e.g. a long-sleeved top, trousers, overalls and suitable footwear (Fig. 14.1). In order to carry out any clinical examination or clinical procedure in the safest possible way, there is a range of recommended handling techniques that should be used.

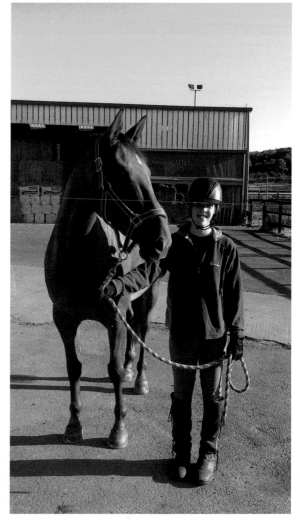

Fig. 14.1 Suitable clothing and personal protective equipment (PPE) for handling the equine patient.

Procedure: Approaching a horse

1. **Action:** Assess the horse's behaviour as you approach.
   Rationale: This will enable you to gauge whether the horse appears relaxed or distressed and adopt an appropriate level of caution.
2. **Action:** Approach from the horse's left side and towards the shoulder.
   Rationale: Horses are generally taught to be handled from the left side, so they are more familiar and therefore more comfortable with being approached from this side.
3. **Action:** Do not approach from directly in front of the horse.
   Rationale: Horses' eyes are located on either side of the head, and they have reduced vision directly in front of the head and behind the body. Providing the horse with the greatest opportunity to see you is safest practice.
4. **Action:** Use verbal communication.
   Rationale: This allows the horse to hear you approaching, particularly if it has not already seen

you, and it is therefore less likely to be surprised by your presence.

Procedure: Putting on a head collar and lead rope

The majority of horses will be familiar with wearing a head collar, which is the most common piece of handling equipment used today.

1. **Action:** Ensure that you have a suitable head collar and lead rope for the size of the horse.
   Rationale: This will ensure that you do not waste time or risk applying a head collar that is too tight or too loose, which may be detrimental to the level of control that you have and to the comfort of the horse.
2. **Action:** Approach the horse as described above.
   Rationale: This is safest practice.
3. **Action:** Stand next to the horse's left shoulder, facing forwards.
   Rationale: Horses are most commonly used to being handled from the left side, and the head collar fastener/buckle will need to be secured on this side.
4. **Action:** Place the lead rope around the horse's neck or over your shoulder.

Rationale: This will prevent the lead rope from hanging on the floor and potentially becoming a dangerous hazard. It will also give you more control if the horse tries to wander off.

5. **Action:** Insert the horse's nose through the nosepiece (Fig. 14.2A) and place the noseband over the nose.
   Rationale: Use both hands to do this as this will give you greater control.
6. **Action:** Using your right hand, take the longest strap up and over behind the ears (Fig. 14.2B) and secure the fastener/buckle on the left side of the horse's cheek.
   Rationale: This will ensure that the head collar is secure and ready for use.
7. **Action:** Ensure that you can fit a hand's width between the noseband and the horse, and that the noseband is approximately two fingers' width below the facial crest.
   Rationale: This will ensure that the head collar is not too tight and is suitably fitted for control (Fig. 14.2C).

Procedure: Putting on a bridle with a bit

Many veterinary practices have a policy that all equine patients are handled using bridles in combination with

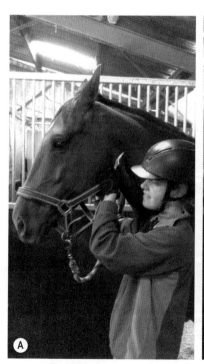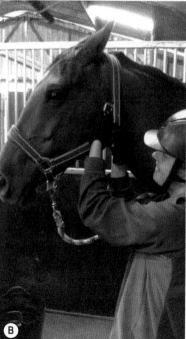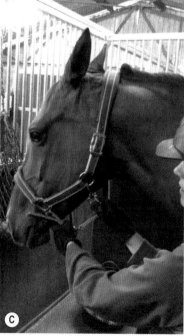

Fig. 14.2 Putting on a head collar. A, Insert the horse's nose through the nosepiece of the head collar. B, Take the longest strap up and behind the horse's ears. C, The head collar and lead rope are now fitted correctly.

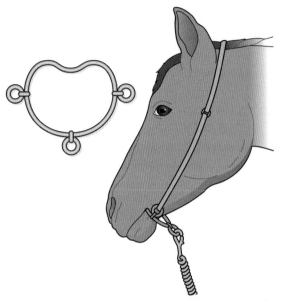

Fig. 14.3 A Chifney bit. (Reproduced, with permission, from Batty-Smith (2008), Shrewsbury.)

a head collar because it gives the handler more control. This is particularly beneficial if dealing with a difficult, excited or enthusiastic patient. The bridle may simply consist of a head piece and a bit or may have a throat lash strap added for extra security.

Some animals may require the use of a Chifney or antirearing bit. This is a bit with a shallow inverted-port mouthpiece that has three rings – two for the cheek pieces and one for the bridle (Fig. 14.3). However, this must only be used by experienced handlers as it can cause injury or damage because of the way that it acts upon the horse's tongue if it tries to rear or pull. Some horses, such as foals and young animals, may not be used to having a bit in their mouth. This must be taken into consideration and the appropriateness of use assessed on an individual basis.

1. **Action:** Approach the horse as described.
   Rationale: This is safest practice.
2. **Action:** Standing at the left shoulder, move your right hand under the horse's mandible and around the front of the head.
   Rationale: This will secure the horse's head in a suitable position.
3. **Action:** Hold the head piece of the bridle up against the front of the head, and with your left hand place

the bit across the horse's mouth (Fig. 14.4A). Then place your thumb in behind the incisors.
   Rationale: This will encourage the horse to open its mouth to accept the bit.
4. **Action:** Gently push the bit into the horse's mouth, ensuring that it sits on top of the tongue.
   Rationale: Do not force the bit into the mouth as this can damage the incisor teeth and may result in the horse refusing the bit in the future.
5. **Action:** Once the bit is in the horse's mouth, carefully place the head piece over and behind the horse's ears (Fig. 14.4B).
   Rationale: This will keep the bit in position.
6. **Action:** Adjust the head piece to fit the horse, ensuring that there are no more than two creases at the edge of the mouth and that the bit is not dangling too low in the mouth.
   Rationale: This will ensure that the bit is comfortable and effective.
7. **Action:** Secure the throat lash (if applicable), ensuring that there is approximately a hand's width of space between the throat lash and the horse.
   Rationale: This will further secure the bridle in place and ensure that it is not too tight or too loose.
8. **Action:** Attach a lead rope to the bit (Fig. 14.4C).
   Rationale: This will allow you to lead and restrain the horse safely and effectively.
9. **Action:** To remove the bridle, undo the throat lash (if applicable), gently push the head piece forwards over the horse's ears, and slowly allow the bit to drop out of the mouth. A hand should be used to catch the bit as it leaves the horse's mouth.
   Rationale: This prevents the bit from causing damage to the incisor teeth.

Procedure: Holding a horse for examination

1. **Action:** Apply the head collar and/or bridle as described.
   Rationale: This is safest practice.
2. **Action:** Using a lead rope, stand at the horse's shoulder and, where possible, on the same side as the person carrying out the examination or procedure.
   Rationale: If the horse moves or jumps, it is more likely to move away from the person carrying out the examination. By standing on the same side as this person, you reduce the risk of injury to yourself.

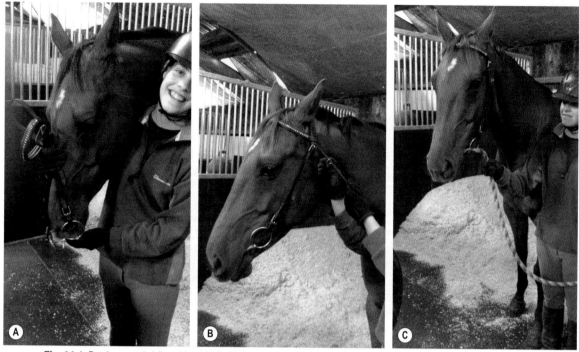

Fig. 14.4 Putting on a bridle with a bit. A, Using the left hand, place the bit across the horse's mouth, then place your thumb behind the incisors to encourage the horse to open its mouth. B, Take the head piece over the horse's ears and secure the throat lash. C, Attach a lead rope to the bit.

3. **Action:** Face towards the front of the horse or towards the person examining the horse, depending on the procedure being carried out.
   Rationale: *This allows for greater control of the horse but will depend on the procedure being carried out.*
4. **Action:** The rope should be held with the near-side hand below the jaw (approx. 20 cm) and the remaining rope in the other hand.
   Rationale: *Holding the remaining rope in the other hand will prevent it from dangling on the floor and becoming a potential hazard.*
5. **Action:** The remaining rope should never be wrapped around the hand.
   Rationale: *This could cause serious damage to your hand if the horse pulls or rears.*

Procedure: Leading a horse

For the purposes of a clinical examination and investigation, the veterinary nurse may be required to lead the horse in both walk and/or trot.

1. **Action:** Apply the head collar or bridle as described.

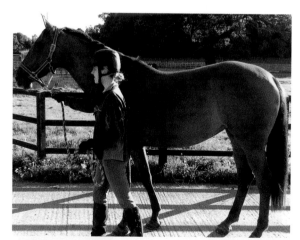

Fig. 14.5 Leading a horse.

   Rationale: *This is safest practice.*
2. **Action:** Using a lead rope, the handler should face forwards and lead the horse from its left shoulder (Fig. 14.5).

Rationale: The horse may run off if it gets too far ahead and is unlikely to move forwards if the handler is positioned too far forwards.

3. **Action:** The rope should be held with the right hand below the jaw (approx. 20 cm). Hold the remaining rope in the left hand.

   Rationale: Holding the remaining rope in the left hand will prevent the lead rope from dangling on the floor and becoming a trip hazard.

4. **Action:** The remaining rope should never be wrapped around the hand.

   Rationale: This can cause serious damage to your hand if the horse pulls or rears.

5. **Action:** Walk the horse out slowly and, if necessary, increase the pace to a trot. If you are on the left side, the vet will observe the horse from the right side, then as it walks towards him or her and then from back view.

   Rationale: This enables the veterinary surgeon to observe the action of the horse from all sides. Some conditions do not show up until the horse is going faster.

6. **Action:** To turn the horse, steady to a walk and turn it away from you in a fairly wide circle.

   Rationale: This gives a greater degree of control and prevents the horse standing on your heels or feet.

Procedure: Tying up a horse using a quick-release knot

It is important to be able to tie a horse up securely to prevent escape, e.g. during grooming, but it should always be tied using a 'quick-release' knot, which can be more easily released if an emergency arises.

1. **Action:** Fold the lead rope, thread it through baler twine (or a similar commercial product) that has been attached to a secure metal ring and create a small loop (Fig. 14.6A).

   Rationale: Tying the horse to something that does not break can be extremely dangerous. Baler twine will break if the horse panics, reducing the risk of injury.

2. **Action:** Twist the loop and thread the lead rope through the loop (Fig. 14.6B).

   Rationale: This will produce a second loop.

3. **Action:** Pull the knot (Fig. 14.6C).

   Rationale: This will secure the knot.

4. **Action:** Do not leave the horse completely unsupervised.

   Rationale: Although the remaining end can be threaded through the second loop to prevent the horse from untying itself, the resulting knot is no longer quick-release. It is safer practice to leave the end unthreaded and the horse supervised. Supervision is always recommended for any horse that is tied up.

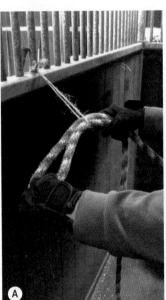
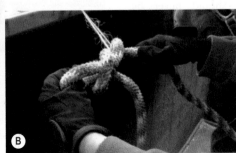
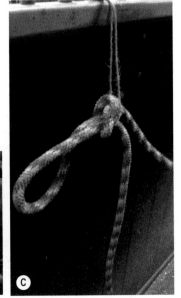

Fig. 14.6 A–C Stages in tying a 'quick-release' knot (see text).

Procedure: Lunging a horse

Being able to lunge a horse is a vital skill for those working in equine practice. Observation of a horse moving on the lunge is a common part of lameness investigation and allows the veterinary surgeon to see the horse moving in a circle at a walk, trot or canter.

When lunging, the handler should stand in the centre of the circle slightly behind the level of the horse's shoulder, which encourages the horse to move forward (Fig. 14.7).

1. **Action:** Prepare the equipment and the horse ready for lunging. Equipment should include your own PPE, i.e. hat, gloves and sensible footwear, and a lunge whip. The horse may be fitted with a lightweight lunging cavesson, which should have adequate padding to the noseband. A long lunge rein is attached by means of a swivel joint and clip.

   Rationale: A bridle with a bit is recommended for safety and control. (Other types of reins, e.g. side reins, may be used to achieve better balance and increase the degree of control.)

2. **Action:** Move the horse to the designated lunging area.

   Rationale: This must be a flat area large enough for the lunging circle, with a suitable non-slip surface.

3. **Action:** Position yourself in the centre of the area (Fig. 14.7). If you are lunging to the left, hold the lunge rein in your left hand and the whip in your right hand.

   Rationale: You should be forming a triangle with the horse's body, the lunge rein and the whip.

4. **Action:** Hold the lunge rein with the excess held in loops in your hand.

   Rationale: This will prevent the lunge rein from dangling on the floor and allow you to lengthen or shorten the rein easily if necessary.

5. **Action:** Carry the whip pointing slightly behind the horse and down when not in use. Keep your wrists, arms and shoulders relaxed and supple.

   Rationale: This will encourage the horse to remain relaxed but continue to move forwards. You may raise the whip (if required) to encourage the horse to continue to move forwards or to increase the pace.

6. **Action:** Control the horse's speed and pace with voice aids, using commands such as 'stand', 'walk on', 'trot on', 'canter', 'steady'.

   Rationale: If the horse is being a little sluggish, you should move a little sideways so that you are further behind the horse; if the horse is going too fast, you should position yourself more towards the head, raising the lunge whip in front of the nose as a barrier.

7. **Action:** Keep the horse from turning in on the circle by pointing the whip at the horse's shoulder.

   Rationale: This will ensure that the horse remains on a circle and will allow the veterinary surgeon to assess the horse's movement and identify any evidence of lameness.

8. **Action:** To stop the horse, ask the horse to slow and point the whip in front of the horse.

   Rationale: This will encourage the horse to slow down and eventually stop.

9. **Action:** Lunge the horse on the opposite rein to the one that you have started on.

   Rationale: The horse will now go in the opposite direction so that the veterinary surgeon can observe all the facts of the case.

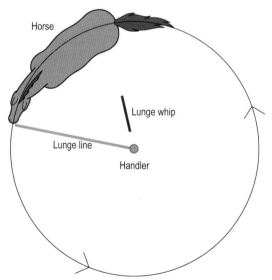

Fig. 14.7 Position of the handler in relation to the horse when lunging.

ADDITIONAL METHODS OF RESTRAINT

Sometimes additional restraint may be required. For a number of procedures, it is extremely important that the patient stands as still as possible. Additional restraint may be achieved using a device such as stocks or by lifting and holding a leg so that the horse finds it difficult to move around. Sometimes restraint may need to be more invasive, with the application of a twitch or the use of chemical sedation.

The use of twitches, which are a means of providing a low-grade pain to a horse, are thought to distract a horse while a minor procedure is being performed. Research has now shown that twitches initiate the release of natural endorphins from the brain, which have a short-term analgesic and sedative effect.

Twitches must always be used with care and must not be left in place for more than 5 minutes at a time. If used for too long, a twitch may cause detrimental effects and could result in permanent scarring. Ear twitches are not recommended as they may result in the horse becoming headshy.

A skin twitch applied to the neck, by firmly grasping a small amount of skin cranial to the shoulder, can encourage the horse to stand still for a procedure. A nose twitch (Fig. 14.8) is made of a length of wood, metal or rubber with a loop of rope attached at one end. Commercial humane twitches are also available but tend to have less effective results.

Procedure: Applying a nose twitch

1. **Action:** Ask a handler to restrain the horse.
   Rationale: Restrain the horse as previously described.
2. **Action:** Stand on the same side as the handler.

Rationale: This will prevent the horse jumping onto you and the handler. If the horse moves, it will probably move away from you.

3. **Action:** Place one hand on the handle of the twitch and the other hand on the rope loop.
   Rationale: This prepares you for applying the twitch.
4. **Action:** Holding the upper lip, place the rope loop over the horse's upper lip (Fig. 14.8). Ensure that you have a firm grip on the handle of the twitch and on the horse's nose at this point.
   Rationale: A firm grip will reduce the risk of the horse being able to move away, potentially causing the handle of the twitch to be thrust into the air.
5. **Action:** Twist the handle until a firm amount of the skin has been gripped by the rope loop (Fig. 14.8).
   Rationale: This will ensure that the desired effect can be achieved and reduce the risk of the rope loop falling off or becoming loose.
6. **Action:** Hold the handle firmly or twist the horse's lead rope over the handle.
   Rationale: This will secure the twitch in place and prevent the handle from causing injury to the horse or handler if the horse throws its head in the air.
7. **Action:** Monitor the horse's behaviour carefully throughout and remove the twitch immediately if there are any concerns.
   Rationale: Some horses will suddenly react or strike out when twitched.

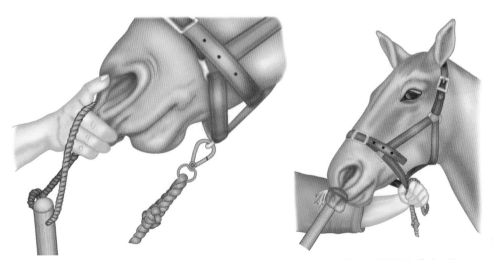

Fig. 14.8 Application of a nose twitch. (Reproduced, with permission, from Aspinall (2011), Oxford.)

8. **Action:** To remove the twitch, slowly unwind it and gently release the horse's upper lip, ensuring that the handle is held firmly at all times.

 Rationale: Some horses may throw their heads in the air at this stage, so it is important not to let go of the twitch as this could cause injury.

Procedure: Lifting a forelimb to examine the foot

1. **Action:** Ensure that the horse is adequately restrained.

 Rationale: The horse may be tied up, but for safety reasons, it is also advisable to use an extra handler, where possible.

2. **Action:** Allow and encourage the horse to stand square and weight-bear on all four limbs.

 Rationale: This allows the horse to balance and enables it to be physically able to lift up a leg when requested.

3. **Action:** Stand at the horse's shoulder, beside the appropriate leg and facing the tail (Fig. 14.9).

 Rationale: This is the safest position to be in for this procedure as you can stay close to the horse and anticipate any movement that may take place.

4. **Action:** Place your hand on the horse's shoulder and then run it down the back of the forelimb until you reach the fetlock.

 Rationale: This allows the horse to recognize that you are there and prepares the horse for the process of lifting the leg.

5. **Action:** Apply gentle pressure to the fetlock and encourage the horse to lift the limb. You may use your voice for encouragement.

 Rationale: Horses generally respond well to the combination of pressure and a low voice at this stage.

6. **Action:** As the limb is lifted, support and hold the horse's foot by moving your hand to the dorsomedial aspect of the foot (Fig. 14.9).

 Rationale: When you support the foot appropriately, the horse is less likely to resist you holding up the limb.

7. **Action:** Keep in close contact with the horse's shoulder whilst the foot is held and stay slightly ahead of the horse.

 Rationale: This allows you to anticipate any movement from the horse and reduces the risk of injury if the horse strikes out.

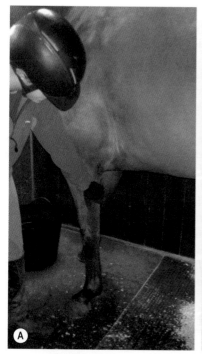 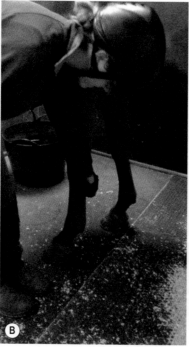 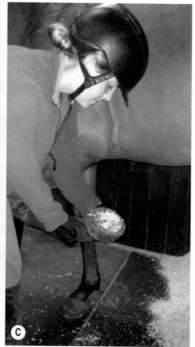

Fig. 14.9 Picking up a forelimb and foot. A, Run your hand down the back of the leg. B, Apply gentle pressure to the back of the leg to encourage the horse to pick up its foot. C, Support the hoof in the palm of your hand.

8. **Action:** Cradle the foot in your hand, using your other hand to clean out the sole with a hoof pick.

   Rationale: This enables you to examine the clean surface of the sole and the hoof wall.

Procedure: Lifting a hindlimb to examine the foot

Holding up a hindlimb is not a normally recognized method of additional restraint as it is both dangerous for the handler and uncomfortable for the horse. However, it is important to know how to lift a hindlimb as it may be a requirement during other procedures, e.g. picking out a foot.

1. **Action:** Ensure that the horse is adequately restrained.

   Rationale: The horse may be tied up, but for safety reasons, it is also advisable to use an extra handler, where possible.

2. **Action:** Allow and encourage the horse to stand square and weight-bear on all four limbs.

   Rationale: This allows the horse to balance and enables it to be physically able to lift up a leg when requested.

3. **Action:** Place your hand on the horse's shoulder and then run it along the back to the hindquarters. Continue down the back and then medial side of the distal limb until you reach the fetlock.

   Rationale: This allows the horse to recognize that you are there and prepares it for the process of lifting the leg.

4. **Action:** Apply gentle pressure to the fetlock and encourage the horse to lift the limb. You may use your voice for encouragement.

   Rationale: Horses generally respond well to the combination of pressure and a low voice at this stage.

5. **Action:** As the limb is lifted, support the horse's foot by moving your hand to the dorsomedial aspect of the foot.

   Rationale: When you support the foot appropriately, the horse is less likely to resist you holding up the limb.

6. **Action:** Keep in close contact with the horse whilst the foot is supported.

   Rationale: This allows you to anticipate any movement from the horse and reduces the risk of being kicked.

7. **Action:** Cradle the foot in your hand, using your other hand to clean out the sole with a hoof pick.

Rationale: This enables you to examine the clean surface of the sole and the hoof wall.

RESTRAINING FOALS

Foals should be fitted with a foal slip (first head collar) as soon as they are used to being approached and touched. When dealing with a foal, it is advisable to use as little restraint as possible; gentle but positive handling is important as foals may react suddenly and be unpredictable, which could result in injury to both the foal and the handler.

Procedure: Catching and restraining a foal

1. **Action:** If the foal is still with its dam, then it is always advisable to catch and restrain the mare first but keep her in close proximity.

   Rationale: Mares can be very protective of their foals and may become distressed or aggressive if they think that they are in danger. Keeping the mare in close proximity will reduce the stress levels of both mare and foal.

2. **Action:** Approach the foal slowly and quietly or let the foal come to you.

   Rationale: Foals have a curious nature and will often approach you when you enter the stable.

3. **Action:** Carefully catch the foal by the head collar or foal slip. Avoid using the head collar to restrain the foal.

   Rationale: Restraint by the head collar is not recommended because foals have a tendency to pull away and flip over backwards.

4. **Action:** Hold the foal with one arm firmly around its chest and one arm firmly around the hindquarters.

   Rationale: Being firm will help the foal to feel more secure and reduce the risk of it panicking. In this position, the foal will find it difficult to move forwards or backwards and the clinical procedure, e.g. a health check, can then be performed.

5. **Action:** When finished, release the foal and then the mare.

   Rationale: This will allow you time to move away from the foal before the mare is released.

MEASURING CLINICAL PARAMETERS

As a veterinary nurse, it is important to be able to recognize, report and record signs of ill health and disease.

TABLE 14.1 Normal clinical parameters in the horse

Clinical parameter	Normal range
Body temperature	37.9–38.5°C
Pulse rate/heart rate	30–40 beats/min
Respiratory rate	8–20 breaths/min
Capillary refill time	<2 seconds

Both subjective and objective assessments should be made, and any concerns or changes reported to the veterinary surgeon in charge of the case. Subjective assessments are non-measurable and may be a matter of opinion, whereas objective assessments can be measured and are based on accepted facts, e.g. body temperature. Table 14.1 lists the most commonly used clinical parameters in equine practice.

Procedure: Making a subjective assessment of a horse's state of health

1. **Action:** Initially observe the horse from outside the stable (Fig. 14.10).
   Rationale: *This will indicate how the horse is behaving on your approach and before you enter the stable. As soon as you interact with the horse, you alter the 'evidence'.*
2. **Action:** Observe the horse's demeanour, attitude, response, behaviour and interest in its surroundings.
   Rationale: *This may indicate if there is some form of problem.*
3. **Action:** Observe other parameters such as physique, the brightness of the eyes and the appearance of the horse's coat.
   Rationale: *These are all indicators of good or poor health.*
4. **Action:** Note whether the horse is standing up or lying down.
   Rationale: *Lying down may indicate that the horse is unable to stand or that the horse is relaxed. Horses will not usually lie down unless they are relaxed in their surroundings.*
5. **Action:** Check that the horse has been eating and defecating normally.
   Rationale: *Assessment of eating and defecation is particularly important in the horse because of the complex anatomy and physiology of its digestive tract. Abnormalities may be an indication of*

serious problems such as colic. The normal horse defecates approximately 8–12 times every 24 hours, and the faeces should be in firm balls that break when they hit the ground.

6. **Action:** Check that the horse has been drinking and urinating normally.
   Rationale: *The normal horse will produce 1–2 ml/kg/h of urine (approx. 10–20 litres in 24 hours). Check the bedding for signs of moisture. Normal horse urine is yellow in colour and is cloudy due to the presence of calcium carbonate crystals.*
7. **Action:** Record your findings on the hospital chart or patient record.
   Rationale: *This can be used to monitor the progress of the case and identify the need for treatment.*

Procedure: Measuring the body temperature

1. **Action:** Ensure that the horse is adequately restrained.
   Rationale: *The horse should be kept as still as possible during the procedure to prevent injury.*
2. **Action:** Approach the horse calmly, ensuring that it sees you and that it is aware that you are going to approach its back end.
   Rationale: *Horses may react and kick out if they are not aware that you are there.*
3. **Action:** Stand to one side of the hind legs.
   Rationale: *This will reduce the risk of being kicked.*
4. **Action:** Hold the tail to one side.
   Rationale: *This allows you a better view of the anus.*
5. **Action:** Using a well-lubricated digital or mercury thermometer, insert it through the anal sphincter into the rectum, using a gentle twisting motion.
   Rationale: *Lubricant will facilitate the passage of the thermometer and reduce the risk of damaging the mucosa.*
6. **Action:** Position the tip of the thermometer against the dorsal rectal wall.
   Rationale: *This will avoid insertion into faeces, which could give an inaccurate reading.*
7. **Action:** Never let go of the thermometer during the procedure.
   Rationale: *Loss of a thermometer into the rectum, particularly a mercury thermometer, can be very dangerous, and if it falls out on to the floor it may break.*
8. **Action:** Leave the thermometer in place until it beeps (digital) or for 1 minute (mercury).

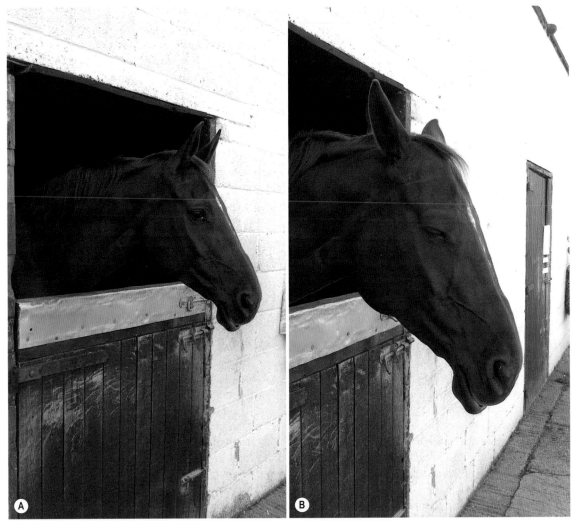

Fig. 14.10 Making a subjective assessment of the patient. A, The horse is alert and aware of its surroundings. B, The horse is relaxed and sleepy. Note the drooping lower lip.

Rationale: This provides sufficient time for the rectal temperature to register on the thermometer.

9. **Action:** Gently and slowly remove the thermometer and clean it on a piece of tissue.
   Rationale: This prevents disease transmission to another patient and makes it easier to read the thermometer.

10. **Action:** Read and record the temperature on the hospital chart or patient record.
    Rationale: This can be used to monitor the progress of the case and identify the need for treatment.

11. **Action:** Reset the digital thermometer and shake down the mercury thermometer.
    Rationale: This will leave the thermometer ready to use again.

Procedure: Measuring the pulse rate by digital palpation of the submandibular artery

1. **Action:** Approach the horse calmly and quietly.
   Rationale: This should reduce the risk of false elevation as a result of fear.

2. **Action:** Ensure that the horse is adequately restrained.

Rationale: The horse should be kept as still as possible during the procedure.

3. **Action:** Locate the submandibular artery, which is palpable as it passes over the ventral ramus of the mandible.

   Rationale: Other arteries can be used, e.g. transverse facial or digital, but this artery is the easiest to detect and the simplest to use for counting heart beats.

4. **Action:** Partially occlude the artery with gentle pressure from your second and third fingers and feel the pulse.

   Rationale: The tips of the fingers are more sensitive to touch and do not have a pulse of their own, so will not be mistaken for the horse's pulse.

5. **Action:** Count the number of beats for 1 minute. Alternatively, you can count the number of beats for 15 seconds then multiply the result by four to give the total number of beats in 1 minute.

   Rationale: You can count the number of beats for 1 minute, but this requires the horse standing still for that period – in some cases this may be difficult. One minute is an appropriate time to obtain an accurate result.

6. **Action:** Record the pulse rate on the hospital chart or patient record.

   Rationale: This can be used to monitor the progress of the case and identify the need for treatment.

Procedure: Measuring the heart rate by auscultation using a stethoscope

1. **Action:** Approach the horse calmly and quietly.

   Rationale: This should reduce the risk of false elevation as a result of fear.

2. **Action:** Ensure that the horse is adequately restrained.

   Rationale: The horse should remain as still as possible during the procedure.

3. **Action:** Place the stethoscope earpieces into your ears and the stethoscope head on the left side of the chest, directly behind the elbow.

   Rationale: This is close to the left ventricle of the heart, where the heart beat can be heard at its strongest.

4. **Action:** Count the number of beats for 1 minute. Alternatively, you can count the number of beats for 15 seconds then multiply the result by four to give the total number of beats in 1 minute. Note the rhythm, intensity and clarity of the heartbeat.

Rationale: You can count the number of beats for 1 minute, but this requires the horse standing still for that period – in some cases this may be difficult. One minute is an appropriate time to obtain an accurate result.

5. **Action:** Record the heart rate on the hospital chart or patient record.

   Rationale: This can be used to monitor the progress of the case and identify the need for treatment.

Procedure: Measuring the respiration rate by direct observation – method 1

1. **Action:** If possible, observe the horse from outside the stable.

   Rationale: Horses tend to be more relaxed when you are not in the stable with them and entering the stable may cause the respiration rate to increase.

2. **Action:** Carefully observe the horse's rib movements.

   Rationale: The chest expands and contracts with each breath.

3. **Action:** Count the number of inspirations or expirations over 1 minute. You can observe the horse for 15 seconds and then multiply by four to give the total number of breaths in 1 minute.

   Rationale: One minute is an appropriate time to obtain an accurate result. Concentrated observation for longer than 15 seconds may be quite difficult as the horse may move around, or you may become distracted.

4. **Action:** Record the respiration rate on the hospital chart or patient record.

   Rationale: This can be used to monitor the progress of the case and identify the need for treatment.

Procedure: Measuring the respiration rate by direct observation – method 2 (during cold weather)

1. **Action:** If possible, observe the horse from outside the stable.

   Rationale: Horses tend to be more relaxed when you are not in the stable with them and entering the stable may cause the respiration rate to increase.

2. **Action:** Carefully observe the horse's nose for exhaled breaths.

   Rationale: In cold weather, the exhaled breaths can be seen as vapour leaving the nostrils and counted.

3. **Action:** Count the number of expirations over 1 minute. You can observe the horse for 15 seconds

and then multiply by four to give the total number of breaths in 1 minute.

Rationale: One minute is an appropriate time to obtain an accurate result. Concentrated observation for longer than 15 seconds may be quite difficult.

4. **Action:** Record the respiration rate on the hospital chart or patient record.

    Rationale: This can be used to monitor the progress of the case and identify the need for treatment.

Procedure: Measuring the respiration rate by direct observation – method 3

1. **Action:** Approach the horse calmly and quietly.

    Rationale: This should reduce the risk of false elevation as a result of fear.

2. **Action:** Ensure that the horse is adequately restrained.

    Rationale: The horse should be kept as still as possible during the procedure.

3. **Action:** Put the palm of your hand below one of the horse's nostrils and feel for exhaled breaths.

    Rationale: The exhaled breaths will feel warm and moist.

4. **Action:** Count the number of expirations over 1 minute. You can count for 15 seconds and then multiply by four to give the total number of breaths in 1 minute.

    Rationale: One minute is an appropriate time to obtain an accurate result. Concentrated observation for longer than 15 seconds may be quite difficult.

5. **Action:** Record the respiration rate on the hospital chart or patient record.

    Rationale: This can be used to monitor the progress of the case and identify the need for treatment.

Procedure: Assessment of the colour of the mucous membrane and capillary refill time (CRT)

1. **Action:** Ensure that the horse is adequately restrained.

    Rationale: The horse should be kept as still as possible during the procedure.

2. **Action:** Standing to one side, carefully lift the horse's top lip.

    Rationale: This will allow for observation and assessment of the colour of the mucous membranes.

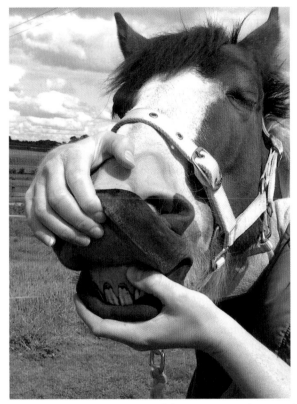

Fig. 14.11 Assessing the colour of the mucous membrane and the capillary refill time.

3. **Action:** Assess the colour of the mucous membrane and then gently press on the gum with the ball of your thumb (Fig. 14.11).

    Rationale: Normal healthy mucous membranes are salmon-pink in colour, but in sick horses they may vary from white to dark grey, with all variations in between. Pressing the gum will blanch it as the blood is pushed out of the area.

4. **Action:** Release your thumb.

    Rationale: This allows the blood to return to the area.

5. **Action:** Count how long the gum takes to return to the original colour.

    Rationale: This indicates how long the capillaries are taking to refill and should take less than 2 seconds.

6. **Action:** Record the mucous membrane colour and CRT on the hospital chart or patient record.

    Rationale: This can be used to monitor the progress of the case and identify the need for treatment.

Procedure: Abdominal assessment using a stethoscope

The equine abdomen is divided into four quarters or quadrants (left upper and lower, and right upper and lower). As food and liquid move through the digestive tract, gurgling sounds, known as borborygmi, may be audible. The right upper quadrant, the location of the caecum, should make gentle mixing sounds before making a sound similar to a flushing toilet. These gut sounds should be checked regularly to ensure that they are not abnormally increased or decreased as this could indicate serious problems such as gut hypermotility, impaction or gut stasis, all of which are potentially life-threatening in an animal that cannot vomit. Gut sounds should be considered in conjunction with the appearance of the faeces and the frequency of their production.

1. **Action:** Ensure that the horse is adequately restrained.
   Rationale: The horse should be kept as still as possible during the procedure.
2. **Action:** Place the stethoscope earpieces into your ears and the stethoscope head on the horse's abdomen.
   Rationale: This is where the small and large intestine are located and where, in the normal horse, gut sounds can be detected.
3. **Action:** Listen to all four quadrants of the abdomen by moving the head of the stethoscope to the appropriate area.
   Rationale: It is important to listen to all quadrants to make an informed assessment.
4. **Action:** Record the regularity and intensity of the gut sounds in each of the quadrants on the hospital chart or patient record (Table 14.2).
   Rationale: This can be used to monitor the progress of the case and identify the need for treatment.

TABLE 14.2 **An example of how equine gut sounds may be recorded**	
Upper left quadrant	Upper right quadrant
++	+
Lower left quadrant	Lower right quadrant
++	+/−

+ indicates the presence of gut sounds (the more + s recorded, the more gut sounds that are heard). − indicates a lack of gut sounds.

BANDAGING

The general principles of wound care and bandage management in horses are similar to those of other species (see Chapter 8) and will largely depend upon the location and the severity of the wound. Bandaging materials are also similar to those used in small animal practice, although larger sizes are generally required for equine patients. Light and simple bandages are used for shorter-term use, e.g. following nerve or joint blocks, or for more superficial wounding. Larger bandages are used for more serious injuries and wounds, e.g. those that are exudative or those that require added support.

There are various bandaging techniques in use, but by far the most common are those that are used on a horse's limbs. Depending on the purpose, limb bandages will either be:

- **Half-limb** – extending from the floor up to the proximal metacarpus (forelimb) or proximal metatarsus (hindlimb)
- **Full-limb** – extending from the floor up to the elbow (forelimb) or stifle (hindlimb).

Procedure: Applying a multilayered bandage to the horse's limb

1. **Action:** Prepare all of the necessary equipment.
   Rationale: This will save time and allow you to complete the bandage without having to leave the horse.
2. **Action:** Ensure that the horse is adequately restrained.
   Rationale: This will ensure that the horse is appropriately controlled and kept as still as possible during the procedure.
3. **Action:** Ideally, the bandage should be applied from the distal to the proximal limb.
   Rationale: This will achieve an even pressure and reduce the risk of swelling below the bandage.
4. **Action:** Using the initial padding layer (soft cotton bandage), secure the primary layer/sterile dressing (if required) in place (Fig. 14.12).
   Rationale: This will secure the dressing over the wounded area and prevent it from slipping or becoming dislodged.
5. **Action:** Apply a second padding layer (cotton wool) to the limb (Fig. 14.12).
   Rationale: This will provide support and absorb any exudates.

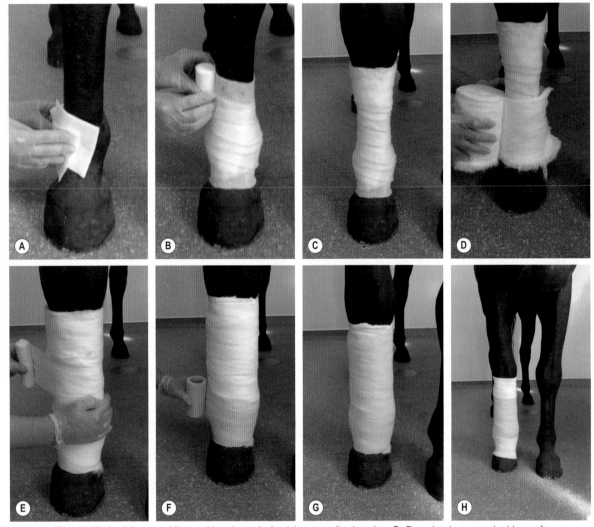

Fig. 14.12 Applying a multilayered bandage. A, Applying a sterile dressing. B, Dressing is covered with a soft cotton bandage. C, Soft bandage in place. D, Cotton-wool padding is applied. E, Conforming bandage is applied over the top. F, Cohesive bandage is used to cover the absorbent layers of the bandage. G, Cohesive bandage in place. H, Adhesive bandage secures the final layers to prevent slippage.

6. **Action:** Apply conforming bandage (crepe or knit bandage), ensuring that appropriate pressure is applied (Fig. 14.12).
   Rationale: This should be applied firmly and evenly to provide the added support required to promote healing.
7. **Action:** Repeat layers described in steps 5 and 6 if required.
   Rationale: This can be repeated multiple times, depending on the support and size of the bandage required.

8. **Action:** Finally, apply the tertiary/outer layer (self-adherent/cohesive bandage) (Fig. 14.12).
   Rationale: This will provide the protective outer layer of the bandage.
9. **Action:** Check the tension of the bandage.
   Rationale: Ensure that the bandage is not so tight that it will cause damage, or so loose that it provides little pressure or support or results in the bandage slipping.
10. **Action:** Use an adherent or adhesive material such as Elastoplast to secure the bandage at the top and bottom (Fig. 14.12).

Rationale: Ensure that these materials are not applied too tightly. When this layer is removed, do so very carefully, so as not to damage the patient's skin. The application of this material will prevent the bandage from moving or slipping, as well as preventing any debris (such as bedding) from entering the bandage and causing irritation.

11. **Action:** If bandaging over the carpus, *carefully* relieve pressure over the accessory carpal bone with a scalpel blade (Fig. 14.13).

    Rationale: This will prevent trauma to the thin skin over the accessory carpal bone, which can become damaged by the pressure of the covering.

12. **Action:** Check that the patient is comfortable and that it can move easily. Check the bandage at regular intervals and change when required.

    Rationale: Ensure that the bandage is intact and has not become wet, soiled, displaced or smelly.

N.B.: Some areas of the limb are particularly vulnerable to trauma if an inappropriate or over-tight bandage is applied:

1. **Hindlimb** – these areas are the common calcanean tendon area, the dorsal aspect of the hock below the tarsometatarsal joint and the point of the hock. To reduce trauma to these areas, a figure-of-eight bandaging technique can be utilized so that there is no tension on the calcanean tendon area, and the point of the hock is left as free as possible.

2. **Forelimb** – although horses tend to tolerate immobilization of the carpus better than the hock, it is still regarded as a vulnerable area because the skin covering the bone in this area is very thin. The skin over the accessory carpal bone is particularly prone to damage if it is covered because of the pressure that is put upon it during movement of the carpus. Trauma caused by bandaging can be prevented by ensuring that the accessory carpal is left uncovered, or by relieving pressure over the area (Fig. 14.13). A figure-of-eight bandaging technique may also be utilized here as this allows the accessory carpal to remain uncovered.

To reduce the risk of damage to these vulnerable areas, it may sometimes be more appropriate to utilize a pressage bandage.

PRESSAGE BANDAGE

The pressage bandage is a reusable elasticated stocking that has a zip fastening that applies even pressure over the dressing and padding layers to reduce oedema, wound exudation and proud flesh. These bandages are available in a range of sizes for the equine hock, carpus and fetlock regions. In the area of the hock and carpus, it is also useful to apply a stable bandage below the pressage bandage and an adherent/adhesive bandage, e.g. Elastoplast, above the pressage bandage to hold it in place and prevent slipping. Pressage bandages are particularly useful for more superficial wounds and following surgical procedures where there is minimal wounding and exudate.

ROBERT JONES BANDAGE

A Robert Jones bandage is applied by the same process as that described for a multilayered limb bandage (Fig. 14.12), and is similar to that described in the dog (see Chapter 8). It provides increased limb immobilization, stability and protection. It can be used with or without a splint support placed over the top of the outside of the bandage, depending on the required degree of immobilization and support. A Robert Jones bandage is multilayered to increase rigidity and spread even pressure over the whole limb. The finished bandage should

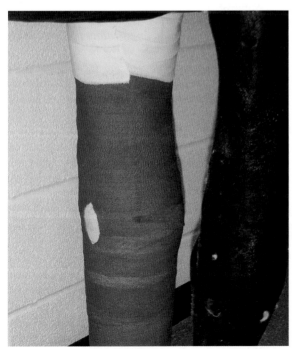

Fig. 14.13 A full-limb multilayered bandage with pressure relieved over the accessory carpal bone.

TABLE 14.3 Suggested bandage requirements for an equine Robert Jones bandage

Bandaging material	No. of rolls in a half-limb bandage	No. of rolls in a full-limb bandage
Cotton wool	4–5	10
Conforming bandage	8–10	20
Self-adherent/ cohesive bandage	2–3	4–6

result in a firm bandage that is three times the diameter of the normal leg. The amount of bandaging material used depends on the size of the patient and the size of the bandage (Table 14.3).

SPLINTING

Splints can be used in combination with a Robert Jones bandage to aid immobilization of wounds, to support fractures and to stabilize limbs prior to travelling and/or surgery. They are applied over the top of the Robert Jones bandage and secured in place with an adhesive bandage. A splint should immobilize the joints above and below the area that is damaged. Equine practices often utilize materials such as wood or plastic guttering to act as splints, and these usually work well, provided that an appropriate-length splint is used and the ends are padded to provide protection. Commercial splints are also available to aid stabilization of fractures below the distal metacarpus/metatarsus, e.g. Kimzey splint, monkey splint.

FOOT BANDAGE

Procedure: Applying a foot bandage

1. **Action:** Prepare all of the necessary equipment.
   Rationale: This will save time and allow you to complete the bandage without having to leave the horse.
2. **Action:** Make sure that the horse is adequately restrained.
   Rationale: This will ensure that the horse is appropriately controlled and kept as still as possible during the procedure.

3. **Action:** Begin the secondary layer of material below the fetlock and apply proximally as this will allow you to incorporate a primary dressing if appropriate.
   Rationale: This will keep the dressing in place and provide an initial layer of padding.
4. **Action:** Continue distally, bringing the dressing several times under the bulbs of the heel, then lift the foot and bring the bandage several times over the palmar third of the sole.
   Rationale: To reduce the risk of the bandage moving upwards over the pastern area and becoming useless, you should incorporate both the heel and sole of the foot.
5. **Action:** Apply the outer/tertiary layer over the secondary layer.
   Rationale: This will provide an initial protective layer and hold the secondary layer/s in place.
6. **Action:** Using strong tape, e.g. duct tape/nylon tape, tape over the solar margin of the hoof and heels (do not allow the tape to contact the skin). It may be useful to use a layered pad of tape to strengthen and protect the sole before placing the encircling tape.
   Rationale: Strong tape will reinforce the bandage, which should stop the horse wearing through the bandage. It is important that the skin and coronet band are not incorporated into such taping as this can result in trauma and irritation to these areas.
7. **Action:** Check the tension of the bandage.
   Rationale: If the bandage is too tight, it will cause damage by interfering with the circulation to the area. If it is too loose, it will slip or become dislodged.
8. **Action:** Use an adherent/adhesive material such as Elastoplast to secure the bandage at the top. Ensure that these materials are not applied too tightly and are removed very carefully, so as not to damage the patient's skin.
   Rationale: This will prevent movement or slippage and prevent any debris from entering the bandage and causing irritation.
9. **Action:** Check patient comfort and the bandage regularly and change the bandage when required.
   Rationale: Ensure that the bandage is intact and has not become wet or soiled or worn at the toe or sole.

In some circumstances, the use of a hospital plate fitted to an egg bar shoe may make the application of solar dressings much easier and also reduce the cost by reducing the number of times the bandage needs changing.

ADMINISTERING MEDICATION

Medication may be administered via a number of different routes; the choice depends on whether the desired effect is local or systemic. It is important to ensure that all medications are administered via the correct route to ensure the efficacy of the drug and the safety and wellbeing of the patient.

LOCAL/TOPICAL ADMINISTRATION

When administering local or topical medications, e.g. ointments and creams, it is essential that the patient is appropriately restrained by one of the methods described at the beginning of this chapter. Great care must be taken during administration to prevent injury to either the horse or the handler.

ORAL ADMINISTRATION

Oral medication can be added to the horse's feed, but it is important to check that the horse has eaten all the medication. Some horses will spill their food onto the floor and into their bedding, and this may not be noticed. Hiding the taste of oral medication can be achieved with the use of palatable feed, molasses and garlic; if in doubt, it may be easier to syringe feed the horse using an oral dosing syringe. Medications that are not available in a paste form are less easy to syringe feed, but water can be added to the majority of oral preparations, e.g. powder and granules, to make a more paste-like substance.

Procedure: Oral dosing of medication

1. **Action:** Make sure that the horse is adequately restrained.
   Rationale: This will ensure that the horse is appropriately controlled and kept as still as possible during the procedure.
2. **Action:** Check that the mouth is empty.
   Rationale: An empty mouth will allow for easier administration of the medication and reduce the risk of the horse being able to spit out the medication.
3. **Action:** Standing to one side of the horse, lift the horse's head and insert the tip of the syringe into

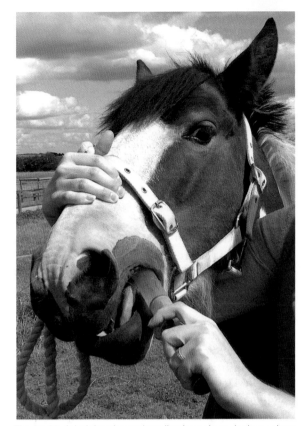

Fig. 14.14 Administering oral medication using a dosing syringe.

the side of the mouth, pointing upwards towards the back of the tongue (Fig. 14.14).
   Rationale: This will reduce the risk of the medication running back out of the mouth and allow it to be introduced directly onto the tongue.
4. **Action:** Push the plunger of the dosing syringe by applying firm continuous pressure with the palm of your hand.
   Rationale: This should ensure a continuous flow into the mouth until the dose is finished.
5. **Action:** Hold the horse's head up for as long as possible.
   Rationale: To prevent the horse spitting out the medication as it should naturally flow back towards the pharynx.
6. **Action:** Continue to hold the head up and insert your thumb behind the incisor teeth or gently massage the throat area.

Rationale: This will encourage the horse to swallow the medication.

PARENTERAL ADMINISTRATION

Procedure: To give a subcutaneous injection

1. **Action:** Ensure that the horse is adequately restrained.
   Rationale: This will ensure that the horse is appropriately controlled and kept as still as possible during the procedure.
2. **Action:** Locate a suitable area for injection.
   Rationale: This should be on the side of the neck, just cranial to the leading edge of the shoulder blade.
3. **Action:** Pinch a fold of skin in this area using your left hand (if you are right-handed).
   Rationale: Subcutaneous injections are given under the skin, and this tents the skin, ready for the injection.
4. **Action:** Using your right hand, introduce the point of the needle into the tented skin.
   Rationale: Be careful not to push the needle too far in as this risks penetration of the underlying muscle.
5. **Action:** Draw back the plunger slightly.
   Rationale: To make that you have not penetrated a blood capillary.
6. **Action:** If there is no blood in the hub of the needle, push the plunger to inject the contents into the subcuticular space.
   Rationale: Blood in the hub of the needle indicates that you may have penetrated a blood capillary. If this happens, reposition the needle and repeat.
7. **Action:** Withdraw the needle and gently massage the site.
   Rationale: To disperse the drug that has been injected.

INTRAMUSCULAR INJECTION

There are three common sites used for intramuscular injection:
- Pectoral muscles, known as the brisket
- Neck
- Gluteal muscles, known as the rump.

In equine veterinary practice, the neck and rump seem to be used most frequently, but the muscles on either side of the horse can also be utilized. It is advisable to rotate sites when a patient is receiving regular doses of intramuscular medication so that the muscles do not become sore or overused. It is imperative to monitor patients for stiffness, pain and possible abscessation during these times.

There are two main techniques in current use.

Procedure: Intramuscular injection into the neck and pectoral muscles

1. **Action:** Make sure that the horse is appropriately restrained.
   Rationale: This will ensure that the horse is fully controlled and kept as still as possible during the procedure. Intramuscular injections can be quite painful, especially if the horse moves.
2. **Action:** Identify the injection site.
   Rationale: The choice of site is related to using a muscle that is easily reached while the horse is properly restrained.
3. **Action:** Ensure the site is free from organic matter.
   Rationale: This is important to minimize the risk of infection.
4. **Action:** Pinch the skin and then introduce the needle at a right angle. The needle may or may not be attached to the syringe.
   Rationale: Pinching the skin may distract the horse and allow the needle to be introduced more smoothly. Separating the needle from the syringe may make it easier to place the needle more accurately.
5. **Action:** If not already attached, firmly attach the syringe, then draw back the plunger.
   Rationale: To check that you have not penetrated a blood capillary. Muscle tissue has a good blood supply, so vascular penetration is a slight risk, and injection of some drugs into a blood vessel could result in anaphylaxis.
6. **Action:** Slowly inject the contents into the muscle.
   Rationale: Administering the medication too quickly is normally difficult because muscle is dense tissue. Slow administration is recommended to allow the drug to disperse and to reduce any discomfort to the patient.
7. **Action:** Withdraw the needle and gently massage the site.
   Rationale: To disperse the drug that has been injected.

Procedure: Intramuscular injection into the neck, pectoral or gluteal muscles

1. **Action:** Make sure that the horse is appropriately restrained.

Rationale: This will ensure that the horse is fully controlled and kept as still as possible during the procedure. Intramuscular injections can be quite painful, especially if the horse moves.

2. **Action:** Identify the injection site.

   Rationale: The choice of site is related to using a muscle that is easily reached while the horse is properly restrained.

3. **Action:** Ensure the site is free from organic matter.

   Rationale: This is important to minimize the risk of infection.

4. **Action:** It is particularly important when injecting into the gluteal muscles to stand facing the caudal end of the horse, i.e. with your back towards the head end, and as far forwards towards the head end as possible.

   Rationale: The gluteal muscles are located in close proximity to the hindlimbs of the horse – standing as far forwards as possible reduces the risk of being kicked.

5. **Action:** Detach the needle from the syringe. Thump the site once or twice with your closed fist and then rapidly and firmly introduce the needle, perpendicular to the skin, right up to the hub.

   Rationale: This prepares the muscle and distracts the horse, allowing for quick, uninterrupted and smooth introduction of the needle. Detaching the needle from the syringe enables the needle to be placed more accurately.

6. **Action:** Attach the syringe to the needle and draw back the plunger.

   Rationale: To check that you have not penetrated a blood capillary. Muscle tissue has a good blood supply, so vascular penetration is a slight risk, and injection of some drugs into a blood vessel could result in anaphylaxis.

7. **Action:** Slowly inject the contents into the muscle and then withdraw the needle.

   Rationale: Administering the medication too quickly is normally difficult because muscle is dense tissue. Slow administration is recommended to allow the drug to disperse and to reduce any discomfort to the patient.

8. **Action:** Withdraw the needle and gently massage the site.

   Rationale: To disperse the drug that has been injected.

INTRAVENOUS INJECTION

Medication can be administered into a number of superficial veins in the horse, including the jugular, cephalic, saphenous and lateral thoracic veins; however, by far the most commonly used and readily accessible vein is the jugular (Fig. 14.15). The left jugular is the side of choice, unless there is reason why this side cannot be used. Intravenous medication may be given via a catheter or via an injection using a needle and syringe.

Procedure: Intravenous injection using the left jugular vein

1. **Action:** Ensure that the horse is appropriately restrained.

   Rationale: This will ensure that the horse is fully controlled and kept as still as possible during the procedure. Transfixing the vein because of accidental movement could result in haemorrhage.

2. **Action:** Have all the equipment ready.

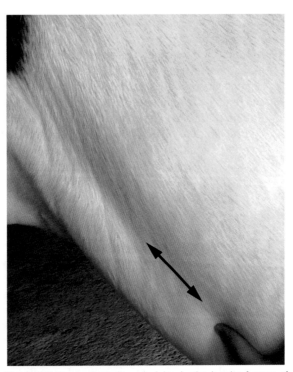

Fig. 14.15 A raised jugular vein lying in the jugular furrow of the neck.

Rationale: This will save time and ensure that the procedure can be carried out as quickly as possible, reducing stress for the patient.

3. **Action:** Locate the jugular vein and the site for needle placement (approx. one-third of the way down the neck).

   Rationale: A jugular vein runs on either side of the neck in the jugular furrow (Fig. 14.15).

4. **Action:** Ensure that the vein is suitable for use.

   Rationale: If there is any doubt about using the vein because it has been previously compromised, then use another vein. It is vital to avoid jugular thrombosis.

5. **Action:** It is preferable to clip the area in horses with a thick coat, and aseptic skin preparation is advised. Ensure the site is free from organic matter by wiping with a spirit swab.

   Rationale: Aseptic technique is important to minimize the risk of infection.

6. **Action:** Using your left hand, apply gentle pressure by putting your thumb in the jugular furrow below the site of the intended venepuncture.

   Rationale: Occluding the vein close to the thoracic inlet will prevent blood flow towards the heart, causing the vein to dilate, which is known as 'raising the vein'.

7. **Action:** With your right hand, insert the needle with its bevel side uppermost. Direct it upwards at a slight angle from the skin surface and into the skin and underlying vein, until a lack of resistance is felt.

   Rationale: This requires great care as there are some structures that must be avoided during insertion of the needle. Be careful not to insert the needle too deeply or at too steep an angle as accidental injection into the carotid artery can have damaging results. Injection of irritant chemicals around the neurovascular bundle can also result in damage. Any damage to the recurrent laryngeal nerve or sympathetic nerves can result in development of iatrogenic laryngeal hemiplegia or Horner's syndrome.

8. **Action:** If the syringe is not attached, then venous blood should be seen slowly oozing from the hub of the needle; if the syringe is attached, draw back on the plunger until you see a little venous blood appearing in the syringe.

   Rationale: This is done to ensure that the needle is in the vein. The carotid artery lies close by, and injection into this could have fatal consequences. If the artery is penetrated, blood will flow into the syringe under pressure.

9. **Action:** Once the needle is in the vein, lift your thumb to release the pressure on the vein and inject the medicine slowly, with intermittent drawing back of the plunger.

   Rationale: To check that the needle is still in the vein.

10. **Action:** Slowly remove the needle from the neck and apply pressure to the vein for 2 minutes.

    Rationale: To prevent perivascular haemorrhage into the area and the risk of haematoma.

COLLECTING BLOOD SAMPLES

Blood is commonly taken for laboratory analysis, i.e. biochemistry and haematology, and can be used to provide an overall picture of the horse's health. Blood may be collected from a number of veins in the horse, including the jugular, cephalic and saphenous veins; however, by far the most commonly used and readily accessible vein is the jugular vein. Samples for blood gas analysis can also be taken from arteries, but this is normally limited to use during anaesthesia.

Blood is easily collected using a Vacutainer kit, but an ordinary hypodermic needle and syringe may also be used. The size of needle and syringe will depend on the size of the patient and the number of samples required. A Vacutainer is an evacuated glass tube sealed at one end with a rubber bung (Fig. 14.16). The rest of the kit consists of a holder with a double-ended needle, one end of which is placed in the vein while the other end pierces the bung. Blood is drawn into the tube by the vacuum. Vacutainers are available as plain tubes or containing different anticoagulants indicated by the colour of the bung (Table 14.4). Plain tubes (red) and those containing ethylene diamine tetra acetic acid (EDTA: purple) and heparin (green) are used most

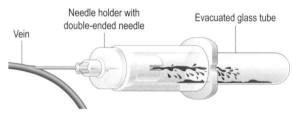

Vein — Needle holder with double-ended needle — Evacuated glass tube

Fig. 14.16 A Vacutainer. (Reproduced, with permission, from Aspinall (2011), Oxford.)

TABLE 14.4 Vacutainer tube top colour related to use and type of anticoagulant

Vacutainer colour	Anticoagulant	Use
Red	None (plain)	Serum collection Biochemistry
Purple	Ethylene diamine tetra acetic acid (EDTA)	Haematology
Green	Heparin	Biochemistry
Grey	Fluoride/oxalate	Assessing glucose concentration
Blue	Sodium citrate	Coagulation studies
Yellow	Acid citrate dextrose	Cross-matching, blood typing

commonly for routine testing, and the other types are used for more specialized analyses.

Procedure: Collecting a blood sample from the left jugular vein using a Vacutainer

1. **Action:** Ensure that the horse is appropriately restrained.
   Rationale: This will ensure that the horse is fully controlled and kept as still as possible during the procedure. Transfixing the vein with the needle may occur if the horse moves suddenly.
2. **Action:** Have all the equipment ready.
   Rationale: This will save time and ensure that the procedure can be carried out as quickly as possible, reducing stress for the patient.
3. **Action:** Locate the jugular vein and the site for needle placement (approx. one-third of the way down the neck).
   Rationale: A jugular vein runs on either side of the neck in the jugular furrow (Fig. 14.15).
4. **Action:** It is preferable to clip the area in horses with a thick coat, and aseptic skin preparation is advised. Ensure the site is free from organic matter by wiping the area with a spirit swab.
   Rationale: Aseptic technique is important to minimize the risk of infection.
5. **Action:** Using your left hand, apply gentle pressure by putting your thumb in the jugular furrow below the site of the intended venepuncture.

Rationale: Occluding the vein close to the thoracic inlet will prevent blood flow towards the heart, causing the vein to dilate, which is known as 'raising the vein'.
6. **Action:** With your right hand, insert the needle with its bevel side uppermost at a slight angle from the skin surface and into the skin and underlying vein until a lack of resistance is felt. Venous blood should then drip from the other end of the needle.
   Rationale: Ensure that this is venous blood, which should drip rather than spurt out of the blood vessel.
7. **Action:** Clip the Vacutainer tube into its holder and onto the needle and hold it steady whilst it fills. If multiple samples are needed, detach the needle from the tube and attach a new tube.
   Rationale: The vacuum within each tube draws blood from the vein by suction.
8. **Action:** Remove the Vacutainer from its needle and holder and invert the tube gently. This is not necessary if a plain tube is used.
   Rationale: Inverting the tube allows the blood sample to mix with any anticoagulant in the tube.
9. **Action:** Slowly remove the needle from the neck and apply pressure to the site for 2 minutes.
   Rationale: This prevents perivascular haemorrhage into the area and reduces the risk of haematoma.
10. **Action:** Label each Vacutainer tube with the patient details and the date of collection.
    Rationale: This will ensure that samples are easily identified and that the correct samples are sent for the correct tests and analysis.

REFERENCES AND FURTHER READING

Ackerman, N., 2016. Aspinall's Complete Textbook of Veterinary Nursing, third ed. Elsevier, Oxford.

Aspinall, V. (Ed.), 2008. Clinical Procedures in Veterinary Nursing. second ed. Elsevier, Oxford.

Aspinall, V., 2011. The Complete Textbook of Veterinary Nursing, second ed. Butterworth-Heinemann, Oxford.

Batty-Smith, J., 2008. The BHS Complete Manual of Horse and Stable Management. Kenilworth Press, Shrewsbury.

Cooper, B., Mullineaux, E., Turner, L. (Eds.), 2011. BSAVA Textbook of Veterinary Nursing. fifth ed. BSAVA, Gloucester.

Coumbe, K.M. (Ed.), 2001. Equine Veterinary Nursing Manual. Blackwell Science, Oxford.

Knottenbelt, D.C., 2003. Handbook of Equine Wound Management. Elsevier Science, London.

Note: Page numbers followed by *f* indicate figures, *t* indicate tables, and *b* indicate boxes.